Case Files™:
Emergency Medicine

NOTICE

Medicine is an ever-changing science. As new research and clinical experience broaden our knowledge, changes in treatment and drug therapy are required. The authors and the publisher of this work have checked with sources believed to be reliable in their efforts to provide information that is complete and generally in accord with the standards accepted at the time of publication. However, in view of the possibility of human error or changes in medical sciences, neither the editors nor the publisher nor any other party who has been involved in the preparation or publication of this work warrants that the information contained herein is in every respect accurate or complete, and they disclaim all responsibility for any errors or omissions or for the results obtained from use of the information contained in this work. Readers are encouraged to confirm the information contained herein with other sources. For example and in particular, readers are advised to check the product information sheet included in the package of each drug they plan to administer to be certain that the information contained in this work is accurate and that changes have not been made in the recommended dose or in the contraindications for administration. This recommendation is of particular importance in connection with new or infrequently used drugs.

Case Files™:

Emergency Medicine

EUGENE C. TOY, MD
THE JOHN S. DUNN, SENIOR ACADEMIC CHAIR
AND PROGRAM DIRECTOR
CHRISTUS ST. JOSEPH HOSPITAL OB/GYN
RESIDENCY PROGRAM, HOUSTON, TX
CLERKSHIP DIRECTOR, ASSISTANT CLINICAL
PROFESSOR,
DEPARTMENT OF OBSTETRICS AND
GYNECOLOGY, UNIVERSITY OF
TEXAS–HOUSTON MEDICAL SCHOOL
HOUSTON, TX

BARRY C. SIMON, MD
ASSOCIATE CLINICAL PROFESSOR OF MEDICINE
UCSF MEDICAL CENTER
CHAIRMAN, DEPARTMENT OF EMERGENCY
MEDICINE
ALAMEDA COUNTY MEDICAL
CENTER/HIGHLAND GENERAL HOSPITAL
OAKLAND, CALIFORNIA

KATRIN Y. TAKENAKA, MD
ASSISTANT PROFESSOR, CLERKSHIP DIRECTOR
DEPARTMENT OF EMERGENCY MEDICINE
UNIVERSITY OF TEXAS-HOUSTON MEDICAL
SCHOOL
HOUSTON, TEXAS

BENTON BAKER III, MD
DIRECTOR OF GRADUATE MEDICAL EDUCATION
CHRISTUS ST. JOSEPH HOSPITAL
PROFESSOR OF OBSTETRICS AND GYNECOLOGY
UNIVERSITY OF TEXAS-HOUSTON MEDICAL
SCHOOL
HOUSTON, TEXAS

TERRENCE H. LIU, MD
ASSOCIATE CLINICAL PROFESSOR OF SURGERY
UNIVERSITY OF CALIFORNIA, SAN FRANCISCO
SCHOOL OF MEDICINE
ATTENDING SURGEON AND PROGRAM
DIRECTOR, UCSF-EAST BAY SURGERY
RESIDENCY PROGRAM
OAKLAND, CALIFORNIA

Lange Medical Books/McGraw-Hill

MEDICAL PUBLISHING DIVISION

New York   Chicago   San Francisco
Lisbon   London   Madrid   Mexico City
Milan   New Delhi   San Juan   Seoul
Singapore   Sydney   Toronto

Case Files™: Emergency Medicine

4567890 DOC/DOC 09876

ISBN 0-07-143795-9

This book was set in Times New Roman.
The editor was Catherine A. Johnson.
The production supervisor was Catherine Saggese.
The cover designer was Aimee Nordin.
The index was prepared by Pamela Edwards.
RR Donnelly was printer and binder.

This book is printed on acid-free paper.

Library of Congress Cataloging-in-Publication Data

Case files : Emergency medicine / Eugene C. Toy…[et al].
      p. ; cm.
   Includes index.
   ISBN 0-07-143795-9
   1. Emergency medicine—Case studies.   I. Title: Emergency medicine   II. Toy, Eugene C.
   [DNLM: 1. Emergency medicine—Case Reports.   2. Emergencies—Case Reports   WB
105 C3365 2004]
   RC86.9.C38 2004
   616.02'5—dc22

                                                              2004048485

❖ DEDICATION

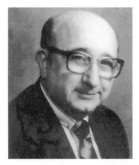

Case Files: Emergency Medicine is the sixth and last planned book in the *Clinical Case Files* series. It is fitting that we take this opportunity to dedicate this series to a great physician, Dr. Joseph A. Lucci, Jr., who has had a tremendous impact on the practice and education in medicine in Houston, particularly at CHRISTUS St. Joseph Hospital. Dr. Lucci was born in Morrone del Sannio, a province of Campobasso in Italy on August 21, 1921. "Dr. Joe" arrived in the United States in 1930 at the age of 9 years. He obtained his medical degree from the Medical College of Wisconsin in 1946. After finishing his internship in 1947, he served as an Air Force base surgeon in Germany during the Berlin Airlift. He then received residency training for 2 years at the Margaret Hague Maternity Hospital in Jersey City, New Jersey. Upon his arrival to Houston, Dr. Lucci received his further training in gynecologic surgery at the MD Anderson Cancer Center. He was appointed as the first academic chair over the department of obstetrics/gynecology at St. Joseph Hospital, and had academic appointments at the MD Anderson Cancer Center, UTMB Galveston Medical School, and later at the University of Texas Houston Medical School. During his 31 years as academic chair, Dr. Joe trained more than 120 excellent residents, revolutionized the education of gynecologic surgery, developed innovative surgical techniques, markedly reduced the maternal mortality, and helped to coordinate the medical education throughout the Houston/Galveston region. He and his wife Joan have five children: Joe, Joan Marie, Jacqueline, Regina Marie, and James, and nine grandchildren. Currently, "Dr. Joe" is academic chief emeritus of the CHRISTUS St. Joseph Hospital Obstetrics-Gynecology Residency. Dr. Lucci has been a true pioneer in many aspects of medicine, touching the lives of thousands of people. We are greatly indebted to this extraordinary man.

To Mabel Wong Ligh whose grace, love, and common sense bind our family together, and in the memory of John Wong, whose smile, integrity, and enthusiasm continue to warm our hearts.

—ECT

To my best friend and wife Zina Rosen-Simon and to my daughters Jamie and Kaylie for teaching me and always reminding me what is most important in life. I would also like to thank my faculty at Highland General Hospital and all the residents and students who have passed through our doors for helping make my career as an academic emergency physician challenging and immensely rewarding.

—BCS

To my parents, who continue to be my guiding light. To my other half, Mark, who knows how to make me smile. And to Clare, who remains my teacher & friend.

—KYT

To my grandchildren, Aidan, John, Joshua, Michael, Noah, Chloe... through whom I see the future!

To Eugene Toy, MD who exemplifies why I became an educator.

—BB

To my wife Eileen for her continuous support, love, and friendship. To all the medical students and residents for their dedication to education and improving patient care.

—THL

❖ CONTENTS

❖ CONTRIBUTORS

Linda K. Barry, MD
Clinical Fellow, Tumor & Endocrine
Department of Surgery
University of Southern California
Los Angeles, California
Clinical Fellow
Hepatobiliary Division
Department of Surgery
LAC/USC Medical Center
Los Angeles, California
Approach to Septic Shock

Terry J. Chong, MD
General Surgery Resident
General Surgery
Alameda County Medical Center
UCSF-East Bay Surgery Residency Program
Oakland, California
Approach to Hemorrhagic Shock

Elizabeth Brand, MD
Resident, Emergency Medicine Department
Alameda County Medical Center/Highland Campus
Oakland, California
Approach to Syncope

Wendy Cole, MD
Co-Director of Medical Student Clerkships, Emergency Medicine Department
Alameda County Medical Center/Highland Campus
Oakland, California
Approach to Meningitis

Eileen T. Consorti, MD, MS
Assistant Clinical Professor of Surgery
Department of Surgery
UCSF-East Bay
Oakland, California
Approach to Intestinal Obstruction

Justin O. Cook, MD
Chief Resident, Department of Emergency Medicine
Alameda County Medical Center/Highland Hospital
Oakland, California
Approach to Pharyngitis/Epiglottitis

Adam R. Corley, MD
Resident, Emergency Medicine Department
University of Texas-Houston Medical School
Houston, TX
Approach to Swallowed Foreign Body
Approach to Headache
Approach to Scrotal Pain

Michael Cripps, MD
Resident, Department of Surgery
UCSF-East Bay Surgery Residency Program
Oakland, California
Approach to Drowning and Near-Drowning

DeShawndranique Gray, MD
Chief Resident, Obstetrics and Gynecology
CHRISTUS St. Joseph Hospital
Houston, Texas
Approach to Frostbite
Approach to Disseminated Gonococcal Disease

Karen Dixon, MD
Department of Emergency Medicine
Inova Fairfax Hospital
Falls Church, Virginia
Approach to Atrial Fibrillation

David K. English, MD
Assistant Clinical Professor, Division of Emergency Medicine
University of California, San Francisco
San Francisco, California
Informatics Director
Department of Emergency Medicine
Alameda County Medical Center
Oakland, California
Approach to Diabetic Ketoacidosis

Juan M. Franco, MD
Resident, Obstetrics and Gynecology
CHRISTUS St. Joseph Hospital
Houston, Texas
Approach to Acute Urinary Retention
Approach to Nephrolithiasis

Bradley W. Frazee, MD
Attending Physician, Department of Emergency Medicine
Alameda County Medical Center/Highland Campus
Oakland, California
Assistant Clinical Professor
Department of Medicine
University of California, San Francisco
San Francisco, California
Approach to Acute Chest Pain

Rose B. Ganim, MD
Clinical Instructor, Department of Surgery
University of California, San Francisco, East Bay
Oakland, California
Approach to Penetrating Trauma

Jocelyn Freeman Garrick, MD
ALS Base Director, Emergency Medicine Department
Alameda County Medical Center/Highland Campus
Oakland, California
Approach to the Child With a Limp

Cherie Hargis, MD
Faculty Physician, Emergency Medicine Department
Alameda County Medical Center/Highland Campus
Assistant Clinical Professor
University of California, San Francisco
Oakland, California
Approach to the Red Eye

Herbert Hern, MD
Associate Residency Director, Emergency Medicine Department
Alameda County Medical Center/Highland Campus
Oakland, California
Assistant Clinical Professor of Medicine
University of California, San Francisco
San Francisco, California
Approach to Pharyngitis/Epiglottitis

Catherine A. Holt, MD
Resident, Obstetrics and Gynecology
CHRISTUS St. Joseph Hospital
Houston, Texas
Approach to Acute Pelvic Inflammatory Disease
Approach to Ectopic Pregnancy

Irfan Hydari, MD
Attending Physician, Emergency Medicine Department
Las Colinas Medical Center
Irving, Texas
Approach to Congestive Heart Failure

Joseph Bram Johns, MD
Department of Obstetrics and Gynecology
CHRISTUS St. Joseph Hospital
Houston, Texas
Approach to Rabies and Animal Bites

Anjali S. Kumar, MD, MPH
Research Fellow
Breast Care Center
Department of Surgery
University of California, San Francisco
San Francisco, California
Resident Physician, Department of Surgery
University of California, San Francisco, East Bay
Oakland, California
Approach to DVT/Pulmonary Embolism

Dustin G. Mark, MD
Resident, Department of Emergency Medicine
Hospital of the University of Pennsylvania
Philadelphia, Pennsylvania
Approach to Acute Transfusion Reaction

Jose Medina, MD
Emergency Medicine Department
University of Texas-Houston
Memorial Hermann Hospital
Houston, Texas
Approach to Acetominophen Toxicity
Approach to Heat-related Illnesses
Approach to Sickle Cell Crises

Amy Moore, BS, MD
Resident Physician, Department of Medicine
Highland General Hospital
Oakland, California
Approach to Drowning and Near-Drowning

Nikole A. Neidlinger, MD
Surgical Resident, Department of Surgery
University of California, San Francisco
San Francisco, California
Approach to Lightning and Electrical Injury

Christopher R. Newton, MD
Critical Care Fellow, Department of Surgery
Children's Memorial Hospital
Chicago, Illinois
Approach to Pediatric Trauma

Amanda Parker, MD
Chief Resident Emergency Medicine
University of Texas Medical School, Department at Houston
Memorial Hermann Hospital
Houston, Texas
Approach to Acute Pneumocystis Pneumonia
Approach to Acute Upper and Lower GI Bleeding
Approach to Cerebrovascular Accidents and Transient Ischemic Accidents

Dolar S. Patolia, MD
Voluntary Faculty, Department of Obstetrics and Gynecology
CHRISTUS St. Joseph Hospital
Houston, Texas
Approach to Herpes Zoster
Approach to Bell Palsy

Molly A. Phelps, MD
Emergency Medicine Department
Alameda County Medical Center
Oakland, California
Approach to Altered Level of Consciousness

Steven G. Pilkington, MD
Resident, Obstetrics and Gynecology
CHRISTUS St. Joseph Hospital
Houston, Texas
Approach to Cocaine Intoxication

Jason Quinn, BS, MD
Resident, Emergency Medicine Department
Alameda County Medical Center/Highland Campus
Oakland, California
Approach to Acute Chest Pain
Approach to Anaphylaxis

Andrea Richter-Werning, MD
Resident, Obstetrics and Gynecology
CHRISTUS St. Joseph Hospital
Houston, Texas
Approach to Preeclampsia/Malignant Hypertension

Adam J. Rosh, MD
Medical Resident
Department of Emergency Medicine
NYU/Bellevue
New York, New York
Approach to the Emergency Medicine Patient

Amandeep Singh, MD
Assistant Clinical Professor of Medicine, Emergency Medicine Department
University of California, San Francisco
San Francisco, California
Staff Physician, Department of Medicine
Highland General Hospital
Oakland, California
Approach to Asthma

Eric R. Snoey, MD
Program Director, Emergency Medicine Department
Alameda County Medical Center
Oakland, California
Approach to Atrial Fibrillation

John C. Stein, MD
Assistant Clinical Professor, Emergency Medicine Department
University of California, San Francisco
Oakland, California
Approach to Syncope

Michael Stone, MD
Resident, Emergency Medicine Department
Alameda County Medical Center/Highland Campus
Oakland, California
Approach to Meningitis

Gary W. Tamkin, MD, FACEP
Assistant Clinical Professor of Medicine, Department of Emergency Medicine
University of California, San Francisco
San Francisco, California
Attending Physician, Department of Emergency Medicine
Alameda County Medical Center
Oakland, California
Approach to Seizure Disorder

Alvin Tang, MD
Physician, Emergency Medicine Department
Alameda County Medical Center, Highland Campus
Oakland, California
Approach to the Child with a Limp

Nicole N. Tran, MD
Physician, Obstetrics and Gynecology
Houston Women's Care Associates
The Women's Hospital of Texas
Houston, Texas
Approach to Lyme Disease

Jorge D. Trujillo, MD
Director, Emergency Services
CHRISTUS St. Joseph Hospital
Houston, Texas
Approach to Facial Lacerations
Approach to Infectious Diarrhea

Gregory P. Victorino, MD
Assistant Professor of Surgery
Department of Surgery
UCSF-East Bay
Oakland, California
Trauma Director, Department of Surgery
Alameda County Medical Center
Oakland, California
Approach to Hemorrhagic Shock

Thomas G. Weiser, MD
Resident, Department of Surgery
UC-Davis Medical Center
Sacramento, California
Approach to DVT/Pulmonary Embolism

Charlotte Wills, MD
Clinical Instructor in Medicine, Division of Emergency Medicine
University of California, San Francisco
San Francisco , California
Director of Medical Student Education
Department of Emergency Medicine
Alameda County Medical Center, Highland Hospital
Oakland, California
Approach to Anaphylaxis

Robert Yetman, MD
Professor of Pediatrics
Director, Division of Community and General Pediatrics
Department of Pediatrics
University of Texas-Houston Medical School
Houston, Texas
Approach to Neonatal Sepsis

❖ INTRODUCTION

Mastering the cognitive knowledge within a field such as emergency medicine is a formidable task. It is even more difficult to draw on that knowledge, procure and filter through the clinical and laboratory data, develop a differential diagnosis, and finally to form a rational treatment plan. To gain these skills, the student often learns best at the bedside, guided and instructed by experienced teachers, and inspired toward self-directed, diligent reading. Clearly, there is no replacement for education at the bedside. Unfortunately, clinical situations usually do not encompass the breadth of the specialty. Perhaps the best alternative is a carefully crafted patient case designed to stimulate the clinical approach and decision-making. In an attempt to achieve that goal, we have constructed a collection of clinical vignettes to teach diagnostic or therapeutic approaches relevant to emergency medicine. Most importantly, the explanations for the cases emphasize the mechanisms and underlying principles, rather than merely rote questions and answers.

This book is organized for versatility: to allow the student "in a rush" to go quickly through the scenarios and check the corresponding answers, as well as the student who wants thought-provoking explanations. The answers are arranged from simple to complex: a summary of the pertinent points, the bare answers, an analysis of the case, an approach to the topic, a comprehension test at the end for reinforcement and emphasis, and a list of resources for further reading. The clinical vignettes are purposely placed in random order to simulate the way that real patients present to the practitioner. A listing of cases is included in Section III to aid the student who desires to test his/her knowledge of a certain area, or to review a topic including basic definitions. Finally, we intentionally did not primarily use a multiple choice question (MCQ) format because clues (or distractions) are not available in the real world. Nevertheless, several MCQ's are included at the end of each scenario to reinforce concepts or introduce related topics.

HOW TO GET THE MOST OUT OF THIS BOOK

Each case is designed to simulate a patient encounter with open-ended questions. At times, the patient's complaint is different from the most concerning issue, and sometimes extraneous information is given. The answers are organized in four different parts.

PART I:

1. **Summary**—The salient aspects of the case are identified, filtering out the extraneous information. The student should formulate his/her summary

from the case before looking at the answers. A comparison to the summation in the answer will help to improve one's ability to focus on the important data, while appropriately discarding the irrelevant information, a fundamental skill in clinical problem solving.

2. A **straightforward answer** is given to each open-ended question.

3. The **Analysis of the Case**, which is comprised of two parts:

    a. **Objectives of the Case**—A listing of the two or three main principles that are crucial for a practitioner to manage the patient. Again, the student is challenged to make educated "guesses" about the objectives of the case upon initial review of the case scenario, which help to sharpen his/her clinical and analytical skills.

    b. **Considerations**—A discussion of the relevant points and brief approach to the **specific** patient.

PART II:

Approach to the Disease Process, which has two distinct parts:

    a. **Definitions or pathophysiology**—Terminology or basic science correlates pertinent to the disease process.

    b. **Clinical Approach**—A discussion of the approach to the clinical problem in general, including tables, figures, and algorithms.

PART III:

Comprehension Questions—Each case contains several multiple-choice questions that reinforce the material, or introduce new and related concepts. Questions about material not found in the text will have explanations in the answers.

PART IV:

Clinical Pearls—A listing of several clinically important points, which are reiterated as a summation of the text and to allow for easy review such as before an examination.

❖ ACKNOWLEDGMENTS

The curriculum that evolved into the ideas for this series was inspired by two talented and forthright students, Philbert Yau and Chuck Rosipal, who have since graduated from medical school. It has been a pleasure to work with Dr. Barry Simon, a wonderfully skilled and compassionate emergency room physician, and Dr. Kay Takenaka, who is as talented in her writing and teaching as she is in her clinical care. It has been like a dream to once again work with my mentor, friend, and colleague, Dr. Benton Baker III, who in addition to being an excellent obstetrician-gynecologist is also well-versed in emergency and trauma care. Likewise, I have cherished working together with my friend since medical school Terry Liu, who initially suggested the idea of this book. I am greatly indebted to my editor, Catherine Johnson, whose exuberance, experience, and vision helped to shape this series. I appreciate McGraw-Hill's believing in the concept of teaching through clinical cases. At CHRISTUS St. Joseph Hospital, I applaud the finest administrators I have encountered: Jeff Webster, Janet Matthews, Michael Brown, and Dr. Benton Baker III for their commitment to medical education, and Dorothy Mersinger for her sage advice and support. I thank Adam Rosh MS IV for his excellent review of the manuscript. Without my dear colleagues, Drs. Que Tranvan, Jacqueline Brown, Sterling Weaver, Michael Leung, Carl Lee, and Robert Hilliard, this book could not have been written. Most of all, I appreciate my ever-loving wife Terri, and four wonderful children, Andy, Michael, Allison, and Christina for their patience, encouragement, and understanding.

Eugene C. Toy

How to Approach Clinical Problems

PART 1. APPROACH TO THE PATIENT

Applying "book learning" to a specific clinical situation is one of the most challenging tasks in medicine. To do so, the clinician must not only retain information, organize the facts, and recall large amounts of data but also apply all of this to the patient. The purpose of this text is to facilitate this process.

The first step involves **gathering information**, also known as establishing the database. This includes taking the history, performing the physical examination, and obtaining selective laboratory examinations, special studies, and/or imaging tests. Sensitivity and respect should always be exercised during the interview of patients. **A good clinician also knows how to ask the same question in several different ways, using different terminology.** For example, patients may deny having "congestive heart failure" but will answer affirmatively to being treated for "fluid on the lungs."

❖ **CLINICAL PEARL**

The **history** is usually the **single most important tool** in obtaining a diagnosis. The art of seeking this information in a nonjudgmental, sensitive, and thorough manner cannot be overemphasized.

History

1. Basic information:
    a. Age: Some conditions are more common at certain ages; for instance, chest pain in an elderly patient is more worrisome for coronary artery disease than the same complaint in a teenager.
    b. Gender: Some disorders are more common in men such as abdominal aortic aneurysms. In contrast, women more commonly have autoimmune problems such as chronic immune thrombocytopenic purpura or systemic lupus erythematosus. Also, the possibility of pregnancy must be considered in any woman of child-bearing age.
    c. Ethnicity: Some disease processes are more common in certain ethnic groups (such as type II diabetes mellitus in the Hispanic population).

❖ **CLINICAL PEARL**

The possibility of pregnancy must be entertained in any woman of child-bearing age.

---

2.   Chief complaint: What is it that brought the patient into the hospital? Has there been a change in a chronic or recurring condition or is this a completely new problem? The duration and character of the complaint, associated symptoms, and exacerbating/relieving factors should be recorded. The chief complaint engenders a differential diagnosis, and the possible etiologies should be explored by further inquiry.

CLINICAL PEARL

❖   The first line of any presentation should include *Age, Ethnicity, Gender, and Chief Complaint.* Example: A 32-year-old white male complains of lower abdominal pain of 8 hours duration.

3.   Past medical history:
   a.   Major illnesses such as hypertension, diabetes, reactive airway disease, congestive heart failure, angina, or stroke should be detailed.
      i.   Age of onset, severity, end-organ involvement.
      ii.   Medications taken for the particular illness including any recent changes to medications and reason for the change(s).
      iii.   Last evaluation of the condition (example: when was the last stress test or cardiac catheterization performed in the patient with angina?).
      iv.   Which physician or clinic is following the patient for the disorder?
   b.   Minor illnesses such as recent upper respiratory infections.
   c.   Hospitalizations no matter how trivial should be queried.

4.   Past surgical history: Date and type of procedure performed, indication, and outcome. Laparoscopy versus laparotomy should be distinguished. Surgeon and hospital name/location should be listed. This information should be correlated with the surgical scars on the patient's body. Any complications should be delineated including, for example, anesthetic complications, or difficult intubations.

5.   Allergies: Reactions to medications should be recorded, including severity and temporal relationship to medication. Immediate hypersensitivity should be distinguished from an adverse reaction.

6.   Medications: A list of medications, dosage, route of administration and frequency, and duration of use should be developed. Prescription, over-the-counter, and herbal remedies are all relevant.

If the patient is currently taking antibiotics, it is important to note what type of infection is being treated.

7.   Social history: Occupation, marital status, family support, and tendencies toward depression or anxiety are important. Use or abuse of illicit drugs, tobacco, or alcohol should also be recorded.

8.   Family history: Many major medical problems are genetically transmitted (e.g., hemophilia, sickle cell disease). In addition, a family history of conditions such as breast cancer and ischemic heart disease can be a risk factor for the development of these diseases.

9.   Review of systems: A systematic review should be performed but focused on the life-threatening and the more common diseases. For example, in a young man with a testicular mass, trauma to the area, weight loss, and infectious symptoms are important to note. In an elderly woman with generalized weakness, symptoms suggestive of cardiac disease should be elicited, such as chest pain, shortness of breath, fatigue, or palpitations.

Physical Examination

1.   General appearance: Is the patient in any acute distress? The emergency physician should focus on the **ABCs (Airway, Breathing, Circulation).** Note cachectic versus well-nourished, anxious versus calm, alert versus obtunded.

2.   Vital signs: Record the temperature, blood pressure, heart rate and respiratory rate. An oxygen saturation assessment is useful in a patient with respiratory symptoms. Height and weight are often placed here.

3.   Head and neck examination: Evidence of trauma, tumors, facial edema, goiter and thyroid nodules, and carotid bruits should be sought. In patients with altered mental status or a head injury, pupillary size, symmetry, and reactivity are important. Mucous membranes should be inspected for pallor, jaundice, and evidence of dehydration. Cervical and supraclavicular nodes should be palpated.

4.   Breast examination: Inspection for symmetry and skin or nipple retraction, as well as palpation for masses. The nipple should be assessed for discharge, and the axillary and supraclavicular regions should be examined.

5.   Cardiac examination: The *point of maximal impulse* (PMI) should be ascertained, and the heart auscultated at the apex as well as the base. It is important to note whether the auscultated rhythm is regular or irregular. Heart sounds (including S3 and S4), murmurs, clicks, and rubs should be characterized. Systolic flow murmurs are fairly common in

pregnant women because of the increased cardiac output, but significant diastolic murmurs are unusual.

6. Pulmonary examination: The lung fields should be examined systematically and thoroughly. Stridor, wheezes, rales, and rhonchi should be recorded. The clinician should also search for evidence of consolidation (bronchial breath sounds, egophony) and increased work of breathing (retractions, abdominal breathing, accessory muscle use).

7. Abdominal examination: The abdomen should be inspected for scars, distension, masses, and discoloration. For instance, the Grey-Turner sign of bruising at the flank areas may indicate intraabdominal or retroperitoneal hemorrhage. Auscultation should identify normal versus high-pitched and hyperactive versus hypoactive bowel sounds. The abdomen should be percussed for the presence of shifting dullness (indicating ascites). Then one should carefully palpate, beginning away from the area of pain and progressing to include the whole abdomen to assess for tenderness, masses, organomegaly (i.e., spleen or liver), and peritoneal signs. Guarding and whether it is voluntary or involuntary should be noted.

8. Back and spine examination: The back should be assessed for symmetry, tenderness, or masses. The flank regions particularly are important to assess for pain on percussion that may indicate renal disease.

9. Genital examination
    a. Female: The external genitalia should be inspected, then the speculum used to visualize the cervix and vagina. A bimanual examination should attempt to elicit cervical motion tenderness, uterine size, and ovarian masses or tenderness.
    b. Male: The penis should be examined for hypospadias, lesions, and discharge. The scrotum should be palpated for tenderness and masses. If a mass is present, it can be transilluminated to distinguish between solid and cystic masses. The groin region should be carefully palpated for bulging (hernias) upon rest and provocation (coughing, standing).
    c. Rectal examination: A rectal examination will reveal masses in the posterior pelvis and may identify gross or occult blood in the stool. In females, nodularity and tenderness in the uterosacral ligament may be signs of endometriosis. The posterior uterus and palpable masses in the cul-de-sac may be identified by rectal examination. In the male, the prostate gland should be palpated for tenderness, nodularity, and enlargement.

10.   Extremities/ skin: The presence of joint effusions, tenderness, rashes, edema, and cyanosis should be recorded. It is also important to note capillary refill and peripheral pulses.

11.   Neurological examination: Patients who present with neurological complaints require a thorough assessment including mental status, cranial nerves, strength, sensation, reflexes, and cerebellar function. In trauma patients, the Glasgow Coma Score is important (Table I-1).

Table I-1
GLASGOW COMA SCALE

ASSESSMENT AREA	SCORE
Eye Opening	
Spontaneous	4
To speech	3
To pain	2
None	1
Best motor response	
Obeys commands	6
Localizes pain	5
Withdraws to pain	4
Decorticate posture (abnormal flexion)	3
Decerebrate posture (extension)	2
No response	1
Verbal response	
Oriented	5
Confused conversation	4
Inappropriate words	3
Incomprehensible sounds	2
None	1

CLINICAL PEARL

❖ A thorough understanding of anatomy is important to optimally
   interpret the physical examination findings.

Laboratory Assessment

1. Laboratory assessment depends on the circumstances

2. CBC (complete blood count) can assess for anemia, leukocytosis
    (infection) and thrombocytopenia.

3. Basic metabolic panel: Electrolytes, glucose, BUN (blood urea nitro-
    gen) and creatinine (renal function).

4. Urinalysis and/or urine culture: To assess for hematuria, pyuria, or bac-
    teriuria. A pregnancy test is important in women of child-bearing age.

5. AST (aspartate aminotransferase), ALT (alanine aminotransferase),
    bilirubin, alkaline phosphatase for liver function; amylase and lipase
    to evaluate the pancreas.

6   Cardiac markers (CK-MB [creatine kinase myocardial band], tro-
    ponin, myoglobin) if coronary artery disease or other cardiac dys-
    function is suspected.

7. Drug levels such as acetaminophen level in possible overdoses.

8. Arterial blood gas measurements give information about oxygena-
    tion, but also carbon dioxide and pH readings.

Diagnostic Adjuncts

1. Electrocardiogram if cardiac ischemia, dysrhythmia, or other cardiac
    dysfunction is suspected.

2. Ultrasound examination: useful in evaluating pelvic processes in
    female patients (e.g., pelvic inflammatory disease, tubo-ovarian
    abscess) and in diagnosing gall stones and other gallbladder disease.
    With the addition of color-flow Doppler, deep venous thrombosis
    and ovarian or testicular torsion can be detected.

3. Computed tomography (CT): Useful in assessing the brain for mass-
    es, bleeding, strokes, skull fractures. CT of the chest can evaluate for
    masses, fluid collections, aortic dissections, and pulmonary emboli.
    Abdominal CT can detect infection (abscess, appendicitis, divertic-
    ulitis), masses, aortic aneurysms, and ureteral stones.

4. Magnetic resonance imaging (MRI) helps to identify soft tissue
    planes very well. In the emergency department (ED) setting, this is
    most commonly used to rule out spinal cord compression, cauda
    equina syndrome, and epidural abscess or hematoma.

PART 2. APPROACH TO CLINICAL PROBLEM-SOLVING

Classic Clinical Problem-Solving

There are typically five distinct steps that an ED clinician undertakes to systematically solve most clinical problems:

1. Addressing the ABCs and other life-threatening conditions
2. Making the diagnosis
3. Assessing the severity of the disease
4. Treating based on the stage of the disease
5. Following the patient's response to the treatment

Emergency Assessment and Management

Patients often present to the ED with life-threatening conditions that necessitate **simultaneous evaluation and treatment**. For example, a patient who is acutely short of breath and hypoxemic requires supplemental oxygen and possibly intubation with mechanical ventilation. While addressing these needs, the clinician must also try to determine whether the patient is dyspneic because of a pneumonia, congestive heart failure, pulmonary embolus, pneumothorax, or for some other reason.

As a general rule, **the first priority is stabilization of the ABCs** (see Table I-2). For instance, a comatose multi-trauma patient first requires intubation to protect the airway. See Figures I-1 through I-3 regarding management of airway and breathing issues. If the patient has a tension pneumothorax (breathing problem), (s)he needs an immediate needle thoracostomy. If (s)he is hypotensive, large-bore IV access and volume resuscitation are required for circulatory support. Pressure should be applied to any actively bleeding region. Figures I-4 through I-6 outline the key algorithms for cardiac dysthythmias. Once the ABCs and other life-threatening conditions are stabilized, a more complete history and head-to-toe physical exam should follow.

CLINICAL PEARL

❖ Because emergency physicians are faced with unexpected illness and injury, they must often perform diagnostic and therapeutic steps simultaneously. **In patients with an acutely life-threatening condition, the first and foremost priority is stabilization—the ABCs.**

Making the Diagnosis

This is achieved by carefully evaluating the patient, analyzing the information, assessing risk factors, and developing a list of possible diagnoses (the differen-

Table I-2
ASSESSMENT OF ABCs

	ASSESSMENT	MANAGEMENT
Airway	Assess oral cavity, patient color (pink vs. cyanotic), patency of airway (choking, aspiration, compression, foreign body, edema, blood), stridor, tracheal deviation, ease of ventilation with bag and mask	Head-tilt and chin-lift. If cervical spine injury suspected, stabilize neck and use jaw thrust. If obstruction, Heimlich maneuver, chest thrust, finger sweep (unconscious patient only). Temporizing airway (laryngeal mask airway). Definitive airway (intubation [nasotracheal or endotracheal], cricothyroidotomy)
Breathing	Look, listen, and feel for air movement and chest rising. Respiratory rate and effort (accessory muscles, diaphoresis, fatigue). Effective ventilation (bronchospasm, chest wall deformity, pulmonary embolism)	Resuscitation (mouth-to-mouth, mouth-to-mask, bag and mask). Supplemental oxygen, chest tube (pneumothorax or hemothorax)
Circulation	Palpate carotid artery. Assess pulse and blood pressure. Cardiac monitor to assess rhythm. Consider arterial pressure monitoring. Assess capillary refill	If pulseless, chest compressions and determine cardiac rhythm (consider epinephrine, defibrillation). Intravenous access (central line). Fluids. Consider 5Hs and 5Ts: Hypovolemia, Hypoxia, Hypothermia, Hyper-/Hypokalemia, Hydrogen (acidosis); Tension pneumothorax, Tamponade (cardiac), Thrombosis (massive pulmonary embolism), Thrombosis (myocardial infarction), Tablets (drug overdose).

Source: Reprinted, with permission, from Roman AM. Noninvasive airway management. In: Tintinalli JE, Kelen GD, Stapczynski JS, eds. Emergency medicine, 6th ed. New York: McGraw-Hill, 2004:102–8; and Danzl DE, Vissers RJ. Tracheal intubation. In: Tintinalli JE, Kelen GD, Stapczynski JS, eds. Emergency medicine, 6th ed. New York: McGraw-Hill: 2004,108–24.

tial). Usually a long list of possible diagnoses can be pared down to a few of the most likely or most serious ones, based on the clinician's knowledge, experience, and selective testing. For example, a patient who complains of upper abdominal pain and who has a history of nonsteroidal antiinflammatory drug (NSAID) use may have peptic ulcer disease; another patient who has abdominal pain, fatty

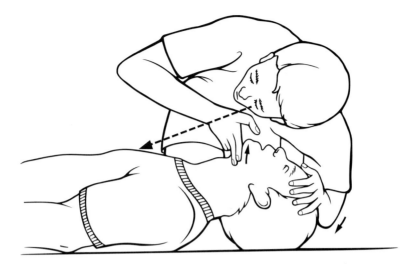

Figure I-1. Determination of breathlessness. The rescuer "looks, listens, and feels" for breath.

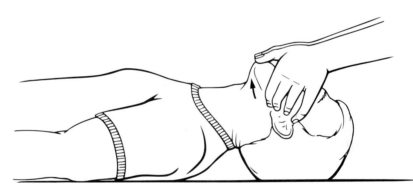

Figure I-2. Jaw-thrust maneuver. The rescuer lifts upward on the mandible while keeping the cervical spine in neutral position.

food intolerance, and abdominal bloating may have cholelithiasis. Yet another individual with a 1-day history of periumbilical pain that now localizes to the right lower quadrant may have acute appendicitis.

CLINICAL PEARL

❖ The second step in clinical problem solving is **making the diagnosis**.

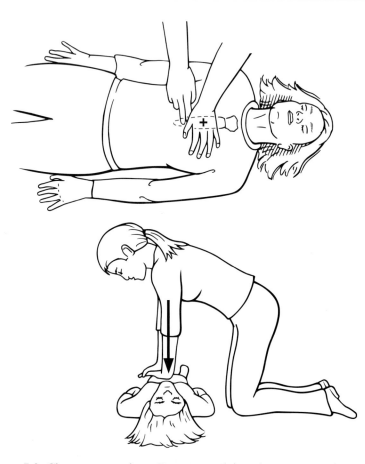

Figure I-3. Chest compressions. Rescuer applying chest compressions to an adult victim.

Assessing the Severity of the Disease

After establishing the diagnosis, the next step is to characterize the severity of the disease process; in other words, to describe "how bad" the disease is. This may be as simple as determining whether a patient is "sick" or "not sick." Is the patient with a urinary tract infection septic or stable for outpatient therapy? In other cases, a more formal staging may be used. For example, the Glasgow coma scale is used in patients with head trauma to describe the severity of their injury based on eye-opening, verbal, and motor responses.

> ### CLINICAL PEARL
> ❖ The third step is to **establish the severity or stage of disease**. This usually impacts the treatment and/or prognosis.

Treating Based on Stage

Many illnesses are characterized by stage or severity because this effects prognosis and treatment. As an example, a formerly healthy young man with pneumonia and no respiratory distress may be treated with oral antibiotics at home. An older person with emphysema and pneumonia would probably be admitted to the hospital for IV antibiotics. A patient with pneumonia and respiratory failure would likely be intubated and admitted to the intensive care unit for further treatment.

CLINICAL PEARL

❖ **The fourth step is tailoring the treatment to fit the severity or "stage" of the disease.**

Following the Response to Treatment

The final step in the approach to disease is to follow the patient's response to the therapy. Some responses are clinical such as improvement (or lack of improvement) in a patient's pain. Other responses may be followed by testing (e.g., monitoring the anion gap in a patient with diabetic ketoacidosis). The clinician must be prepared to know what to do if the patient does not respond as expected. Is the next step to treat again, to reassess the diagnosis, or to follow up with another more specific test?

CLINICAL PEARL

❖ **The fifth step is to monitor treatment response or efficacy.** This may be measured in different ways—symptomatically or based on physical examination or other testing. For the emergency physician, the vital signs, oxygenation, urine output, and mental status are the key parameters.

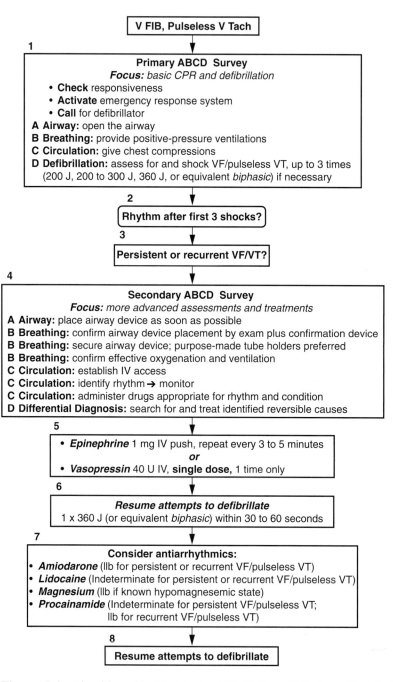

Figure I-4. Algorithm for Ventricular Fibrillation, Pulseless Ventricular Tachycardia. With permission from American Heart Association, ECC Guidelines, 2000. VF = Ventricular Fibrillation; VT = Ventricular Tachycardia.

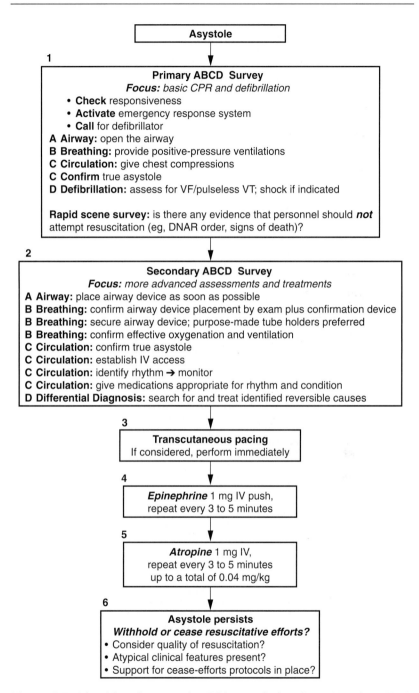

Figure I-5. Algorithm for asystole. With permission from American Heart Association, ECC Guidelines, 2000.

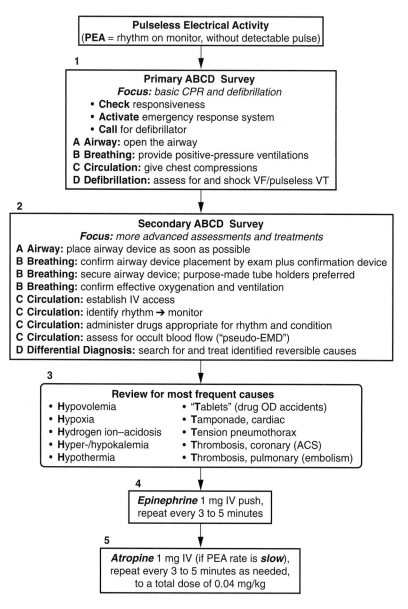

Figure I-6. Algorithm for Pulseless Electrical Activity. With permission from American Heart Association, ECC Guidelines, 2000.

PART 3. APPROACH TO READING

The clinical problem-oriented approach to reading is different from the classic "systematic" research of a disease. Patients rarely present with a clear diagnosis; hence, the student must become skilled in applying textbook information to the clinical scenario. Because reading with a purpose improves the retention of information, the student should read with the goal of answering specific questions. There are seven fundamental questions that facilitate **clinical thinking**.

1. What is the most likely diagnosis?
2. How would you confirm the diagnosis?
3. What should be your next step?
4. What is the most likely mechanism for this process?
5. What are the risk factors for this condition?
6. What are the complications associated with the disease process?
7. What is the best therapy?

CLINICAL PEARL

❖ **Reading with the purpose of answering the seven fundamental clinical questions improves retention of information** and facilitates the application of "book knowledge" to "clinical knowledge."

What Is the Most Likely Diagnosis?

The method of establishing the diagnosis was covered in the previous section. One way of attacking this problem is to develop standard "approaches" to common clinical problems. It is helpful to understand the most common causes of various presentations, such as "the worst headache of the patient's life is worrisome for a subarachnoid hemorrhage." (See the "Clinical Pearls" at end of each case.)

The clinical scenario would be something such as: "A 38-year-old woman is noted to have a 2-day history of a unilateral, throbbing headache and photophobia. What is the most likely diagnosis?"

With no other information to go on, the student would note that this woman has a unilateral headache and photophobia. Using the "most common cause" information, the student would make an educated guess that the patient has a migraine headache. If instead the patient is noted to have "the worst headache of her life," the student would use the Clinical Pearl: "The worst headache of the patient's life is worrisome for a subarachnoid hemorrhage."

> ### CLINICAL PEARL
>
> ❖ The more common cause of a unilateral, throbbing headache with photophobia is a migraine, but **the main concern is subarachnoid hemorrhage**. If the patient describes this as "the worst headache of her life," the concern for a subarachnoid bleed is increased.

How Would You Confirm the Diagnosis?

In the scenario above, the woman with "the worst headache of her life" is suspected of having a subarachnoid hemorrhage. This diagnosis could be confirmed by a CT scan of the head and/or lumbar puncture. The student should learn the limitations of various diagnostic tests, especially when used early in a disease process. The lumbar puncture (LP) showing xanthochromia (lysed red blood cells) is the "gold standard" test for diagnosing subarachnoid hemorrhage, but it may be negative early in the disease course.

What Should Be Your Next Step?

This question is difficult because the next step has many possibilities; the answer may be to obtain more diagnostic information, stage the illness, or introduce therapy. It is often a more challenging question than "What is the most likely diagnosis?" because there may be insufficient information to make a diagnosis and the next step may be to pursue more diagnostic information. Another possibility is that there is enough information for a probable diagnosis, and the next step is to stage the disease. Finally, the most appropriate answer may be to treat. Hence, from clinical data, a judgment needs to be rendered regarding how far along one is on the road of:

(1) Make a diagnosis → (2) Stage the disease → (3) Treat based on stage → (4) Follow response

Frequently, the student is taught "to regurgitate" the same information that (s)he has read about a particular disease, but is not skilled at identifying the next step. This talent is learned optimally at the bedside, in a supportive environment, with freedom to take educated guesses and with constructive feedback. A sample scenario might describe a student's thought process as follows:

1. *Make the Diagnosis:* "Based on the information I have, I believe that Mr. Smith has a small-bowel obstruction from adhesive disease *because* he presents with nausea and vomiting, abdominal distension, high-pitched hyperactive bowel sounds, and has dilated loops of small bowel on x-ray."
2. *Stage the Disease:* "I don't believe that this is severe disease because he does not have fever, evidence of sepsis, intractable pain, peritoneal signs, or leukocytosis."

3. *Treat Based on Stage:* "Therefore, my next step is to treat with nothing per mouth, NG (nasogastric) tube drainage, IV fluids, and observation."

4. *Follow Response:* "I want to follow the treatment by assessing his pain (I will ask him to rate the pain on a scale of 1 to 10 every day), his bowel function (I will ask whether he has had nausea or vomiting, or passed flatus), his temperature, abdominal exam, serum bicarbonate (for metabolic acidemia), and white blood cell count, and I will reassess his status in 48 hours."

In a similar patient, when the clinical presentation is unclear, perhaps the best "next step" may be diagnostic, such as an oral contrast radiological study to assess for bowel obstruction.

CLINICAL PEARL

❖   Usually, the vague query, "What is your next step?" is the most difficult question because the answer may be diagnostic, staging, or therapeutic.

What Is the Likely Mechanism for This Process?

This question goes further than making the diagnosis, but also requires the student to understand the underlying mechanism for the process. For example, a clinical scenario may describe a 68-year-old male who notes urinary hesitancy and retention, and has a nontender large hard mass in his left supraclavicular region. This patient has bladder neck obstruction either as a consequence of benign prostatic hypertrophy or prostatic cancer. However, the indurated mass in the left neck area is suspicious for cancer. The reason that the metastasis occurs in the area of the thoracic duct is because the malignant cells flow in the lymph fluid, which drains into the left subclavian vein. The student is advised to learn the mechanisms for each disease process, and not merely memorize a constellation of symptoms. Furthermore, in emergency medicine, it is crucial for the student to understand the anatomy, function, and how the treatment would correct the problem.

What Are the Risk Factors for This Process?

Understanding the risk factors helps the practitioner to establish a diagnosis and to determine how to interpret test results. For example, understanding the risk factor analysis may help in the management of a 55-year-old woman with anemia. If the patient has risk factors for endometrial cancer (such as diabetes, hypertension, anovulation) and complains of postmenopausal bleeding, she likely has endometrial carcinoma and should have an endometrial biopsy. Otherwise, occult colonic bleeding is a common etiology. If she takes NSAIDs or aspirin, then peptic ulcer disease is the most likely cause.

> ### CLINICAL PEARL
>
> ❖ Being able to assess risk factors helps to guide testing and develop the differential diagnosis.

What Are the Complications to This Process?

Clinicians must be cognizant of the complications of a disease, so that they will understand how to follow and monitor the patient. Sometimes the student will have to make the diagnosis from clinical clues and then apply his or her knowledge of the consequences of the pathological process. For example, "A 26-year-old male complains of right-lower-extremity swelling and pain after a trans-Atlantic flight" and his Doppler ultrasound reveals a deep vein thrombosis. Complications of this process include pulmonary embolism (PE). Understanding the types of consequences also helps the clinician to be aware of the dangers to a patient. If the patient has any symptoms consistent with a PE, a ventilation-perfusion scan or CT scan angiographic imaging of the chest may be necessary.

What Is the Best Therapy?

To answer this question, not only does the clinician need to reach the correct diagnosis and assess the severity of the condition, but the clinician must also weigh the situation to determine the appropriate intervention. For the student, knowing exact dosages is not as important as understanding the best medication, route of delivery, mechanism of action, and possible complications. It is important for the student to be able to verbalize the diagnosis and the rationale for the therapy.

> ### CLINICAL PEARL
>
> ❖ Therapy should be logical based on the severity of disease and the specific diagnosis. An exception to this rule is in an emergent situation such as respiratory failure or shock when the patient needs treatment even as the etiology is being investigated.

SUMMARY

1. The first and foremost priority in addressing the emergency patient is stabilization, first assessing and treating the ABCs (airway, breathing, circulation).
2. There is no replacement for a meticulous history and physical examination.
3. There are five steps in the clinical approach to the emergency patient: addressing life-threatening conditions, making the diagnosis, assessing severity, treating based on severity, and following response.

4. There are seven questions that help to bridge the gap between the textbook and the clinical arena.

REFERENCES

Hamilton GC. Introduction to emergency medicine. In: Hamilton GC, Sanders AB, Strange GR, Trott AT. Emergency medicine: an approach to clinical problem-solving. Philadelphia: Saunders, 2003:3–16.

Hirshop JM. Basic CPR in adults. In: Tintinalli J, Kelen GD, Stapczynski JS, eds.. Emergency medicine, 6th ed. New York: McGraw-Hill, 2004 pp 66–71.

Jeffrey RB. Imaging the surgical patient. In: Niederhuber JE, ed. Fundamentals of surgery. New York: Appleton & Lange, 1998:68–75.

Niederhuber JE. The surgical service and surgery training. In: Niederhuber JE, ed. Fundamentals of surgery. New York: Appleton & Lange, 1998:3–9.

Ornato JP. Sudden cardiac death. In: Tintinalli J, Kelen GD, Stapczynski JS, eds.. Emergency medicine, 6th ed. New York: McGraw-Hill, 2004 pp 61–66.

SECTION II

Clinical Cases

A 13-year-old male presents to the emergency department with a chief complaint of sore throat and fever for the past 2 days. He reports that his younger sister has been ill for the past week with "the same thing." The patient has no other medical problems, takes no medications, and has no allergies. He denies any recent history of cough, rash, nausea, vomiting, or diarrhea. He denies any recent travel and has completed the full series of childhood immunizations.

On examination, the patient has a temperature of 38.5°C (101.3°F), a heart rate of 104 bpm, blood pressure 118/64 mmHg, a respiratory rate of 18 breaths per minute, and an oxygen saturation of 99% on room air. HEENT (head, ears, eyes, nose, throat) exam reveals erythema of the posterior oropharynx with tonsillar exudates, but no uvular deviation or significant tonsillar swelling. Neck exam reveals mild tenderness of anterior lymph nodes. His neck is supple. The chest and cardiovascular exams are unremarkable, and his abdomen is nontender with normal bowel sounds and no hepatosplenomegaly. His skin is without rash.

◆ **What is the most likely diagnosis?**

◆ **What is your next step?**

◆ **What are potential complications?**

ANSWERS TO CASE 1: Streptococcal Pharyngitis ("Strep Throat")

Summary: This is a 13-year-old male with pharyngitis. He has fever, tonsillar exudate, no cough and no tender cervical adenopathy. There is no evidence of airway compromise.

◆ **Most likely diagnosis:** Streptococcal pharyngitis

◆ **Next step:** Evaluate patient for antibiotics (penicillin)

◆ **Potential complications:** Poststreptococcal glomerulonephritis and acute rheumatic fever

Analysis

Objectives

1. Recognize the differential diagnosis for pharyngitis, especially the life-threatening conditions.
2. Be familiar with widely accepted decision-making strategies for the diagnosis and management of group A β-hemolytic streptococcal (GAβS) pharyngitis.
3. Learn about the treatment of GAβS pharyngitis and the sequelae of this disease. Be familiar with appropriate follow-up management of this condition.
4. Recognize acute airway emergencies associated with upper airway infections.

Considerations

This 13-year-old patient presents with a common diagnostic dilemma: sore throat and fever. The first priority for the physician is to assess whether the patient is more ill than the complaint would indicate: **stridorous breathing, air hunger, toxic appearance**, or **drooling with inability to swallow** would **indicate impending disaster**. The ABCs (airway, breathing, circulation) must always be addressed first. This patient does not have those type of "alarms." Thus a more relaxed elicitation of history and examination of the head, neck, and throat can occur. In instances suggestive of epiglottitis such as stridor, drooling, and toxic appearance, examination of the throat (especially with a tongue blade) may cause upper airway obstruction in a child leading to respiratory failure. During the examination, the clinician should be alert for complications of upper airway infection; however, this patient presents with a simple pharyngitis.

Although the most common etiology of pharyngitis is viral organisms over-all, this teenager has several features that make group A streptococcus more likely: **his age being less than 15 years, fever, absence of cough**, and the presence of **tonsillar exudate**. The one criterion he is missing is "tender anterior cervical adenopathy." Thus, the diagnosis is not assured without further testing. Rapid streptococcal antigen testing can give a fairly accurate result immediately and treatment or nontreatment with penicillin can be based on this result. If the rapid streptococcal antigen test is positive, antibiotic therapy should be given; if the rapid test is negative, throat culture should be performed. The **gold standard for diagnosis is bacterial culture**, and if positive, the patient should be notified and given penicillin therapy.

APPROACH TO PHARYNGITIS

The differential diagnosis of pharyngitis is broad and includes **viral etiologies** (rhinovirus, coronavirus, adenovirus, herpes simplex virus [HSV], influenza, parainfluenza, Epstein-Barr virus [EBV] and CMV [cytomegalovirus] [causing infectious mononucleosis], coxsackie virus [causing herpangina], and the human immunodeficiency virus [HIV]), bacterial causes (GAβS, group C streptococci, *Arcanobacterium haemolyticum*, meningococci, gonococci, diphtheria, chlamydia, *Legionella*, and *Mycoplasma* species), specific anatomically related conditions caused by bacterial organisms (peritonsillar abscess, epiglottitis, retropharyngeal abscess, Vincent angina, and Ludwig angina), candidal pharyngitis, aphthous stomatitis, thyroiditis, and bullous erythema multiforme. **Viruses** are **the most common cause of pharyngitis.**

Group A streptococcus causes pharyngitis in 5 to 10 percent of adults and 15 to 30 percent of children who seek medical care with the complaint of sore throat. It is often clinically indistinguishable from other etiologies, yet it is the major treatable cause of pharyngitis. Primary HIV infection may also be a cause of acute pharyngitis, and its recognition can be beneficial because early antiretroviral therapy can be started. Infectious mononucleosis is also important to exclude because of the risk of splenomegaly and splenic rupture. Other **bacterial etiologies** may also be treated with antibiotics. Studies suggest that certain symptoms and historical features are suggestive of streptococcal pharyngitis and may help guide the provider in generating a reasonable pretest probability of GAβS. The Centor criteria, modified by age risk; is helpful in assessing for GAβS (see Table 1-1).

Throat cultures remain the gold standard for the diagnosis of GAβS pharyngitis, but it has several limitations and decreasing utility in daily practice. False-negative throat cultures may occur in patients with few organisms in their pharynx or as a result of inadequate sampling technique (e.g., improper swabbing method, or errors in incubation or reading of plates). Patients may be asymptomatic carriers of GAβS, resulting in false positives. Throat cultures are costly and, perhaps more importantly, 24 to 48 hours are required for results. Although it may be reasonable to delay therapy for this period of time (delay will not increase likelihood of development of rheumatic fever specifically), it requires further communication with the patient and perhaps an uncomfortable latency in therapy from the concerned parent. Nevertheless, a negative throat culture may prompt discontinuation of antibiotics.

Table 1-1

CENTOR CRITERIA FOR PREDICTING STREPTOCOCCAL
PHARYNGITIS

Presence of tonsillar exudates: 1 point

Tender anterior cervical adenopathy: 1 point

Fever by history: 1 point

Absence of cough: 1 point

Age under 15 years*, add 1 point to total score

Age over 45 years*, subtract 1 point from total score.

*Modifications to the original Centor Criteria
Sources: Centor Rm, Witherspoon JM, Dalton HP, et al. The diagnosis of strp throat in adults in
the emergency room. Med Decis making.. 1981;1:239–46; and McIsaac WJ, White D,
Tannenbaum D, Low DE. A clinical score to rduce unnecessary antibiotic use in patients with
sore throat.CMAJ 1998;158(1):75–83.

The rapid-antigen test (RAT) for GAβS, although having some limitations, has been embraced by many experts and has been incorporated into diagnostic algorithms. The **RAT is 80 to 90 percent sensitive** and exceedingly specific when compared to throat cultures, and results are available in minutes at the point-of-care. Again, these tests are somewhat costly, and many experts recommend **confirmation of negative tests with definitive throat cultures**. Individuals with **positive RAT results should be treated**. Newer technologies, such as the optical immunoassay, may prove to be as sensitive as throat cultures while providing results within minutes; its cost-effectiveness has not been established. One widely accepted algorithm is summarized in Figure 1-1.

◆ Patients with 4 points (from the Centor and McIsaac criteria) should be empirically treated, because their pretest probability is reasonably high (although overtreatment may result in as many as 50 percent of patients).

◆ Patients with 0 or 1 points should not receive antibiotics or diagnostic tests (the criteria have been shown here to yield a negative predictive value of roughly 80 percent).

◆ Those with 2 or 3 points should have RAT and those with positive RAT results should be treated. Negative RAT results should be followed with a definitive throat culture.

If rapid antigen testing is unavailable, then one suggested strategy is as follows (see Figure 1-2):

◆ Patients with 3 or 4 points should be empirically treated with antibiotics.

◆ Patients with zero or 1 point should not receive antibiotics or diagnostic tests.

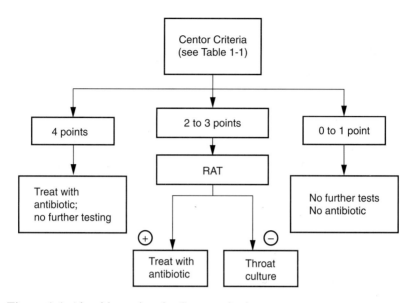

Figure 1-1. Algorithm using the Centor criteria.

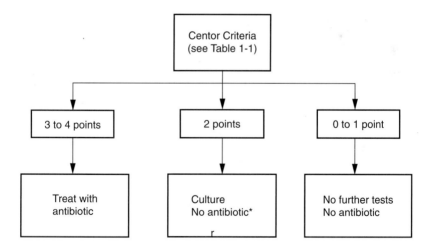

*   Consider antibiotics if in setting of GAβS outbreak, patient had contact with many children, is immunocompromised, or recent exposure to a patient with documented GAβS.

Figure 1-2. Algorithm when RAT unavailable.

◆ Patients with 2 points should *not* receive antibiotics. The possible exceptions to this 2-point rule is in the setting of a GAβS outbreak, patient contact with many children, an immunocompromised patient, or a patient with recent exposure to someone with confirmed GAβS.

Antibiotic therapy in GAβS pharyngitis has been scrutinized because complications have become increasingly rare and the data to support the efficacy of antibiotic therapy in prevention of these complications is sparse and many decades old. The complications of GAβS can be classified into nonsuppurative and suppurative processes. The **nonsuppurative complications of GAβS pharyngitis** include **rheumatic fever, streptococcal toxic shock syndrome, poststreptococcal glomerulonephritis, and PANDAS** (pediatric autoimmune neuropsychiatric disorder associated with group A streptococci). Rheumatic fever is now rare in North America (some sources cite an incidence of 1/100,000 population), and is thought to be caused by only a handful of strains of GAβS. Despite its rarity, rheumatic fever can result in highly morbid cardiac and neurological sequela; it also remains a significant problem in developing countries. Streptococcal toxic shock syndrome is a very rare complication of pharyngitis. Poststreptococcal glomerulonephritis, another feared complication of GAβS pharyngitis, is also very rare, and evidence is mounting that it may occur with equal frequency in both antibiotic-treated and nonantibiotic-treated groups. It is unclear if antibiotic therapy reduces the incidence of **PANDAS**, which is a clinical entity in development and presents with episodes of **obsessive-compulsive behavior.**

Prevention of the suppurative complications of GAβS pharyngitis remains perhaps the most compelling reason for antibiotic therapy, although these conditions are also less frequently encountered. These processes include **tonsillopharyngeal cellulitis, peritonsillar and retropharyngeal abscesses, sinusitis, meningitis and brain abscess, otitis media, and streptococcal bacteremia.** The precise incidence of these complications is unclear, but what remains clear is that these are often preventable sequela that can have devastating consequences. Ultimately, the current practice is to treat suspected GAβS pharyngitis with an appropriate antibiotic.

Treatment of GAβS   **Penicillin is the antibiotic of choice for GAβS pharyngitis**; it is inexpensive, well-tolerated, and has a reasonably narrow spectrum. **Oral therapy requires a ten-day course**, although multiple daily doses for this duration may pose an issue with respect to compliance; penicillin V 500 mg twice-daily dosing for 10 days in adults (as opposed to 250 mg t.i.d. or q.i.d.) is a reasonable alternative. For patients in whom compliance may be a significant issue, **a single IM shot of 600,000 units of penicillin G benzathine for patients weighing <27 kg (1.2 million units if patient weighs >27 kg)** is another option, although it requires an uncomfortable injection and, more significantly, it cannot be reversed or discontinued should an adverse reaction to the agent occur. All patients, regardless of final diagnosis, should be given adequate analgesia and reassurance. Patient satisfaction depends more on the clinician showing concern and reassurance than actually giving antibiotics.

AIRWAY COMPLICATIONS   There are several life-threatening causes of sore throat. Patients may suffer airway obstruction from acute epiglottitis, peritonsillar abscess, retropharyngeal abscess, and Ludwig angina (Table 1-2); although less frequent, airway compromise may also occur with Vincent angina and diphtheric pharyngitis; the latter, although rare, requires prompt diagnosis

Table 1-2
COMPLICATED UPPER AIRWAY INFECTIONS

	CLINICAL PRESENTATION	DIAGNOSIS	TREATMENT
Epiglottitis	Sudden onset of fever, drooling, tachypneic, stridor, toxic appearing	Lateral cervical radiograph (thumb-printing sign)	Urgent ENT (ear, nose, throat) consultation for airway management Helium-O_2 mixture Cefuroxime antibiotic therapy
Retropharyngeal abscess	Usually child or if adult (trauma) Fever, sore throat, stiff neck, no trismus	Lateral cervical radiograph or CT imaging	Stabilize airway Surgical drainage Antibiotics (penicillin and metronidazole)
Ludwig angina	Submaxillary, sub-lingual, or sub-mental mass with elevation of tongue, jaw swell-ing, fever, chills, trismus	Lateral cervical radiograph or CT imaging	Stabilize airway Drain abscess Antibiotics (penicillin and metronidazole)
Peritonsillar abscess	Swelling in the peritonsillar region with uvula pushed aside, fever, sore throat, dys-phagia, trismus	Cervical radio-graph or CT imaging Aspiration of the region with pus	Abscess drainage Antibiotic therapy (penicillin and metronidazole)

and treatment to avoid spread of this highly infectious condition. Management of the airway in these conditions (see Table I-2 in the "Introduction") sometimes necessitates emergency cricothyroidotomy (Figure 1-3), because the pharynx and larynx may be edematous, distorted, or inflamed. Prompt identification of acute retroviral syndrome from recent HIV infection can allow for

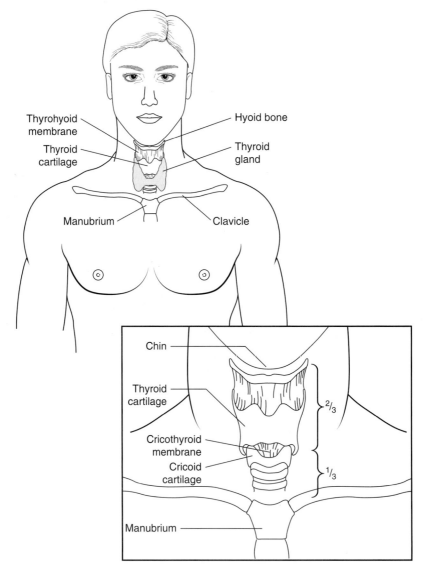

Figure 1-3. Anatomy of the neck for emergency cricothyroidotomy. Note the location of the thyroid and cricoid cartilages.

rapid antiretroviral therapy. Infectious mononucleosis should be identified so that potentially serious sequelae can be considered. These complications include splenomegaly that predisposes the patient to traumatic rupture of the spleen with relatively minor trauma; additionally, this splenomegaly can cause splenic sequestration and thrombocytopenia.

Comprehension Questions

[1.1] A 48-year-old man is noted to have a 2-day history of sore throat, subjective fever at home, and no medical illnesses. He denies cough or nausea. On examination, his temperature is 38.3°C (101°F), and he has some tonsillar swelling but no exudate. He has bilateral enlarged and tender lymph nodes of the neck. The rapid streptococcal antigen test is negative. Which of the following is the best next step?

A. Oral clindamycin
B. Treat based on results from throat culture
C. Observation
D. Begin amantadine

[1.2] Which of the following patients is most likely to have group A streptococcal infection?

A. An 11-month-old male with fever and red throat.
B. An 8-year-old girl with fever and sore throat.
C. A 27-year-old man with a temperature of 38.9°C (102°F), pharyngitis, and cough.
E. A 52-year-old woman who complains of fever of 39.2°C (102.5°F) and sore throat.

[1.3] A 19-year-old college student has had a sore throat, mild abdominal pain, and fever for 5 days. He was playing football with some friends, and was tackled just short of the goal line, hitting the grass somewhat forcibly. He experiences some abdominal pain, and passes out. The EMS (Emergency Medical Services) is called and his vital signs reveal the heart rate as 140 bpm and blood pressure as 80/40 mmHg with a distended abdomen. Which of the following is the most likely etiology?

A. Vasovagal reaction
B. Ruptured aortic aneurysm
C. Complications of Epstein-Barr infection
D. Ruptured jejenum

[1.4]   An 18-year-old female presents with fever and a sore throat. She is sitting up drooling, with some stridor. Her temperature is 39.4°C (103°F) and she appears ill. Which of the following is your next step?

A. Examine the pharynx and obtain a rapid antigen test
B. Empiric treatment with penicillin
C. Throat culture and treat based on results
D. Send the patient to radiology for an anteroposterior (AP) neck radiograph
E. Prepare for emergent airway management

Answers

[1.1]   **B.** This individual has a modified Centor score of 2 (history of fever, tender adenopathy, no cough, age greater than 45 years). The rapid antigen test is negative, but a definitive culture should be performed for a Centor score of 2 or 3, and treatment should be based on culture results.

[1.2]   **B.** GAβS is most common in the younger than 15-year-old age group (although not in infants.) McIsaac added age as a criteria because patients older than age 45 years have a much lower incidence of streptococcal pharyngitis.

[1.3]   **C.** This patient most likely suffered from splenic rupture caused by mononucleosis (EBV). He is hypotensive because of the massive hemoperitoneum.

[1.4]   **E.** Regardless of the etiology, this patient has a clinical presentation alarming for impending respiratory collapse, and preparation for emergent airway management is the most important next step. The drooling and stridor are suspicious for epiglottitis, which can present more insidiously in adults. Examination of the posterior pharynx may induce laryngospasm and airway obstruction, particularly in children; a lateral neck radiograph to assess for a "thumb-printing" of epiglottitis may be helpful in making the diagnosis, but sending the patient with impending respiratory failure to a radiology area is inappropriate.

CLINICAL PEARLS

❖ The most common causes of pharyngitis in general are viruses.
❖ The Centor criteria suggestive of GAβS pharyngitis include tonsillar exudate, tender anterior cervical adenopathy, history of fever, and absence of cough.
❖ GAβS pharyngitis is more common in patients younger than 15 years of age, and less common in those older than 45 years of age.

❖ Overtreatment of pharyngitis with antibiotics is common and is a major source of antibiotic overuse in this country.

❖ Glomerulonephritis is a rare complication of GAβS pharyngitis (but not GAβS infections of other tissues) that is not clearly prevented by antibiotic therapy.

❖ Rheumatic fever is an exceedingly rare complication of GAβS pharyngitis that can be prevented by antibiotic therapy.

❖ Complicated upper airway conditions should be considered when a patient presents with "sore throat."

❖ In general, cricothyroidotomy is the safest method of surgically securing an airway in the ED.

REFERENCES

Bisno AL. Acute pharyngitis. N Engl J Med 2001;344(3):205–11.

Bisno AL, Gerber MA, Gwaltney JM, Kaplan EL, Schwartz RH. Practice guidelines for the diagnosis and management of group A streptococcal pharyngitis. Clin Infect Dis 2002;35:113–125.

Centor RM, Witherspoon JM, Dalton HP, Brody CE, Link K. The diagnosis of strep throat in adults in the emergency room. Med Decis Making, 1981;1:239-46.

Cooper RJ, Hoffman JR, Bartlett, JG, et al. Principles of appropriate antibiotic use for acute pharyngitis in adults: background. Ann Intern Med 2001;134:509–17.

McIsaac WJ, Goel V, To T, Low DE. The validity of a sore throat score in family practice. CMAJ 2000;163(7):811–15.

McIsaac WJ, White D, Tannenbaum D, Low DE. A clinical score to reduce unnecessary antibiotic use in patients with sore throat. CMAJ 1998;158(1):75–83.

Snow V, Mottur-Pison C, Cooper RJ, Hoffman JR. Principles of appropriate antibiotic use for acute pharyngitis in adults. Ann Intern Med 2001;134:506–8.

A 58-year-old man arrives at the emergency department complaining of chest pain. The pain began 1 hour ago, during breakfast, and is described as severe, dull, and pressure-like. It is substernal in location, radiates to both shoulders and is associated with shortness of breath. His wife adds that he was very sweaty when the pain began. The patient has diabetes and hypertension and takes hydrochlorothiazide and glyburide. His blood pressure is 150/100 mmHg, pulse rate is 95 bpm, respirations are 20 breaths per minute, temperature 37.3°C (99.1°F), and oxygen saturation by pulse oximetry is 98 percent. The patient is diaphoretic and appears anxious. On auscultation, faint crackles are heard at both lung bases. The cardiac exam reveals an S_4 gallop and is otherwise normal. The examination of the abdomen reveals no masses or tenderness. An EKG is performed (see Figure 2-1).

◆ **What is the most likely diagnosis?**

◆ **What are the next diagnostic steps?**

◆ **What therapies should be instituted immediately?**

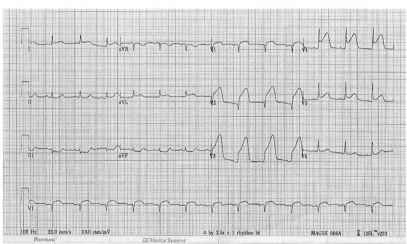

Figure 2-1. EKG. Courtesy of Dr. Bradley Frazee, MD.

ANSWERS TO CASE 2: Myocardial Infarction, Acute

Summary: This is a 58-year-old man presenting with acute severe chest pain, diaphoresis, and dyspnea. The patient has a number of risk factors for underlying coronary artery disease and the history and physical exam are typical of an acute coronary syndrome (ACS). The EKG shows marked ST segment elevation of V3 to V6, I aVL.

 Most likely diagnosis: Acute myocardial infarction, probable anterolateral MI.

 Next diagnostic steps: Place the patient on a cardiac monitor and establish IV access. A chest x-ray and serum levels of cardiac markers should be obtained as soon as possible.

 Immediate therapies: Aspirin is the most important immediate therapy. **Oxygen** and **sublingual nitroglycerin** are also standard early therapies. Emergency reperfusion therapy, such as a thrombolysis, is likely indicated. Intravenous beta blockers, IV nitroglycerin, low-molecular-weight heparin, and additional antiplatelet agents, such as clopidogrel, might also be indicated.

Analysis

Objectives

1. Recognize acute myocardial infarction (MI) and the spectrum of acute coronary syndromes (ACSs).
2. Know the appropriate diagnostic tests and their limitations.
3. Understand the therapeutic approach to ACS.

Considerations

As soon as this patient arrives into the ED with chest pain, immediate triaging is critical, because **"time is myocardium."** As usual, the initial concern is focused on ABCs, and life-threatening complications of MI such as arrhythmias or heart failure. Concurrently, unless contraindicated, the patient should receive **aspirin to chew (162 mg),** be placed on oxygen, cardiac monitors, oxygen saturation monitors, and be given nitroglycerin if the chest pain is still present. IV access should be established, and labs sent for cardiac enzymes, electrolytes, renal function tests, prothrombin time (PT), partial thromboplastin time (PTT), and CBC. An **EKG** should be **performed optimally within 10 minutes of the patient's arrival**. Within minutes, an assessment of risk factors and character of the chest pain, and other less-common **life-threatening diseases** presenting as chest pain, including **aortic dissection, pulmonary embolus, pneumothorax, rupture of the esophagus (Boerhaave syndrome),** should be considered.

This patient is a 58-year-old male, which in itself places him in a category at risk for cardiovascular disease; furthermore, he has diabetes and hypertension, two significant risk factors for coronary heart disease. The description of this patient's chest pain is classic for angina: substernal in nature, associated with diaphoresis and dyspnea; frequently, diabetics will have atypical or subtle chest pain requiring a high index of suspicion. He should be placed into the "cardiac room," and efforts made to save myocardium at risk (by decreasing myocardial demand), monitor for complications, assess for angioplasty or thrombolytic therapy. **Cardiac monitoring is important because sudden death, especially caused by ventricular arrhythmias, is common**; a defibrillator should be nearby, preferably in the room. A portable chest radiograph is vital, because it helps to assess for other causes of chest pain such as aortic dissection (widened mediastinum). **Aortic dissection is a contraindication for thrombolytic therapy**.

APPROACH TO SUSPECTED MYOCARDIAL INFARCTION

Definitions

Myocardial infarction: permanent myocardial damage (muscle necrosis) as evidenced by elevation of cardiac enzymes, subdivided into ST elevation and non-ST elevation.

Acute coronary syndrome: acute chest pain caused by myocardial ischemia encompassing myocardial infarction (permanent heart damage) and unstable angina (reversible heart damage).

Unstable angina: acute chest pain at rest, new-onset, or increasing in severity.

Non-ST elevation myocardial infarction: myocardial infarction, usually associated with incomplete coronary artery occlusion, and usually not resulting in Q-wave formation.

ST elevation myocardial infarction: Cardiac muscle necrosis associated with ST-segment elevation, usually caused by complete coronary artery occlusion, and usually resulting in Q waves on the EKG.

Clinical Approach

Pathophysiology Chest pain accounts for more than 6 million visits every year to emergency departments in the United States. Of these 6 million visits, nearly 800,000 will end with a diagnosis of MI and 1.5 million will be given diagnoses of unstable angina (UA) or non-ST elevation myocardial infarction (NSTEMI). **Coronary heart disease (CHD) is the leading cause of death in adults in the United States.** Furthermore, missed MI accounts for the most money paid in malpractice claims in emergency medicine. Because ACS is common, treatable, and potentially catastrophic both clinically and medicolegally, emergency physicians should be thoroughly familiar with this problem.

Our understanding of the pathophysiology behind cardiac ischemia has evolved from a model of progressive coronary artery narrowing to a current model of **plaque rupture and thrombus formation**. The concept of fixed narrowing explains only stable angina brought on by increased myocardial demand. In contrast, ACS, which encompasses the spectrum of UA, NSTEMI and ST elevation myocardial infarction (STEMI), involves a dynamic process of inflammation and intravascular thrombosis, beginning with coronary artery plaque rupture. The fate of this plaque, in terms of location and extent of subsequent thrombosis, determines the clinical presentation and seems to correlate with the subdivisions of ACS. **STEMI occurs when total occlusion of an epicardial vessel causes transmural infarction,** classically presenting as **unremitting chest pain** and **ST segment elevation on the EKG.** It is **treated with immediate reperfusion therapy**.

The clinical syndromes of **NSTEMI and UA**, in contrast, are caused by **subendocardial infarction or ischemia, respectively**, usually caused by microemboli arising from the ruptured plaque. Chest pain is often stuttering and EKG changes such as ST segment depression may be transient. Although often indistinguishable upon initial presentation, **elevation in cardiac markers** is **what eventually distinguishes NSTEMI from UA.** Immediate therapy for both NSTEMI and UA focuses on halting ongoing thrombosis and reducing myocardial demand. Many patients go on to have percutaneous coronary intervention (PCI), such as stent placement, directed at the unstable plaque.

Evaluation   The cornerstone of diagnosis of coronary syndromes is the **EKG**, and the findings on the initial EKG form a **critical branch point in therapy**; thus, ideally, patients presenting to the emergency department with chest pain suggestive of ACS should have an EKG within 10 minutes of arrival. **Identifying STEMI by EKG as soon as possible is the first step** toward rapidly establishing reperfusion and reducing mortality (the EKG criteria for reperfusion therapy are listed in Table 2-1). In contrast to STEMI, EKG findings may be subtle or absent in NSTEMI and UA, and are not required for diagnosis and initiation of therapy. However, certain findings, such as ST segment depression or deep T-wave inversions, particularly those that change in accord with symptoms, can rapidly establish the diagnosis of UA and NSTEMI. Unfortunately, the **EKG is frequently nondiagnostic in ACS**; it is nondiagnostic in approximately 50 percent and completely normal in up to 8 percent of individuals who eventually are diagnosed with myocardial infarction. Comparing the current EKG to old tracings is crucial, because subtle changes may be seen. Serial EKGs, or continuous ST-segment monitoring may reveal the subtle dynamic changes of UA, or those of an evolving MI (Table 2-2 lists the anatomical locations of MI).

In the face of a **normal or nondiagnostic EKG**, the **pretest probability** (likelihood that the pain is actually of cardiac origin based on the patient's overall risk profile) dictates diagnostic testing. Inquiring about traditional

Table 2-1
KEY EKG FINDINGS IN ACS

STEMI: indications for immediate reperfusion therapy

ST elevation>1 mV (1 mm) in 2 contiguous leads and <12 hours since pain onset	Left bundle-branch block not known to be old with a history suggestive of acute MI

Typical EKG findings in NSTEMI and UA

Horizontal ST segment depression	Deep T-wave inversions
EKG findings change in accord with symptoms	

Source: Hollander JE, Diercks DB. Intervention strategies for acute coronary syndromes. In: Tintinalli JE, Kelen GD, Stapczynski JS, eds. Emergency medicine 6th ed. New York: McGraw-Hill: 2004:108–24.

Table 2-2
FINDINGS AND ANATOMICAL CORRELATION

CORONARY ARTERY	LOCATION	EKG LEADS
LAD	Anteroseptal	V1, V2, V3
LAD	Anterior	V2–V4
LCA	Lateral	I, aVL, V4-6
RCA	Inferior	II, III, aVF
RCA	Right ventricular	V4R (also II, III, aVF)
RCA, LCA	Posterior	R waves in V1, V2

Abbreviations: LAD = left anterior descending artery; LCA = left circumflex artery; RCA = right circumflex artery; V4R = right-sided lead which should be placed any time an inferior MI is suspected.
Source: Hollander JE, Diercks DB. Intervention strategies for acute coronary syndromes. In: Tintinalli JE, Kelen GD, Stapczynski JS, eds. Emergency medicine 6th ed. New York: McGraw-Hill: 2004:108–24.

risk factors (Table 2-3) for CHD remains a standard component of the chest pain evaluation. High risk is easily established if there is a prior history of definite CHD such as prior MI or abnormal coronary angiogram. Characteristics of the history and physical examination that affect the pretest probability are listed in Table 2-4. Patients who are young, without a family history of premature CHD, with an atypical history and a normal or nondiagnostic EKG, can usually be safely discharged without further evaluation for ACS. Prognostic data regarding those with known or suspected UA or NSTE-MI can be calculated with the thrombolytics in myocardial infarction (TIMI) risk score (Table 2-5).

Serum cardiac markers are used to confirm or exclude myocardial cell death, and are considered the **gold standard for the diagnosis of MI.** There are a number of markers currently in wide use, including **myoglobin, CK-MB (creatine kinase myocardial band), and troponin.** While algorithms vary, serum levels of one or more cardiac markers should be obtained initially and

Table 2-3
RISK FACTORS FOR CORONARY HEART DISEASE

Diabetes mellitus

Hypercholesterolemia; high-density lipoprotein (HDL) cholesterol <40 mg/dL

Current tobacco use

Hypertension

Age (male ≥45 years; female ≥55 years or premature menopause)

Family history of premature CHD (MI or sudden death before age 55 years in male first-degree relative; before age 55 years or before age 65 years in female first-degree relative)

Source: Hollander JE, Diercks DB. Intervention strategies for acute coronary syndromes. In: Tintinalli JE, Kelen GD, Stapczynski JS, eds. Emergency medicine 6th ed. New York: McGraw-Hill: 2004:108–24.

Table 2-4
HISTORY AND PHYSICAL IN THE EVALUATION OF POSSIBLE ACS

Increases likelihood that chest pain is from CHD	Decreases likelihood that chest pain is from CHD
Pressure-like quality	Pleuritic quality
Radiation to either arm, neck, or jaw	Constant pain for days
Diaphoresis	Pain lasting less than 2 minutes
Third heart sound	Discomfort localized with one finger
Pain that is similar to prior MI pain	Discomfort reproduced by movement or palpation

Table 2-5
TIMI RISK SCORE*

Age >65 years

Prior documented coronary artery stenosis >50%

Three or more CHD risk factors

Use of aspirin in the preceding 7 days

Two or more anginal events in the preceding 24 hours

ST-segment deviation (transient elevation or persistent depression)

Increased cardiac markers

*One point is assigned to each of the seven components. Risk of death, MI, or revascularization at 2 weeks by score: 1, 5%; 2, 8%; 3, 13%; 4, 20%; 5, 26%; 6, 41%.
Abbreviation:TIMI = thrombolysis in myocardial infarction.
Source: Antman EM, Cohen M, Bernink PJ, et al. The TIMI risk score for UA/NSTEMI. JAMA 2000;284(7):835–42.

then repeated at 4 to 12 hours after presentation. **Troponin I and T levels** are extremely sensitive and specific for cardiac damage; thus an elevated level confirms infarction, whereas a normal level at 8 to 12 hours after the onset of pain essentially excludes infarction. Important limitations of cardiac markers are that levels remain normal in unstable angina and serum elevations are delayed 4 to 12 hours after infarction.

Other studies that are routinely obtained in the work up of ACS include a chest radiograph (CXR), complete blood count, chemistries, coagulation studies, and blood type. The CXR serves to rule out other causes of chest pain, and to identify pulmonary edema. Although not a perfect test, **a normal mediastinum on CXR makes aortic dissection unlikely**. For this reason, a chest radiograph should be performed prior to thrombolytic therapy.

Treatment When ACS is suspected based on history, treatment should be started immediately. The patient should be placed on **a cardiac monitor, IV access established, and an EKG** obtained. Unless allergic, affected patients should be immediately given **aspirin** to chew (162 mg dose is common). Aspirin is remarkably beneficial across the entire spectrum of ACS. For example, in the setting of STEMI, the survival benefit from a single dose of aspirin is roughly equal to that of thrombolytic therapy (but with negligible risk or cost). Other mainstays of initial treatment are **oxygen**, sublingual **nitroglycerin**, which decreases wall tension and myocardial oxygen demand, and **morphine sulfate**. Together with **aspirin** these three therapies make up the mnemonic **MONA**, which is said to "greet chest pain patients at the door." Other important therapies include beta blockers, which decrease myocardial demand and decrease mortality. Based on results of the initial EKG, therapy then progresses in one of two directions: (a) STEMI = reperfusion intervention, or (b) UA/NSTEMI = individualized intervention.

ST Elevation MI   When the EKG reveals **STEMI** and symptoms have been present for **less than 12 hours**, **immediate reperfusion therapy** is indicated. The saying "time is myocardium" is a reminder that myocardial salvage and clinical benefit are critically dependent on the time to restoration of flow in the infarct related artery. There are two ways to achieve reperfusion: primary PCI (angioplasty or stent placement) and thrombolysis: the choice is largely determined by the capabilities of the hospital. Primary PCI is the treatment of choice when it can be performed within 6 hours of presentation (ideal goal is 90 minutes "door to balloon"). Compared to thrombolysis, PCI leads to lower 30-day mortality (4.4% vs. 6.5%), death or nonfatal reinfarction (7.2% vs. 11.9%) and fewer hemorrhagic strokes. Recent studies suggest that transfer to a neighboring facility for primary PCI is superior to thrombolysis if transfer can be accomplished within 2 hours. Administration of low-molecular-weight heparin and a glycoprotein IIB/IIIA inhibitor prior to PCI reduces the risk of reinfarction.

When PCI is not an option, intravenous thrombolytic agents may be used to achieve reperfusion. Studies of thrombolytic therapy versus placebo for STEMI show an absolute mortality reduction of roughly 3 percent. The **benefit of thrombolysis is greatest** when **treatment is begun within 4 hours**, and **benefit approaches that of primary PCI when thrombolytics are begun within 70 minutes.** However, clear benefit extends out to 12 hours. Adjunctive antithrombotic therapy with unfractionated or low-molecular-weight heparin is required with most thrombolytic agents. Recent evidence suggests that a so-called pharmaco-invasive approach to reperfusion, combining primary PCI, thrombolytics, and other drugs, may soon emerge as the therapeutic state of the art. Table 2-6 lists other measures, in addition to **aspirin, beta blockers, and reperfusion therapy**, that **reduce mortality after MI**.

Unstable Angina/Non-ST Elevation MI   Cases of ACS lacking EKG criteria for reperfusion fall into the UA/NSTEMI category. The approach to therapy for UA/NSTEMI tends to be graded, based on EKG findings, cardiac marker results, TIMI risk score, and whether the patient is likely to undergo early angiography and PCI. **Aspirin and nitroglycerin constitute the minimum therapy**. **Beta blockers**, such as IV metoprolol, are usually added for persistent pain, hypertension, or tachycardia. In high-risk patients, a more aggressive approach to halting the thrombotic process is taken, by adding low-molecular-weight or unfractionated heparin and oral clopidogrel, an antiplatelet agent. Patients are considered to be high risk if there are ischemic EKG changes, elevated cardiac markers, or if the TIMI risk score is 3 or greater. Intravenous glycoprotein IIB/IIIA inhibitors, an even more potent and expensive type of antiplatelet drug, are generally reserved for the subset of

Table 2-6
THERAPIES OF PROVEN BENEFIT FOR MI

Aspirin (162 mg, chewed, immediately, then continued daily for life)

Primary percutaneous coronary intervention (angioplasty or stenting the blocked artery)

Thrombolysis (if primary PCI not available; most regiments require heparin therapy)

Beta-blocker (started immediately, if no contraindications, then continued daily for life)

Angiotensin-converting enzyme inhibitor (started within 1-3 days, continued for life)

Cholesterol-lowering drugs (started within 1-3 days and continued daily for life)

Source: American College of Cardiologists. Guidelines for managing patients with AMI, UA, and NSTEMI. J Am Coll Cardiol 2002, 40:1366–74.

high-risk patients who will undergo early angiography and PCI, in whom these agents have been shown to reduce subsequent CHD morbidity.

In the past, angiography was often postponed for a number of days or weeks following an episode of ACS. So-called early invasive strategies, where patients with UA and NSTEMI are taken for angiography and PCI within 24 to 36 hours, may have slightly superior efficacy to medical therapy and delayed angiography. Like primary PCI for STEMI, whether an early invasive strategy is chosen often depends on hospital resources and cardiology expertise.

Complications   Several life-threatening complications of acute MI may arise at any time after presentation (Table 2-7). Serious complications occur most often in the setting of anterior STEMI. MI-associated **ventricular tachycardia and ventricular fibrillation** (sudden death) are the **most frequently encountered complications in the ED** and prehospital setting, occurring in approximately 10 percent of cases. Continuous cardiac monitoring and immediate cardioversion/defibrillation have been the mainstays of cardiac care since the 1960s, and have been shown to save lives on a large scale. **Bradyarrhythmias** may also complicate MI. Heart block developing in the setting of anterior MI generally implies irreversible damage to the His-Purkinje system and is an indication for transvenous pacing. Inferior MI, in contrast, frequently causes atrioventricular (AV) node dysfunction and second-degree block that is transient and may respond to atropine.

Pump dysfunction, leading to pulmonary edema or shock, is an ominous complication of MI that implies a large area of myocardial injury. The left ventricular dysfunction that occurs with anterior MI usually causes recognizable pulmonary edema, with tachypnea, rales, and visible congestion on chest x-ray. A new systolic murmur may be heard when cardiogenic pulmonary edema

Table 2-7
POTENTIAL COMPLICATIONS FROM ACUTE MI

Ventricular fibrillation, ventricular tachycardia		
Heart block	Cardiogenic plumonary edema	Cardiogenic shock
Right ventricular infarction		Mitral regurgitation
Free wall rupture	Ventricular septal defect	Pericarditis
Ventricular aneurysm		Thromboembolism
Hemorrhage secondary to therapy		

Source: Hollander JE, Diercks DB. Intervention strategies for acute coronary syndromes. In: Tintinalli JE, Kelen GD, Stapczynski JS, eds. Emergency medicine, 6th ed. New York: McGraw-Hill: 2004:108–24.

is caused by papillary muscle dysfunction and acute mitral regurgitation. Signs of cardiogenic shock range from frank hypotension to subtle indicators of impaired perfusion such as oliguria, cool extremities, and confusion. **Emergency PCI is the reperfusion strategy of choice for cardiogenic shock,** and, insertion of an **aortic balloon pump** may be indicated in addition to **pressor agents. Right ventricular infarction**, which complicates inferior MI, usually presents as **hypotension without pulmonary congestion**. The diagnosis is confirmed by ST elevation in lead V4 on a right-sided ECG, and the **primary treatment is aggressive volume loading.**

Complications of MI that tend to occur in the intensive care unit several hours to days after presentation include left ventricular free wall rupture causing tamponade, ventricular septal defect, pericarditis, left ventricular aneurysm, and thromboembolism. Finally, iatrogenic complications of MI therapy can occur. Emergency physicians who administer **thrombolytics** for STEMI must consider the risk of serious hemorrhagic complications, particularly **intracranial hemorrhage**, which occurs in 0.5 to 0.7 percent of patients and is usually fatal. Heparin and antiplatelet therapy lead to significant bleeding in up to 10 percent of patients, depending on what agents are given, although life-threatening hemorrhage is rare.

Comprehension Questions

[2.1]   In the initial evaluation of a patient with chest pain, what is the most important diagnostic test?

   A. Chest x-ray
   B. EKG
   C. Serum cardiac markers
   D. Computed tomography
   E. Cholesterol levels

[2.2] A 58-year-old man comes into the physician's office complaining of 2 hours of substernal chest pain and dyspnea. Which of the following is the most important next step in management?

A. Administration of propranolol
B. Aspirin to chew
C. Sublingual nitroglycerin
D. Administration of a diuretic agent
E. Chest radiograph

[2.3] A 45-year-old man is seen the emergency center with a 3-hour history of unremitting substernal chest pain radiating to his left arm. The EKG shows only nonspecific changes. The man wants to go home because of the normal EKG findings. Which of the following statements is most accurate?

A. The patient is correct and may be safely discharged home.
B. The patient should wait an additional 30 minutes for a repeat EKG and if this is normal, myocardial infarction is essentially ruled out.
C. The patient should be advised that half of patients with myocardial infarction will have nonspecific changes on EKG and he should have cardiac enzymes drawn.
D. The patient should have a thallium stress test to further assess for coronary artery disease to help clarify the management.

Answers

[2.1] **B.** The EKG is the crucial first diagnostic test in the evaluation of chest pain. Presence versus absence of ST elevation represents a major branch point.

[2.2] **B.** While all of these therapies are useful, aspirin significantly decreases mortality and should be given immediately.

[2.3] **C.** Roughly half of patients with MI, as defined by a typical rise in cardiac markers, will have a nondiagnostic EKG upon presentation. Thallium stress testing in the acute setting is not helpful and may be dangerous.

CLINICAL PEARLS

❖ Aspirin to chew should be given immediately to the patient presenting to the emergency room with chest pain.

❖ "Time is myocardium." In general, all patients with concerning chest pain should have an EKG immediately.

❖ The EKG will dictate the next step in management: clear evidence of ST elevation MI usually requires reperfusion therapy, whereas unstable angina/non-ST elevation MI may be individualized.

❖ The goals of therapy are restoring blood flow to myocardium as quickly as possible, preventing further clot formation, and controlling pain.

❖ MONA greets chest pain at the door (morphine, oxygen, nitroglycerin, and, most importantly, *aspirin*).

REFERENCES

American College of Cardiology: Guidelines for Managing Patients with AMI, UA, and NSTEMI. Available at: www.acc.org.

Macfarlane T, Snoey ER. Unstable angina and non-ST-segment elevation myocardial infarction. Emerg Med Pract (Accepted).

Panju AA, Hemmelgarn BR. Is this patient having a myocardial infarction? JAMA 1998;280:1256–63.

Ryan TJ, Reeder GS. Evaluation of suspected acute coronary ischemia in the emergency department. Available at: www.uptodate.com.

A 75-year-old female presents to the emergency department with palpitations and mild dyspnea on exertion. Her symptoms began 4 days ago while she was gardening. She is currently taking hydrochlorothiazide and simvastatin for hypertension and hypercholesterolemia respectively. Her family history is remarkable for hyperthyroidism in a maternal aunt. On physical exam she is comfortable, speaking without difficulty. Her temperature is 37°C (98.6°F), heart rate is 144 beats per minute, blood pressure is 110/70 mmHg, respirations 22 breaths per minute. Her head and neck examination is unremarkable. Her lungs are clear to auscultation bilaterally. The heart rate is rapid, irregular, without rub, murmur, or gallop. She has no extremity edema, and no jugular venous distention. The abdominal examination reveals no masses or tenderness. Laboratory studies show a normal CBC, normal electrolytes, BUN, and creatinine. The EKG is shown below (Fig. 3-1).

◆ **What is the most likely diagnosis?**

◆ **What are some of the more common contributing factors?**

◆ **What are some of the more serious complications?**

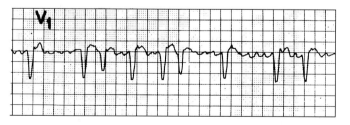

Figure 3-1. EKG. **(Reproduced with permission from Tintinalli JE, Kelen GD, Stapczynski JS, eds. Emergency Medicine, 6th ed. New York: McGraw-Hill, 2004:185.)**

ANSWERS TO CASE 3: Atrial Fibrillation

Summary: A 75-year-old female presents with palpitations and mild dyspnea on exertion. The physical examination reveals a heart rate of 144 beats per minute and irregular.

◆ **Most likely diagnosis**: Atrial fibrillation with rapid ventricular rate.

◆ **Common contributing factors:** Underlying cardiopulmonary disease – age or hypertension related. Also hyperthyroidism, pulmonary embolism, and electrolyte abnormalities may be contributory.

◆ **More serious complications:** Cardiomyopathy, diminished cardiac output, thromboembolism.

Analysis

Objectives
1. Be able to recognize atrial fibrillation on EKG.
2. Know that atrial fibrillation is often a manifestation of serious underlying disease processes.
3. Understand the approach to rhythm and rate control of rapid ventricular response atrial fibrillation.
4. Understand the role of anticoagulation in both the acute and chronic management of atrial fibrillation.

Considerations

This individual is a 75-year-old woman of fairly high function, who is brought into the ED because of palpitations and dyspnea. The initial approach should be to assess ABCs and to address life-threatening concerns. **Upon arrival, this patient should be placed on cardiac and oxygen saturation monitors**. Both the cardiac rhythm and the assessment of pulse will uncover the irregular tachycardia. A focused history and physical examination should target the cardiac and pulmonary status. A fairly broad differential diagnosis should be entertained such as myocardial infarction, pulmonary embolism, stroke, anemia, sepsis, and pneumonia. A workup for myocardial infarction (see Case 2) should be performed.

This patient with risk factors for cardiovascular disease is symptomatic from an **irregularly irregular tachycardia, which is typical for atrial fibrillation**. The **priority** for the management of this **patient is ventricular rate control**. Without rate control, the patient is at risk for hypotension, myocardial infarction, and pulmonary edema. Cardioversion should be considered, but anticoagulation must first be considered, because an intramural thrombus may be dislodged upon conversion to sinus rhythm. The patient's history suggests the atrial fibrillation is of short duration (less than 48 hours), and a reasonable approach would be cardioversion without pretreatment anticoagulation. Likewise, a search for the underlying etiology is important because atrial fibrillation is often a response to underlying disease (see Table 3-1).

APPROACH TO ATRIAL FIBRILLATION

Atrial fibrillation (AF) is the most common treatable arrhythmia seen by emergency medicine physicians. Its management is complex and challenging because AF is often a symptom rather than a disease unto itself—reflecting cardiac and pulmonary disease, endocrine problems, drug effects, and the like. Successful management begins by **addressing the patient's overall clinical status first** and then the atrial fibrillation rhythm as a secondary issue.

AF may be simply a marker for age and underlying cardiovascular or systemic disease. It affects only 0.4 percent of the general population but up to 5 percent of patients older than age 60 years, 9 percent of patients older than age 70 years, and 15 percent of patients older than age 75 years. Among patients with AF, 80 percent have underlying **cardiovascular disease**, most commonly **coronary artery disease** (CAD), **hypertensive heart disease** and **cardiomyopathy**. The remaining causes include **pulmonary disease** (chronic obstructive pulmonary disease [COPD], pulmonary hypertension), **systemic diseases** (thyroid, electrolytes, and toxins), and cases of "lone atrial fibrillation," which is defined as AF in the absence of any identifiable cause.

Pathophysiology

The clinical implications of AF must be viewed in the context of the underlying disease process that initially produced the arrhythmia. The **two most important complications** of AF are **thromboembolism and cardiomyopathy**. **Thromboembolism is increased fourfold in the presence of AF**, and the patient's rate of clot formation varies from 1.5 to 17 percent per year, depending on the age and other risk factors. AF causes progressive electrophysiological and structural changes in the atria that may promote the recurrence of AF.

Table 3-1
DISEASES ASSOCIATED WITH ATRIAL FIBRILLATION

1. Cardiac etiologies such as coronary artery disease, rheumatic heart disease, cardiomyopathy, hypertensive heart disease (approximately 80% of cases)
2. Pulmonary disease such as chronic obstructive pulmonary disease (COPD), pulmonary embolism, or pulmonary hypertension
3. Systemic disease such as thyroid disease, diabetes
4. "Holiday heart" syndrome related to alcohol intoxication
5. Idiopathic or "lone" atrial fibrillation (approximately 10%)

The loss of the "atrial kick" accounts for up to a 15 percent loss of cardiac output (CO). When coupled with a rapid ventricular response and a shortened diastolic filling time, CO may be significantly compromised, particularly in patients with poor left ventricle (LV) function. Lastly, chronic low-level tachycardia may lead to a global cardiomyopathy over time. Because cardiomyopathy predisposes to AF and vice versa, it is said that atrial fibrillation "begets" atrial fibrillation. The mortality and morbidity from atrial fibrillation are based on the underlying etiology.

Treatment

The treatment of stable atrial fibrillation is based on the patient's clinical picture (see Figure 3-2). Options include **rate control or rhythm control,** with or without anticoagulation. In the **acute setting, ventricular rate control is the single most important goal of therapy.** Slowing the ventricular response of AF provides positive hemodynamic effects: increase in diastolic filling time, improved stroke volume and cardiac output, and stabilization of blood pressure. Table 3-2 lists medical agents for rate control. **Patients with unstable AF require direct current cardioversion.**

Cardioversion

Although there is no clear consensus as to an ideal approach, the two essential issues are the need for **anticoagulation** and the **method and timing of cardioversion.** The uncoordinated atrial contractions lead to the intraatrial thrombus formation. The longer the duration of AF, the greater the likelihood of clot formation. Following cardioversion, "atrial stunning" may also lead to thrombogenesis, also affected by duration of AF. Approximately 6% of affected patients will experience a thromboembolic complication within 1 week of cardioversion, either because of the dislodging of an existing clot or the formation of new clot caused by "atrial stunning." This risk increases with the duration of the AF and the underlying disease processes.

Many practitioners use **"the 48-hour rule"** to guide **anticoagulation**: AF of less than 48 hours duration does not generally require acute anticoagulation except when the patient has mitral stenosis or a prior history of embolic stroke; atrial fibrillation exceeding 48 hours duration should generally be anticoagulated *before* cardioversion. The two main methods of precardioversion anticoagulation are Coumadin, or transesophageal echocardiography plus heparin. Coumadin generally requires 3 weeks of therapy, whereas if no clot is seen on echocardiography, heparin may be administered and cardioversion may be immediately performed (Table 3-3 lists anticoagulation options).

The technique of cardioversion begins with the question of whether to use direct current (DC) cardioversion or pharmacologic cardioversion. The **likelihood of success** will be determined less by the method used than by the **characteristics of the patient**, the **etiology** of the AF, and, most importantly, the **duration** of the AF. New-onset AF will spontaneously convert in approximately 70 percent of cases, while cases of longer duration with dilated atria

Table 3-2
THERAPIES FOR RATE CONTROL OF ATRIAL FIBRILLATION

MEDICATION	MECHANISM OF ACTION	COMMENT
Digoxin	Increases parasympathetic tone at the AV node via the vagus nerve	Traditionally used in RVR AF, now limited role in the ED because of its slow onset of action, long half-life, and ineffectiveness as a rate-controlling agent in the typical high sympathetic tone ED patient; has a role in rate control in sedentary patients or those with chronic CHF
Diltiazem	Calcium channel blocker with excellent AV block-ing effects and a relatively mixed profile of vaso-dilation and negative inotropy	A number of small studies suggest that diltiazem may be safe and effective even in patients with moderate to severe LV dysfunction
Verapamil/ beta blockers	Both provide excellent AV nodal blockade and are effective in rate control for RVR AF	Both also have significantly more negative inotropy than diltiazem and carry a greater likelihood of hypo-tension, particularly in patients with borderline low blood pressures or poor LV function
Amiodarone	While essentially an antiarrhythmic agent, amiodarone has beta-blocking activity as well	If cardioversion is the goal, amio-darone may represent a single-agent approach to simultaneous rate and rhythm control (although likely less efficacious than pure rate-control agents above)
Cardioversion	In the acute setting, cardioversion remains an option for management of the unstable patient	

Abbreviations: AF = atrial fibrillation; AV = atrioventricular; CHF = congestive heart failure; ED = emergency department; LV = left ventricle; RVR = rapid ventricular response

may prove refractory to any and all attempts. Regardless of the method used, the thromboembolic considerations are the same. Tables 3-4 and 3-5 list the considerations of DC cardioversion and pharmacologic cardioversion, respectively. The relative efficacy of the most commonly used drugs appears to be similar. to all classes of drugs converting 50 to 70 percent of patients of recent-onset AF and about 30 percent of those with long-term AF.

Table 3-3
ANTICOAGULATION OPTIONS PRIOR TO CARDIOVERSION

Coumadin: Most time-honored method for reduction of thromboembolic risk
  Coumadin therapy (INR 2–3) reduces the risk of post-cardioversion thromboembolism from 6% to 0.8%
  Coumadin must be "on board" for at least 3 weeks to achieve this reduction
  Coumadin must also be continued for $\geq$ 4 weeks postcardioversion

Heparin + transesophageal echocardiography (TEE): Quicker alternative to 3 weeks of outpatient Coumadin therapy. If no clot is seen on echocardiography, heparin may be given and the patient can be immediately cardioverted.
  Appears to be equivalent to 3 weeks of oral Coumadin
  Postconversion Coumadin therapy still necessary because of the "atrial stunning"-induced risk of clot formation
  Low-molecular-weight heparin probably equivalent to unfractionated heparin in this setting

Table 3-4
DC CARDIOVERSION

Preparation: IV, O_2, cardiac monitor—following standard sedation protocols, advanced cardiac life support/airway materials ready and available

Synchronized DC cardioversion: 100–360 Joules, most patients require 200 or greater; for AF <24 hours duration: start with 100J; biphasic cardioversion offers a better success rate with fewer complications; achieves conversion at 50% of monophasic levels

Success rates between 65 and 90%

Complications: The complication rate is ~15%; bradycardia, but also ventricular tachycardia; ventricular stunning with hypotension, etc.

Following cardioversion, antiarrhythmic therapy is often used to maintain normal sinus rhythm (NSR). Only 20 to 30 percent of patients will remain in NSR after conversion without drug therapy. Amiodarone and propafenone are commonly used agents to maintain sinus rhythm. With therapy, approximately 40 percent of patients remain in sinus rhythm at 1 year, and 30 percent at 4 years. Those with large atria or rheumatic heart disease are at greatest risk for recidivism.

Longterm Thromboembolic Risk Reduction
Patients with chronic AF have a fourfold increase in thromboembolic complications compared to the general population. It was previously thought

Table 3-5

AGENTS FOR PHARMACOLOGIC CARDIOVERSION

DRUG CLASS		
Ia	Procainamide (quinidine)	Hypotension, left ventricle depression
Ic	Fleclainide, propafenone	Contraindicated with coronary artery disease, structural heart disease
III	Amiodarone	Well tolerated, agent of choice with left ventricle dysfunction, side effects with long-term use
III	Ibutilide (dofetilide)	Specifically for atrial fibrillation and flutter, risk of torsade de pointes ventricular tachycardia

Table 3-6

ANTICOAGULATION BASED ON AGE

AGE (YEARS)	RISK FACTORS	THERAPY
<65	None	Acetylsalicylic acid (ASA) or none
65–75	None	ASA or Coumadin—assess risk of CVA vs. bleeding
Any	One or more (including age >75 y)	Coumadin (unless strong contraindications)

Risk factors: Mitral stenosis, hypertension (HTN), previous cerebrovascular accident (CVA), left ventricle (LV) dysfunction, age >75 years.

that the use of antiarrhythmic agents to maintain sinus rhythm would reduce this risk. The Atrial Fibrillation Follow-up Investigation of Rhythm Management (AFFIRM) trial, which compared rhythm control to rate control plus Coumadin in 4060 patients, showed the rate control plus Coumadin group had a trend toward better survival, fewer hospitalizations, and better quality-of-life scores. Interestingly, the rhythm control patients not on Coumadin experienced a significantly higher incidence of stroke. This data suggests that even patients with rare or intermittent AF may benefit from Coumadin therapy. The decision to use Coumadin is risk and age based (Table 3-6).

Comprehension Questions

[3.1] What is the most common complication of atrial fibrillation?

    A. Sudden death
    B. Stroke
    C. Shock
    D. Pericardial tamponade

[3.2] A 65-year-old woman presents to the ED with dyspnea, fatigue, and palpitations. Her blood pressure is 85/50 mmHg and her heart rate is 140 beats per minute. Which of the following is the best treatment for this patient?

    A. Diltiazem
    B. Metoprolol
    C. Coumadin
    D. Cardioversion

[3.3] A 62-year-old man is seen in the ED for lower abdominal pain which has since resolved; however, his heart rate is 80 beats per minute and palpates irregularly. On EKG, he is diagnosed with atrial fibrillation with a ventricular response of 114 beats per minute. He does not recall ever being told about this condition. Which of the following is the best initial treatment for this patient?

    A. Diltiazem
    B. Cardioversion
    C. Synthroid
    D. Ibutilide

Answers

[3.1] **B.** There is a fourfold increase in the risk of stroke in patients with atrial fibrillation.

[3.2] **D.** Cardioversion is usually the best treatment for any unstable patient (congestive heart failure [CHF], chest pain, hypotension) with atrial fibrillation.

[3.3] **A.** Diltiazem was the only rate-controlling agent listed, and is very useful in the initial management of atrial fibrillation with rapid ventricular response.

CLINICAL PEARLS

❖ Unstable patients with atrial fibrillation or Wolff-Parkinson-White tachyarrhythmia with atrial fibrillation should undergo cardioversion.

❖ Stable patients with atrial fibrillation of less than 48 hours' duration may be cardioverted.

❖ Stable patients with atrial fibrillation greater than 48 hours' duration or unknown duration may be rate controlled then anticoagulated for 3 weeks prior to cardioversion and 4 weeks after cardioversion, with the addition of an antiarrhythmic. Alternatively, patients may undergo transesophageal echocardiography (TEE) and if negative, be acutely anticoagulated with heparin and cardioverted.

❖ Atrial fibrillation carries a fourfold increased risk of thromboembolism. This risk is independent of whether the AF is paroxysmal, persistent, or chronic.

❖ Longterm anticoagulation is based on patient age and risk factors.

❖ Coumadin therapy with a target international normalized ratio (INR) of 2 to 3 reduces the risk of thromboembolism.

❖ Of new-onset AF cases, 70% will spontaneously convert to sinus rhythm.

❖ The goal of management of atrial fibrillation is ventricular rate control by cardioversion to normal sinus rhythm or blocking of the AV node to decrease the rate of ventricular contraction.

❖ Treatment of the underlying illness is important in the evaluation of atrial fibrillation.

REFERENCES

Albers G, Dalenj E, Laupacis A, et al. Antithrombotic therapy in atrial fibrillation. Chest 2001;119:194S–206S.

Gallagher M, Hennessy BJ, Edvardssonn N, et al. Embolic complications of direct current cardioversion of atrial arrhythmias: association with low intensity of anticoagulation at the time of cardioversion. J Am Coll Cardiol 2002;40:926–33

Fuster V, Ryden LE, Asinger RU, et al. ACC/AHA/ESC Guideline for the management of patients with atrial fibrillation: executive summary. A report of the American College of Cardiology/American Heart Association Task Force on Practice Guidelines and the European Society of Cardiology Committee for Practice Guidelines and Policy Conferences. J Am Coll Cardiol 2001;38:2118–50

Stewart S, Hart CL, Hole DJ, McMurray JJ. A population-based study of the long-term risks associated with atrial fibrillation: 20 year follow-up of the Renfrew/Paisley study. Am J Med 2002;113:359–64

Weigner M, Caulfield TA, Danias PG, et al. Risk for clinical thromboembolism associated with conversion to sinus rhythm in patients with atrial fibrillation lasting less than 48 hours. Ann Intern Med 1997;126:615–200

Wyse D, Waldo AL, DiMarco JP, et al. A comparison of rate control and rhythm control in patients with atrial fibrillation. The atrial fibrillation follow-up investigation of rhythm management (AFFIRM) investigators. N Engl J Med 2002;347:1825–33

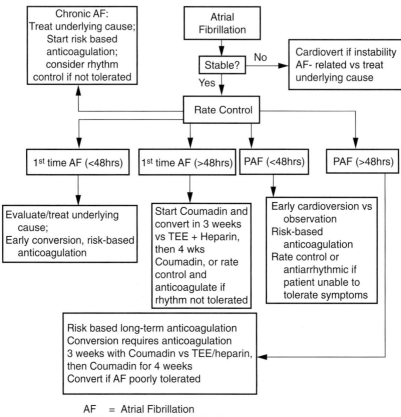

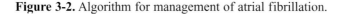

AF = Atrial Fibrillation
PAF = Persistent Atrial Fibrillation
TEE = Transesophageal Echocardiography

Figure 3-2. Algorithm for management of atrial fibrillation.

A 19-year-old man presents to the emergency department with severe abdominal pain and an "altered level of consciousness." The patient's symptoms began approximately 48 hours previously, when he complained of abdominal discomfort and urinary frequency. Today he was found in bed moaning, but otherwise unresponsive. His past medical history is unremarkable, and he is currently not taking any medications. On physical examination, the patient appears pale and ill. His temperature is 36°C (96.8°F), pulse rate is 140 beats per minute, blood pressure is 82/40 mmHg, and the respiratory rate is 40 breaths per minute. His head and neck examination shows dry mucous membranes and sunken eyes; there is an unusual odor to his breath. The lungs are clear bilaterally with increased rate and depth of respiration. The cardiac examination reveals tachycardia, no murmurs, rubs, or gallops. The abdomen is diffusely tender to palpation, with hypoactive bowel sounds and involuntary guarding. The rectal examination is normal. Skin is cool and dry with decreased turgor. On neurological exam the patient moans and localizes pain but does not speak. Laboratory studies: the leukocyte count is 16,000 cells/mm^3, and the hemoglobin and hematocrit levels are normal. Electrolytes show a sodium level of 124 mEq/L, potassium 3.4 mEq/L, chloride 98 mEq/L, and bicarbonate 6 mEq/L. Serum BUN and creatinine are mildly elevated. The serum glucose is 740 mg/dL (41.1 mmol/L). The serum amylase, bilirubin, AST, ALT, and alkaline phosphatase are within normal limits. A 12-lead EKG shows sinus tachycardia. His chest radiograph is normal.

◆ **What is the most likely diagnosis?**

◆ **What is your next step?**

ANSWERS TO CASE 4: Diabetic Ketoacidosis

Summary: This is a 19-year-old man with severe hyperglycemia, anion-gap acidosis, dehydration, hyponatremia, hypotension, altered level of consciousness, and diffuse abdominal pain.

◆ **Most likely diagnosis:** Diabetic ketoacidosis

◆ **Next step:** Management of the ABCs, including fluid resuscitation, the initiation of insulin therapy, correction of electrolyte and metabolic disturbances, and a careful search for any precipitating or concomitant illness.

Analysis

Objectives

1. Recognize the clinical settings, the signs and symptoms, and the complications of diabetic ketoacidosis.
2. Understand the diagnostic and therapeutic approach to suspected diabetic ketoacidosis.

Considerations

This previously healthy 19-year-old man arrives to the ED with numerous "red flags" indicating severe illness. This patient should be of immediate concern to the ED physician, and delay in assessment and therapy will likely increase morbidity and mortality. The severe abdominal pain and altered level of consciousness may be caused by sepsis, intraabdominal infection, ruptured appendicitis, toxic ingestion, illicit substance abuse, or a severe metabolic process. On physical examination, the patient "appears pale and ill." One of the skills that an emergency physician must develop is a **sense of the "sick" patient, to better prioritize assessment and therapy**, and have a higher index of suspicion of severe processes. Furthermore, young, healthy patients generally have excellent reserve and will have mechanisms to compensate for hemodynamic status, until late in the course of the disease process. The fact that this patient is hypotensive indicates that this patient is extremely ill, and necessitates immediate resuscitation and treatment.

    The first priority is the ABCs. Oxygen saturation monitoring and giving oxygen by nasal cannula is a first step. **Intravenous fluids, such as with normal saline,** would resuscitate an obviously volume-depleted patient. The patient should be placed on a **cardiac monitor**. Urine drug screen, CBC, electrolytes, renal and liver function tests, urinalysis, and arterial blood gas tests should be obtained. A fingerstick **blood sugar** can give an immediate answer at the bedside. Before giving an intravenous solution with dextrose, the possibility of alcohol abuse should be entertained, because **alcohol encephalopathy may be exacerbated with glucose in the face of thiamine deficiency.**

This patient's clinical presentation is typical for diabetic ketoacidosis (DKA). Morbidity may result from either underlying precipitating conditions, or from delayed or inadequate treatment. The essential aspects of therapy are prompt recognition, effective resuscitation, and scrupulous attention to fluid, electrolyte, and insulin replacement (Table 4-1 lists typical lab values in DKA). A thoughtful search for associated illnesses along with frequent reassessment of the patient will lead to the best outcome.

APPROACH TO SUSPECTED DIABETIC KETOACIDOSIS

Diabetic ketoacidosis is a metabolic emergency. A delay in treatment leads to increased morbidity and mortality. DKA is the initial presentation in up to 25 percent of type I diabetics, so the lack of a diabetic history does not exclude the diagnosis. Most cases occur in patients with type I diabetes, although occasional patients with type II diabetes may develop DKA during severe physiological stress. Some patients will present with the classic symptoms of diabetes, such as polyuria, polydipsia, and fatigue. Others will complain more of **dyspnea related to the metabolic acidosis**, or of the idiopathic, but **severe, abdominal pain** that often accompanies DKA. Patients with an underlying infection or other precipitating illness may have symptoms predominantly from that process. Some patients have such altered sensorium that a history is entirely unobtainable. The physical examination is

Table 4-1
TYPICAL LABORATORY VALUES IN DIABETIC KETOACIDOSIS

LAB TEST	MODERATE	SEVERE
Glucose (mq/dL)	500–700	900 or higher
Sodium (mEq/L)	130	125
Potassium (mEq/L)	4–6	5–7
HCO_3 (mEq/L)	6–10	<5
BUN (mg/dL)	20–30	30+
pH	7.1	6.9
pCO_2 (mmHg)	15–20	>20 (respiratory failure)

Abbreviations: BUN = blood urea nitrogen; HCO_3 = bicarbonate; pCO_2 = partial pressure of carbon dioxide.

directed at **searching for a source of infection** that might have been the precipitant for the DKA. **Infectious processes, such as pneumonia and urinary tract infections, are the most common,** but close inspection of the skin is important to look for an occult cellulitis, especially in unusual locations such as the perineum and in other intertriginous areas.

DKA results from an **absolute or severe relative lack of insulin,** leading to a starvation state at the cellular level. Gluconeogenesis is stimulated even as glucose utilization falls. **Hyperglycemia and ketoacidosis** cause a **profound osmotic diuresis and massive fluid shifts**. The diuresis and acidosis cause severe electrolyte disturbances, with wasting of sodium, potassium, magnesium, and phosphate. **Acidosis and dehydration** can lead to **potassium shifts** into the extracellular space, so **patients may have significant hyperkalemia at presentation, even with massive total body deficits of potassium**. Nausea and vomiting can be severe and further cloud the clinical picture with variable superimposed acid–base and electrolyte disturbances.

Diagnosis is based on the triad of **hyperglycemia, ketosis, and metabolic acidosis**. The major differential diagnosis is hyperosmolar nonketotic (HONK) hyperglycemia, which can present with very high glucose but slight or no acidosis. Starvation, pregnancy, alcoholic ketoacidosis, and various toxic ingestions can present with elevated serum ketones, but the glucose is normal or low. Patients can be rapidly screened for DKA with a bedside blood glucose measurement and a dipstick urinalysis. Except for the rare anuric patient, the absence of ketones in the urine reliably excludes the diagnosis of DKA. Consideration for the precipitating cause (such as MI, stroke, pregnancy, or gastrointestinal [GI] bleeding) of DKA behooves one to order studies to help rule out the presence of infection and myocardial infarction (Table 4-2 is a guide to the differential diagnosis of DKA).

Patients in DKA can have massive fluid deficits, sometimes as much as 5 to 10 L. **Shock** is fairly common, and must be **promptly treated with crystalloid infusion** to prevent further organ damage. An adult in clinical shock should receive an **initial 2-L bolus of normal saline** with frequent reassessment. In children, shock is treated with boluses of 20 mL/kg of normal saline. Although overaggressive hydration can present substantial complications later in the course of treatment, this concern takes a back seat to the reversal of shock. **Untreated shock promotes multiple-organ dysfunction and contributes further to the severe acidosis seen in DKA**.

Insulin is absolutely required to reverse ketoacidosis. Regular insulin is usually given by continuous IV infusion, although frequent IV boluses may be nearly as effective. Intramuscular injections are painful and less reliably absorbed when the patient is in shock. There is no role for long-acting insulin, or for subcutaneous injection, until the ketoacidotic state has resolved. The combination of rehydration and insulin will commonly lower the serum glucose much faster than ketones are cleared. Regardless, **insulin infusion should continue until the anion gap has returned to normal. Dextrose should be added to the IV infusion when the serum glucose falls to 200 to**

Table 4-2

DIFFERENTIAL DIAGNOSIS OF DIABETIC KETOACIDOSIS

HYPERGLYCEMIA	ACIDOSIS	KETOSIS
Diabetes	Hyperchloremic acidosis	Starvation
Stress hyperglycemia	Salicylate poisoning	Pregnancy
Nonketotic hyperosmolar coma	Uremia	Alcoholic ketoacidosis
Impaired glucose tolerance	Lactic acidosis	Isopropyl alcohol ingestion
Dextrose infusion	Other drugs	
DKA	DKA	DKA

300 mg/dL (11.1 to 16.7 mmol/L) to prevent hypoglycemia, a common complication of treatment.

An **insulin dose of 0.1 U/kg/h (5 to 10 U/h in the adult)** is adequate for almost all clinical situations. This is sufficient to achieve maximum physiological effect. Higher doses used in the past were no more effective, but did cause a higher rate of hypoglycemia. An initial bolus of insulin, equal to 1 hour's infusion, is commonly given, but does not hasten recovery. Insulin does bind readily to common medical plastics, so IV tubing should be thoroughly flushed with the drip solution at the start of therapy.

Patients in DKA generally have massive total body deficits of water, sodium, potassium, magnesium, phosphate, and other electrolytes. Specific laboratory values may vary widely depending on the patient's intake, gastrointestinal and other losses, medications, and comorbid illnesses; generally, electrolytes, BUN, creatinine, serum ketones, and arterial blood gas levels need to be monitored. The sodium level can sometimes measure low as a consequence of hyperglycemia—Na is spuriously lowered 1.6 mEq/L for each 100 mg/dL of glucose above 100 mg/dL. It is not usually necessary to calculate exact sodium and water deficits and replacements, except in cases of severe renal failure. Simply reversing the shock with normal saline, then continuing an infusion of half-normal saline at two to three times maintenance is generally sufficient. A glucose solution should be initiated *before* the serum glucose falls to the normal range.

Potassium deficits are usually quite large, yet the serum potassium at presentation may be low, normal, or even high. If the potassium is elevated initially, **hyperkalemic changes** on the **ECG** should be identified and treated. Fluids without potassium should be used until the serum potassium level reaches the normal range, and then potassium can be added to the IV infusion. If the initial serum potassium is normal or low, then potassium should be added immediately. Magnesium supplementation may be necessary to help the patient retain potassium. For patients with extremely low phosphate levels (which can cause muscle breakdown), some of the potassium can be given in the form of potassium phosphate.

Because metabolic acidosis is such a prominent feature in DKA, many clinicians have administered substantial doses of sodium bicarbonate. Many studies have failed to demonstrate any improvement from this treatment even at surprisingly low serum pH values. There are multiple theoretical and observed complications from bicarbonate, including hypernatremia, hypokalemia, paradoxical cerebrospinal fluid (CSF) acidosis, and residual systemic alkalosis. Therefore as a **general rule, bicarbonate should not be used to treat patients in DKA** even when there is a severe acidosis. Of course, in the case of hyperkalemia, bicarbonate can be lifesaving and should not be withheld.

Cerebral edema is a rare, but devastating, complication of DKA, seen more often and more severely in **children**. It almost always occurs during treatment, and is a leading cause of morbidity and mortality in pediatric DKA. It has been ascribed to the development of cryptogenic osmoles in the central nervous system (CNS) to counter dehydration, which then draw water intracellularly during treatment. It has been variously associated with overhydration and vigorous insulin therapy, leading many pediatric centers to use extremely conservative, slow and low-dose treatment protocols for DKA. However, one large, well-controlled study has shown that the only reliable predictor of cerebral edema is the severity of metabolic derangements at presentation. Concern for cerebral edema should never be used as an excuse for the undertreatment of clinical shock.

Comprehension Questions

[4.1]   A 14-year-old type I diabetic male is brought into the emergency room for the suspected diagnosis of DKA. Which of the following would provide the strongest evidence of the diagnosis?

    A. Polyuria, polydipsia, fatigue
    B. Hypotension, dehydration, fruity breath odor
    C. Hyperglycemia, ketosis, metabolic acidosis
    D. Elevated HCO_3 and elevated glucose levels

[4.2]   A 25-year-old male is diagnosed with DKA. His blood pressure is 80/50 mmHg and heart rate is 140 beats per minute. His glucose level is 950 mg/dL, potassium level is 6 mEq/L, and bicarbonate level is 5 mEq/L. Which of the following is the best initial therapy for this patient?

    A. Give 20 units regular insulin intramuscularly followed by D_5W (dextrose 5% in water) at 200 mL/h
    B. Initiate a dopamine drip to raise blood pressure above 90 mmHg
    C. Administer 2 L of normal saline with KCl 20 mEq/L intravenously
    D. Give two ampules of sodium bicarbonate
    E. Give normal saline 2 L as a intravenous bolus and insulin intravenous infusion at 0.1 U/kg/h

[4.3] A 57-year-old man is noted to have an arterial pH of 7.46, pCO_2 of 24 mmHg, pO_2 of 110 mmHg, and HCO_3 level of 16 mEq/L with an anion gap of 18 mEq/L. His blood sugar is 90 mg/dL. Which of the following is the most likely etiology of his condition?

    A. Severe chronic obstructive pulmonary disease with carbon dioxide retention
    B. Acute diarrhea
    C. Renal tubular acidosis
    D. Salicylate ingestion

[4.4] A 16-year-old woman is noted to have a diagnosis of moderately severe DKA. The initial blood sugar is 680 mg/dL and pH is 7.21. After 10 hours of intravenous saline therapy and continuous insulin infusion, her blood sugar is now 240 mg/dL but serum ketones are still high and pH is still low at 7.24. Which of the following is the best management?

    A. Consider other causes of metabolic acidosis such as lactic acidemia or ingestion
    B. Increase the rate of insulin infusion
    C. Add dextrose to the intravenous fluid and continue insulin infusion
    D. Initiate a bicarbonate infusion

Answers

[4.1] **C.** The triad of hyperglycemia, ketosis, and acidosis is diagnostic of DKA. Many other conditions cause one or two of the triad, but not all three. Although a fruity breath odor may suggest acetone, it is not reliably present and not all clinicians can distinguish it.

[4.2] **E.** Fluid resuscitation to reverse shock and IV insulin to reverse ketoacidosis are the mainstays of therapy. The blood pressure will almost always respond to intravenous isotonic saline replacement. Although most patients will require potassium, it should not be given while the serum K is elevated. Pressors have no role until volume is restored.

[4.3] **D.** Salicylates may lead to an increased anion gap acidemia, although early on, it may induce a respiratory alkalosis. This mixed respiratory alkalosis (evidenced by low pCO_2 caused by increasing minute ventilation), and metabolic acidosis (indicated by low bicarbonate level and elevated anion gap) is typical of aspirin intoxication.

[4.4] **C.** The serum glucose often drops much more rapidly than the ketoacidosis resolves; insulin is necessary to metabolize the ketone bodies but dextrose prevents hypoglycemia. Potassium replacement is usually necessary, but should be delayed until hyperkalemia is excluded. Bicarbonate does not hasten resolution of DKA and can cause complications.

CLINICAL PEARLS

❖ Hyperglycemia, ketosis, and acidosis confirm the diagnosis of DKA and are enough to start isotonic fluids and insulin.

❖ Patients in DKA are almost always volume depleted and have significant sodium and potassium deficits, regardless of their specific laboratory values.

❖ The cornerstones of therapy of DKA are fluid and electrolyte replacement, intravenous insulin, and identification and treatment of the precipitating etiology.

❖ Abdominal pain is a common feature in DKA and is usually idiopathic, especially in younger patients.

❖ Most morbidity in DKA is iatrogenic.

❖ Anion gap acidosis is usually caused by renal failure, lactic acidosis, ketoacidosis (diabetic, starvation, alcohol), and ingestions (methanol, ethylene glycol, salicylates).

REFERENCES

Kitabchi AE, Wall BM. Diabetic ketoacidosis. Med Clin North Am 1995;79(1):9–37. Review.

Marcin JP, Glaser N, Barnett P, et al. Factors associated with adverse outcomes in children with diabetic ketoacidosis-related cerebral edema. J Pediatr 2002;141(6):793–7.

Umpierrez GE, Khajavi M, Kitabchi AE. Review: diabetic ketoacidosis and hyperglycemic hyperosmolar nonketotic syndrome. Am J Med Sci 1996;311:225–33.

A 73-year-old woman is brought to the emergency center from an assisted-living facility, where she resides. The patient has a history of mild dementia, hypertension, hypothyroidism, and type II diabetes mellitus. By report, the patient has refused ambulation and food consumption for the past 24 hours. No cough, diarrhea, hematochezia, nor hematemesis have been reported. The physical examination reveals a well-nourished, elderly woman who is somnolent but arousable. Her temperature is 36.0°C (96.8°F) taken rectally, pulse rate is 90 beats per minute, blood pressure is 84/50 mmHg, and respiratory rate is 25 breaths per minute. Her mucous membranes are dry. The lungs are clear bilaterally with good air entry. Her abdomen is soft, mildly distended, and minimally tender throughout. The extremities are cool with cyanotic discoloration over the knees. The patient is confused, moving all extremities, and without focal deficits. The thyroid-stimulating hormone (TSH) level is normal and the serum glucose level is 140 mg/dL.

◆ **What is the most likely diagnosis?**

◆ **What is the most likely etiology for this condition?**

ANSWERS TO CASE 5: Sepsis

Summary: A 73-year-old woman presents from an assisted-living facility with dehydration, lethargy, and hypotension of unknown etiology. The TSH and glucose levels are normal.

◆ **Most likely diagnosis:** Sepsis.

◆ **Most likely etiology:** Urinary tract infection or urosepsis.

Analysis

Objectives

1. Learn to recognize the clinical presentations of sepsis and the possible atypical presentations in children and elderly patients.
2. Learn the pathophysiology, systemic effects, and management of sepsis.
3. Become familiar with the role of biological response modifiers in the treatment of sepsis.

Considerations

This 73-year-old woman has a definite change in mental status, and is both hypothermic and hypotensive. The blood pressure is especially bothersome considering older individuals usually have blood pressures higher than normal. The cyanotic extremities are consistent with vascular insufficiency. **Elderly patients may have subtle signs of sepsis, and thus a high index of suspicion is critical in their evaluation.** Other diseases that must be considered include myxedema coma, stroke, pulmonary embolism, electrolyte or metabolic abnormalities, hypoxemia, or myocardial infarction. Whatever the process, this is a very serious illness, and aggressive action for diagnosis and management is paramount. Upon entry to the emergency room, the patient should have intravenous access, EKG, cardiac enzymes, CBC, arterial blood gas, electrolytes, renal and liver function tests, and glucose level performed. A urinalysis and urine and blood cultures should be obtained. A chest radiograph is important to assess for pneumonia. An efficient but fairly complete history and physical examination should be performed; often **querying family members or personnel at the assisted-living facility is helpful**. Judicious intravenous fluids should be administered to support the blood pressure.

Because the **most common sources of sepsis in the elderly** (especially those in long-term care facilities) are **urosepsis and pneumonia**, the urinalysis and chest x-ray are usually helpful. Unlike younger patients, elderly patients with sepsis may not demonstrate fever and leukocytosis. They often present as either hypothermic or normothermic, altered mental status, and with either normal white count or leukopenia. Patients with diabetes mellitus or glucose intolerance may present with hyperglycemia and/or diabetic ketoacidosis.

With this patient it is important to consider the potential microbial organisms associated with urosepsis in order to select the most appropriate empiric antibiotic regimen. Inappropriate initial antibiotic selection in patients admitted to the ICU is associated with increased patient mortality. For this patient, the most likely organisms are gram-negative bacteria such as *E. coli* or *Proteus* species. Traditionally, for the empiric coverage of urinary tract-related infections, aminoglycosides have been effectively used because of the high concentrations achieved in the urine. Ampicillin is frequently added in these settings for the synergism toward enterococci. With the availability of the newer antimicrobial agents, including the quinolones, other agents are increasingly used as first-line therapy for the treatment of urosepsis. Once the results of the urine culture become available, the antibiotics can be changed accordingly. Urosepsis may occur in patients with obstructive uropathy or other barriers preventing antibiotic penetration (such as renal and perinephric abscess); therefore, if the patient does not improve clinically within 48 hours, CT scan evaluation and additional treatment may be needed.

APPROACH TO SEPSIS

Definitions

Sepsis: host response to infection.
Systemic inflammatory response syndrome (SIRS): systemic inflammation independent of etiology.
Septic shock: sepsis complicated by refractory hypotension.
Multiorgan dysfunction syndrome (MODS): dysfunction of organs not involved in the original infectious process.

Clinical Approach

Pathophysiology   Initiated by an infectious source, sepsis is actually part of a continuum of ongoing inflammation marked by progressive clinical deterioration. The sepsis syndrome is a reflection of the host inflammatory response. Generally, cell components of bacteria or bacterial product, such as lipopolysaccharide (LPS) from gram-negative bacteria are capable of eliciting the primary responses in specific immune cells (macrophages, neutrophils, monocytes). A secondary response is induced with amplification of the inflammatory response, modulated by proinflammatory cytokines. Notably, interleukin (IL)-1 causes fever via prostaglandin E_2, increases production of neutrophils, and inhibits apoptosis (programmed cell death). IL-6 induces hepatocyte production of acute phase proteins, such as C-reactive protein. Finally, tumor necrosis factor (TNF) increases the production of IL-1 and IL-6, which upregulate adhesion molecules on vascular endothelial cells, and increase nitric oxide production to cause vasodilation.

During the evolution of the inflammatory process, the host counterregulatory responses to the proinflammatory changes include upregulation of antiinflammatory cytokines such as IL-10, IL-1 receptor antagonist, and transforming growth factor. Additional host antiinflammatory responses include the production and release of endogenous glucocorticoids that downregulate cytokine synthesis. **It is currently believed that severe sepsis, septic shock, and MODS are the end-results of an overabundance of host proinflammatory responses and/or insufficient counter-regulatory inflammatory responses.**

Because the inflammatory pathways and coagulation pathways are intimately involved, sepsis is also marked by derangement of the coagulation cascade leading to a procoagulation state. As a consequence of the **systemic prothrombotic state, microvascular thrombosis, consumption of clotting factors, and disseminated intravascular coagulation** occurs. Clinically, **low levels of protein C and antithrombin III** correlate with increased mortality in septic patients.

Vitamin K-dependent protein C becomes activated by binding to a thrombin–thrombomodulin complex, and the activated form of protein C, using protein S as a cofactor, inactivates factor Va and VIIIa to inhibit thrombin generation. For a variety of reasons, some patients with sepsis have a reduction in protein C production as well as decreased production of activated protein C. With depletion of the physiologic anticoagulants antithrombin III and protein C, thrombin formation continues unchecked. Thrombin activates platelets, recruits neutrophils, and causes degranulation of mast cells. These proinflammatory properties of thrombin enhance the inflammatory response of the host.

Clinical Presentation of Sepsis Sepsis can be divided clinically into an **early** (hyperdynamic) phase and a **late** (hypodynamic) phase. The hemodynamic response predominates in both settings. During the **hyperdynamic** phase, the **increased capillary leakage and increased peripheral vasodilation result in decreased systemic vascular resistance** and **decreased venous return, i.e., hypotension.** As a compensatory mechanism, **cardiac output is increased** to maintain cardiac-filling pressures. Diarrhea, vomiting, insensible losses, and dehydration further exacerbate the decreased intravascular volume. During the **hyperdynamic phase**, patients present with **tachycardia, tachypnea, and warm extremities**. Altered level of consciousness in the guise of **disorientation, confusion, or encephalopathy** is an early sign, especially in the elderly. While fever is common in sepsis, neonates, elderly, alcoholics, and uremic patients may present as normothermic or hypothermic.

Amplification of the inflammatory response fuels the progression from a hyperdynamic to a hypodynamic state. This heralds significant dysregulation of homeostatic mechanisms and clinically presents as **septic shock and MODS. Cardiac output is decreased as myocardial function is depressed.** A large tissue perfusion deficit develops with poor oxygen extraction. The increased tissue hypoxia results in increased **lactate production**, connoting a predominance of **metabolic acidosis**. Hyperglycemia is commonly found and is more pronounced in diabetics.

Leukocytosis is frequently seen; however, children and the elderly who present with leukopenia or normal leukocyte count, invariably have a left shift associated with it. Thrombocytopenia may worsen as sepsis progresses. In the **hyperdynamic phase, hyperventilation can cause a respiratory alkalosis**. Because hypotension, followed by hypoperfusion, is predominant in the hypodynamic phase, anaerobic metabolism results in elevated lactate levels. **Late sepsis is marked by a metabolic acidosis**.

MODS   Later in the course of sepsis, the decreased cardiac output, peripheral vasoconstriction, and microvasculature thromboses contribute further to end-organ perfusion defects. Clinically, the patients may be found to have **skin and extremities that are cool, mottled, and cyanotic**. The pulmonary manifestation may include pulmonary edema from alveolar capillary leak leading to decreased pulmonary compliance and increased work of breathing. During this process, the formation of nonsegmental pulmonary infiltrates develops with further decrease in oxygenation, as measured by diminished arterial oxygen pressure (PaO_2)/fraction of inspired oxygen (FiO_2). The culmination of these pulmonary abnormalities generally leads to the need for mechanical ventilation at this stage. Either acute tubular necrosis induced by hypotension or capillary injury can cause renal failure. The gastrointestinal tract is vulnerable to decreased perfusion with the risks of stress ulceration, ischemia and acute hepatic injury among the possibilities. Patients can develop a polyneuropathy or distal motor weakness.

Therapy   **Resuscitation** to **restore organ perfusion** and **control of the infectious source** are the cornerstones of initial therapy. The patient should be monitored closely for organ dysfunction so that appropriate organ support may be initiated as needed. The goal of initial fluid therapy is to correct the sepsis-induced hypotension by restoring intravascular volume. **Normal saline or lactated Ringer solution is administered until the blood pressure responds or normovolemia is achieved**. Urine output (0.5 mL/kg/h) and central venous pressure are monitored to evaluate the adequacy of resuscitation. If **hypotension persists despite fluids,** then vasopressor agents such as **dopamine** should be given.

The source of infection must be controlled systemically and locally. Broad-spectrum systemic antibiotics are given to cover the suspected organisms associated with the infection. When cultures are available, the antibiotics can be changed to target the identified organisms. Thorough examination of the patient will identify if the infectious etiology is an abscess requiring drainage or devitalized tissue such as sacral ulcer requiring debridement or foreign body needing removal. Sometimes a more definitive surgical intervention may be necessary if the septic nidus is related to anatomical pathology, such as sigmoid diverticulitis with perforation or acute cholecystitis. Thus, the combination of systemic antibiotics and surgical management may be required for adequate control of some infections.

Despite early administration of antibiotics, resuscitation and surgery, the patient may still progress to MODS. In these patients, an organ-based approach of supportive therapy is required, where respiratory failure is managed with appropriate mechanical ventilation. Cardiac dysfunction is supported by appropriate vasopressors and inotropes. The fluid and metabolic abnormalities associated with renal insufficiency can be addressed with diuretics and/or renal replacement therapy (hemodialysis and ultrafiltration). Nutritional support via enteral or parental route is also important for promotion of the healing process and enhancement of immune function.

Newer Therapies **Human recombinant activated protein C** (drotrecogin alfa) is the first physiologic antiinflammatory agent proven to be effective in the treatment of sepsis. The **Protein C Worldwide Evaluation in Severe Sepsis (PROWESS) prospective trial** demonstrated a 20 percent decrease in the 28-day mortality rate in septic patients. The efficacy of activated protein C lies in its anticoagulation and antiinflammatory characteristics. It inhibits the formation of thrombin, reducing mast cell degranulation, neutrophil recruitment and platelet activation. It also has direct antiinflammatory effects by preventing monocyte production of inflammatory cytokines (TNF-α, IL-6, IL-1) and limiting cell adhesion to endothelium. As an antiapoptotic agent, it may maintain the survival of lymphocytes. **Only patients with severe sepsis involving multiorgan dysfunction and a high likelihood of mortality are eligible for activated protein C.** Because the **major risk in using activated protein C is bleeding,** adequate hemostasis must be achieved in surgical patients prior to its use. Patients with INR >3.0 or platelet counts <30,000/mm^3 should not receive this agent. The efficacy of the drug is seen when therapy is initiated within the first 24 hours of diagnosis.

Recent studies have suggested that **early goal-directed therapy** may improve outcome in severely septic individuals. This strategy uses hemodynamic targets to guide fluid resuscitation and optimize cardiac function in the septic patient. Conventional management end-point parameters include the clinical exam and the physiologic parameters of **mean arterial pressure of 65 mmHg, central venous pressure of 8 to 12 mmHg,** and **urine output of 0.5 mL/kg/h.** The goal-directed therapy, initiated within the first 6 hours in the emergency room, involved several approaches: maintaining **central venous oxygen saturation of 70 percent**, using a protocol with the sequential administration of fluid, vasopressors, blood transfusions, and mechanical ventilation as needed. Mortality was reduced by about one-third in the early, goal-directed therapy group. The difference between the two groups lies with earlier receipt of treatment and more blood transfusions given to the goal-directed group. Vasopressors and mechanical ventilation were used less in this group. The benefit of goal-directed treatment in the septic patient relies on the early initiation of therapy and reestablishing the balance between oxygen delivery and demand. **Monitoring lactate, mixed venous oxygen saturation, pH, and base deficits** can provide direction in achieving this balance via resuscitation.

Intensive Glucose Control **Hyperglycemia, even in nondiabetics, correlates with adverse outcomes in critically ill** patients. **Strict glycemic control to a range of 80 to 110 mg/dL** appears to lead to a decreased incidence of sepsis; similarly, the mortality associated with MODS is reduced among the septic patients. The presumed benefit of intensive glucose control is the reversal of hyperglycemia-associated leukocyte dysfunction. While the mechanism remains unknown, **tight control of blood glucose** does appear to **improve survival** among **septic patients. Frequent testing of blood glucose and appropriate administration of insulin are indicated.**

Corticosteroids The benefit of corticosteroid therapy in the treatment of sepsis is unclear. Low-dose corticosteroids may improve survival in septic patients requiring vasopressors and mechanical ventilation, perhaps correcting the relative adrenal insufficiency in these patients. Nevertheless, other studies have demonstrated that high-dose corticosteroids do not improve survival in septic patients and may be associated with increased infections.

Comprehension Questions

[5.1] A 32-year-old woman is noted to have persistent hypotension from suspected toxic shock syndrome despite 3 L of normal saline given intravenously. Which of the following is the best next step?

A. Use antishock military anti-shock trousers (MAST) suit
B. Initiate dopamine infusion
C. Administer corticosteroid therapy
D. Transfuse with fresh-frozen plasma
E. Administer activated protein C

[5.2] A 45-year-old man with acute cholecystitis is noted to have a fever of 38.3°C (101°F), hypotension, and altered sensorium. Broad-spectrum antibiotics and intravenous saline are administered. Which of the following is most likely to be beneficial?

A. Initiate corticosteroids
B. Tight glucose control
C. Plasmapheresis
D. Antithrombin III infusion
E. Lithotripsy

[5.3] A 32-year-old woman is admitted to the hospital for acute pyelonephritis. The patient is treated with oral ciprofloxacin. After 4 days of therapy, she returns to the ED with persistent fever to 38.9°C (102°F) and flank tenderness. The urine culture reveals *E. coli* greater than 100,000 colony-forming units sensitive to ciprofloxacin. Which of the following is the best next step?

A. Order an intravenous pyelogram
B. Add anaerobic coverage with additional antibiotic therapy
C. Initiate a workup for fictitious fever
D. Consult a surgeon for possible appendicitis
E. Add anti-fungal therapy

[5.4] A 66-year-old female is noted to have acute pneumococcal pneumonia and is being treated with antibiotics, and with dopamine and dobutamine to maintain her blood pressure and urine output. Which of the following is a bad prognostic sign?

A. Urine output of 1 mL/kg/h
B. Mean arterial blood pressure of 80 mmHg
C. Decreased arterial-venous oxygen gradient
D. Serum bicarbonate level of 22 mEq/L

Answers

[5.1] **B.** A vasopressor agent such as dopamine is the treatment of choice for hypotension that is unresponsive to intravenous saline infusion.

[5.2] **B.** Tight glucose control decreases mortality in septic patients. Activated protein C started within 24 hours of diagnosis of sepsis decreases mortality by 20 percent.

[5.3] **A.** Many orally and parenterally administered antibiotics can achieve high concentrations in the urinary tract, leading to rapid improvements in most patients. Obstructive uropathy, such as a result of a renal or ureteral stone, is a leading cause of slow response to appropriate antibiotics therapy. Intravenous pyelogram (IVP) would identify such an obstruction.

[5.4] **C.** The decreased arterial-venous oxygen gradient connotes less extraction of oxygen from the tissues, meaning multiorgan failure. Dying organs do not use oxygen. Simultaneously, the lactate levels are likely elevated.

CLINICAL PEARLS

❖ The most common causes of sepsis in older patients are urosepsis and pneumonia.

❖ Older or immunocompromised individuals may present with subtle signs such as lethargy, decreased appetite, or hypothermia.

❖ Therapy for sepsis includes restoration of organ perfusion, usually by intravenous fluids, and infection source control.

❖ A vasopressor agent such as dopamine is the next step in treating hypotension that persists despite intravenous isotonic fluids.

❖ Tight glucose control may lead to better outcomes in individuals with severe sepsis.

REFERENCES

Ambrose PG, Owens RC Jr, Quintiliani R, et al. Antibiotics use in the critical care unit. Crit Care Clinics 1998;14:283–308.

Annane D. Corticosteroids for septic shock. Crit Care Med 2001;29(Supple): S117–20.

Annane D, Sebille V, Charpentier G, et al. Effect of treatment with low doses of hydrocortisone and fludrocortisone on mortality in patients with septic shock. JAMA 2002;288:862–71.

Bernand GR, Vincent JL, Laterre P, et al. Efficacy and safety of recombinant human activated protein C for severe sepsis. N Engl J Med 2001;344:699–709.

Hotchkiss R, Karl I. The pathophysiology of sepsis. N Engl J Med 2003;348:138–50.

Marshall JC, Papia G. The septic response. In: Cameron JL, ed. Current surgical therapy, 7th ed. St. Louis: Mosby, 2001:1327–32.

Rivers E, Nguyen B, Havstad S, et al. Early goal-directed therapy in the treatment of severe sepsis and septic shock. N Engl J Med 2001;345:1368–77.

Schein RMH, Kinasewitz GT. Risk-benefit analysis for drotrecogin alfa (activated). Am J Surg 2002;184(Suppl):25S–38S.

Van den Berghe G, Wouters P, Weekers F, et al. Intensive insulin therapy in the critically ill patients. N Engl J Med 2001;345:1359–67.

A 23-year-old man is transported to your emergency department (ED) from the scene of a single-car motor vehicle crash. The patient's car apparently veered off the highway resulting in rollover and ejection of the patient from the car. He was found approximately 1 hour after the incident. At the scene, the patient was awake and complained of pain in his back and legs. In the ED, his temperature is 35.6°C (96.1°F) rectally, pulse rate is 106 beats per minute, blood pressure is 110/88 mmHg, respiratory rate is 24 breaths per minute, and Glasgow Coma Scale score is 15. Multiple abrasions are noted over the neck, shoulders, abdomen, and legs. His chest wall is nontender with normal breath sounds over both lung fields. His abdomen is mildly tender. The pelvis is stable. Bony deformity, extensive swelling and tenderness of the right thigh are present. A focused abdominal sonographic examination for trauma (FAST) was performed revealing free fluid in Morrison pouch and no other abnormalities. The patient's initial CBC revealed white blood cell count (WBC) of 14,800 cells/mm^3, hemoglobin of 11.2 g/dL, and hematocrit of 34.4%.

◆ **What are the next steps in the evaluation of this patient?**

◆ **If this patient becomes hypotensive, what is the most likely cause?**

ANSWERS TO CASE 6: Hemorrhagic Shock

Summary: A healthy 23-year-old man presents following a motor vehicle accident with mild tachycardia, femur fracture, and possible intra-abdominal injury.

◆ **Next steps: The ABCs (airway, breathing, circulation) are always the first steps in the evaluation of a trauma patient.** Intraabdominal blood loss has been already been identified by the FAST examination, and because the patient is stable hemodynamically, a computed tomography (CT) scan of the abdomen should be done to help identify and quantify the injuries. The CT scan is useful to estimate the amount of intraperitoneal free fluid, and if severe intravascular volume depletion is present, collapse of the inferior vena cava (IVC) may be visualized.

◆ **Most likely cause of hypotension:** Hemorrhagic shock. The key areas of blood loss in this patient are intraabdominal and in his femur.

Analysis

Objectives

1. Learn the definition of hemorrhagic shock.
2. Learn the clinical manifestations of hemorrhagic shock, and the limitations of clinical parameters for the recognition of shock.
3. Learn the advantages and disadvantages of base deficit, serum lactate, central venous measurement, and pulmonary artery catheter application for shock identification and patient resuscitation.

Considerations

The **first priorities in the evaluation of any trauma patient are the ABCs**. Next, the history and physical examination should be quickly elicited. This patient was apparently ejected from a vehicle involved in a collision at high-speed, which suggests multisystem injuries, and significant kinetic energy transfer. The history of having been found 1 hour after the injury should raise concern for possible delayed treatment of shock and for hypothermia with diminished ability to respond to hemorrhagic shock.

A thorough patient survey should assess for blood loss from various sites. Special attention to signs of shock, such as skin pallor/coolness, delayed capillary refill, weak distal pulses, low blood pressure, elevated heart rate, increased respiratory rate, and anxiousness are important to facilitate early recognition of shock. The clinician, however, must not rely solely on vital signs, because patients with limited amount of hemorrhage (≤ 15 percent total intravascular volume loss) can present without clinical signs of shock because the body compensates for intravascular volume loss (Table 6-1). This patient obviously has had some blood loss from his femur fracture, and the **focused abdominal sono-**

graphic examination for trauma (FAST) suggests intra-abdominal solid organ injury associated with additional hemorrhage. Nevertheless, he has a normal blood pressure and only a slightly elevated heart rate, which places him in the category of potentially having Class II hemorrhagic shock.

During the secondary survey, the clinician assesses for fractures by inspecting and palpating the chest, shoulder, extremities, and pelvis. Fractures are not only associated with blood loss from the bone and adjacent soft tissue, but their presence are signs of significant energy transfer and should increase the clinical suspicion for intraabdominal and retroperitoneal bleeding and injuries. Typically, tibial or humeral fractures can be associated with 750 mL of blood loss (1.5 units of blood), whereas femur fractures can be associated with up to 1500 mL of blood (3 units of blood) in the thigh. Pelvic fractures may result in even more blood loss: up to several liters in a retroperitoneal hematoma.

In this patient with suspected class II hemorrhagic shock, the possibility of bleeding should be assessed in **five areas**: (a) **external bleeding** (scalp/extremity lacerations); (b) **pleural cavity** (hemothorax); (c) **peritoneal cavity** (bleeding from intraabdominal injuries; (d) **pelvic girdle** (pelvic fractures); and (e) **soft-tissue compartments** (long-bone fractures). Adjunctive studies that should be obtained in this patient early during the evaluation include chest and pelvic roentgenograms and computed tomography (CT) scan of the abdomen and pelvis. Chest roentgenograms may help to identify hemothorax and potential mediastinal bleeding. Pelvic films may help detect pelvic

Table 6-1
HEMORRHAGIC SHOCK CLASSIFICATION

	CLASS I	CLASS II	CLASS III	CLASS IV
Blood loss (mL)	<750	750–1500	1500–2000	>2000
Blood loss (%)	<15	15–30	30–40	>40
Pulse rate (beats/min)	<100	>100	>120	>140
Blood pressure	Normal	Normal	↓	↓↓
Pulse pressure	Normal/↑	↓	↓	↓↓
Capillary refill	Normal	Delayed	Delayed	Absent
Respirations (per min)	14–20	20–30	30–40	>35
Urine (mL/h)	>30	20–30	5–15	0
Mental status	Normal	Anxious	Confused	Lethargic

fractures and a source of pelvic blood loss. Uncontrolled blood loss leads to shock and early death. Less-profound blood loss that is unrecognized or uncorrected can be associated with inadequate tissue perfusion (tissue hypoxia) and cellular responses predisposing to the development of multiple organ dysfunction syndrome (MODS).

APPROACH TO HEMORRHAGIC SHOCK

Definitions

Shock: the cardiovascular system's inability to deliver sufficient oxygen to the tissues.

Hemorrhagic shock: inadequate tissue oxygenation resulting from a blood volume deficit. In this situation, the loss of blood volume decreases venous return, cardiac filling pressures, and cardiac output. End-organ perfusion is subsequently decreased as blood flow is preferentially preserved to the brain and heart.

Glasgow Coma Scale: scoring system based on eye-opening response, verbal response, and motor response ranging from 3 to 15 (see also Table I-2 in Section I).

Clinical Approach

Mild hemorrhage may not usually affect the vital signs. **Tachycardia does not occur unless more than 750 mL of blood is lost, whereas blood pressure does not drop until hemorrhage exceeds 1.5 L.** Laboratory studies that aid (but are not very useful) in evaluating blood loss are base deficit, lactate, hemoglobin, and hematocrit levels. With continued blood loss, patients suffer from decreased delivery of oxygen to the tissues, leading to metabolic acidosis that increases base deficit and lactate levels. Some evidence suggests that the presence of lactate elevation and increased base deficit may serve as early laboratory indicators of hypovolemia and underresuscitation. Persistent elevation of these values during resuscitation may help identify patients with ongoing hemorrhage.

In the setting of acute **hemorrhage, hemoglobin and hematocrit levels may or may not be decreased.** These are values that measure concentration, not absolute amounts. Hemoglobin is grams of red blood cells per deciliter of blood; hematocrit is the percentage of blood volume that is composed of red blood cells. Loss of whole blood will not decrease the red blood cell concentration or the percentage of red cells in blood.

The initial minor drops in hemoglobin and hematocrit levels are the results of mechanisms that compensate for blood loss by drawing fluid into the vascular space. To see significant decreases in these values, blood loss must be replaced with crystalloid solution; therefore, most decreases in hemoglobin and hematocrit values are not seen until patients have received large volume of crystalloid fluid for resuscitation.

As blood loss continues, shock progresses from a *compensated stage,* which requires no outside therapy for full recovery, to a *progressive stage,* where aggressive therapy is critical in preventing the development of irreversible shock and death. Patients who survive the initial hemorrhage but who remain underresuscitated may later succumb to systemic inflammatory response syndrome (SIRS) and MODS. **Because hemorrhage is the number one cause of preventable death in the early postinjury period,** the clinician must be vigilant and dexterous at identifying and aggressively treating all sources of blood loss. Normal vital signs do not rule out the presence of hemorrhagic shock. In the early stages of shock, the compensatory mechanisms can mask hypovolemia. The heart rate may be normal in mild to moderate shock. Careful evaluation and a high index of suspicion for occult injuries are essential.

Stages of Shock   **Shock is divided into three stages:** *compensated, progressive,* **and** *irreversible.* Shock is initially compensated by control mechanisms that return cardiac output and arterial pressure back to normal levels. Within seconds, baroreceptors and chemoreceptors elicit powerful sympathetic stimulation that vasoconstricts arterioles, and increases heart rate and cardiac contractility. After minutes to hours, angiotensin and vasopressin constrict the peripheral arteries and veins to maintain arterial pressures and improve blood return to the heart, respectively. Angiotensin and vasopressin also increase water retention, thereby improving cardiac filling pressures. Locally, vascular control preferentially dilates vessels around the hypoxic tissues to increase blood flow to injured areas. The **normal manifestations of shock do not apply** to **pregnant** women, **athletes,** and individuals with **altered autonomic nervous systems** (older patients, those taking beta blockers).

As shock progresses into the *progressive stage,* **arterial pressure falls.** This leads to cardiac depression from decreased coronary blood flow, and, in turn, further decreases arterial pressure. The result is a feedback loop that becomes a vicious cycle toward uncontrolled deterioration. Inadequate blood flow to the nervous system eventually results in complete inactivation of sympathetic stimulation. In the microvasculature, low blood flow causes the blood to sludge, amplifying the inadequate delivery of oxygen to the tissues. This ischemia results in increased microvascular permeability, and large quantities of fluid and protein move from the intravascular space to the extravascular compartment, which exacerbate the already decreased intravascular volume. The **systemic inflammatory response syndrome caused by severe injury and shock may progress to multiple-organ failure.** Lung, cardiac, renal, and liver failures ensue. This leads to pulmonary edema, adult respiratory distress syndrome, poor cardiac contractility, loss of electrolyte and fluid control, and inability to metabolize toxins and waste products. Cells lose the ability to maintain electrolyte balance, metabolize glucose, maintain mitochondrial activity, and prevent lysosomal release of hydrolases. Resuscitation during this *progressive* stage of tissue ischemia can cause reperfusion injury from the burst of oxygen free radicals. Finally, the patient enters the *irreversible stage* of shock, and any therapeutic efforts become futile. Despite transiently elevating arterial pressures and cardiac output, the body is unable to recover, and death becomes inevitable.

Serum Lactate and Base Deficits   Both lactate and base deficit levels are laboratory values that indicate systemic acidosis, not local tissue ischemia. They are global indices of tissue perfusion and normal values may mask areas of under perfusion as a consequence of normal blood flow to the remainder of the body. These laboratory tests are not true representations of tissue hypoxia. It is, therefore, not surprising that lactate and base deficit are poor prognostic indicators of survival in patients with shock. Although absolute values of these laboratory results are not predictors of survival in patients with shock, the baseline value and trends can be used to determine the extent of tissue hypoxia and adequacy of resuscitation. Normalization of base deficit and serum lactate within 24 hours after resuscitation is a good prognostic indicator of survival.

Base deficits measured in cardiac arrest patients show near-normal values from the arterial system, while base deficits are increased by 400% from the venous system. In patients in cardiac arrest, the venous base deficits may more accurately reflect the patient's acidotic state. Also, because lactate is metabolized in the liver, lactate is not a reliable value in patients with liver dysfunction.

Central Venous Catheters   Cardiac filling pressures to determine intravascular volume status may lead to inaccurate assessment in the critically ill patient population. The intended purpose of central venous pressure measurements is to determine the cardiac preload, because the preload is the driving force behind cardiac output as defined by the Starling curve. Strictly defined, **preload is the end-diastolic sarcomere length**, which cannot be measured clinically. Therefore, the clinician indirectly calculates preload from a measurement that is four steps removed from end-diastolic sarcomere length. At the bedside, the placement of a pulmonary artery catheter has provided the clinician with the ability to indirectly assess preload by measuring (a) pulmonary capillary occlusion (wedge) pressure that represents the (b) left atrial pressure. Left atrial pressure is the indirect measurement of (c) left ventricular end diastolic pressure, which is finally correlated to (d) left ventricular end-diastolic volume (which approximates the end-diastolic sarcomere length). **Left ventricular end-diastolic volume is our best clinical estimate of preload.** After making all these assumptions, it is the pulmonary artery occlusion pressure that is the surrogate preload on which intervention is based.

The pulmonary artery catheter, however, is able to provide the clinician with more than pulmonary capillary occlusion pressure. The cardiac output, systemic vascular resistance, oxygen consumption, oxygen delivery, and mixed venous oxygen saturation can all be measured or calculated. Trends or changes in the baseline hemodynamic parameters are probably the most useful information that the clinician can use to determine the adequacy and success of resuscitation. Because the needs of a human body in shock exceed those in a normal healthy state, it has been suggested that adequate resuscitation in the critically injured should reach "supranormal" cardiovascular endpoints. Patients who spontaneously obtain supranormal hemodynamic parameters may have improved outcomes; however, resuscitating patients with the goal of achieving supranormal cardiovascular endpoints does not appear to improve survival.

Treatment The **most common and easily available fluid for replacement is isotonic crystalloid solution** such as normal saline or lactated Ringer solution. For each liter of these solutions, about 300 mL stays in the intravascular space, and the remainder leaks into the interstitial space, leading to the guideline of **3 mL crystalloid replacement for each 1 mL of blood loss.** When the patient persists in shock despite the rapid infusion of 2 to 3 L of crystalloid solution, or if the patient has had such severe blood loss that cardiovascular collapse is imminent, then a blood transfusion is indicated. When possible, typed and cross-matched blood is optimal; however, in the acute setting, this is often unfeasible. Type-specific unmatched blood is the next best option, followed by O-negative blood. Blood is generally administered as packed erythrocytes with crystalloids, and fresh-frozen plasma and/or platelets may need to be transfused if massive blood volumes have been given. Colloid solutions such as albumin and hetastarch or dextran are not superior to crystalloid replacement in the acute setting and have the potential for large fluid shifts and pulmonary or bowel wall edema. Hypertonic solutions such as 7.5% saline have the advantage of retaining as much as 500 mL in the intravascular space and may be useful in trauma situations remote from blood products such as in military field circumstances.

Comprehension Questions

[6.1] A 32-year-old male was involved in a knife fight and is brought into the emergency room with a heart rate of 110 beats per minute and blood pressure of 84/50 mmHg. How much acute blood loss has he experienced?

A. 250 mL
B. 500 mL
C. 1000 mL
D. 1500 mL

[6.2] What is an advantage of diagnostic peritoneal lavage (DPL) and FAST when examining a patient in hemorrhagic shock?

A. Can identify retroperitoneal hematomas
B. Can be performed quickly at beside
C. Can identify the specific site of injury
D. Can quantify the exact amount of blood loss

[6.3] A 20-year-old man involved in a motor vehicle accident is brought into the emergency department having lost much blood at the accident scene. His initial blood pressure is 80/40 mmHg and heart rate 130 beats per minute. He is given 3 L of normal saline and is still hypotensive. Which of these statements most accurately describes the pathophysiology of his condition?

A. Insufficient cardiac preload
B. Insufficient myocardial contractility
C. Excessive systemic vascular resistance
D. Excessive IL-6 and leukotrienes

[6.4] In hypotensive patients, where is the *least* likely source of potentially significant blood loss that could account for the hypotension?

A. Chest and abdomen
B. Pelvic girdle and soft-tissue compartments
C. External bleeding
D. Intracranial bleeding

Answers

[6.1] **D.** Blood pressure does not decrease until class III hemorrhagic shock, when 1500 to 2000 mL of blood is lost (30 to 40% of blood volume)

[6.2] **B.** DPL and FAST cannot rule out retroperitoneal injury or identify the specific site of injury, but they can be performed quickly at bedside on unstable trauma patients. To find the specific site of injury and rule out retroperitoneal injury, a CT scan can be done; however, the trauma patient must be hemodynamically stable to be transported to the CT scan suite.

[6.3] **A.** Preload is end-diastolic sarcomere length, and insufficient circulating volume does not allow for sufficient venous return or cardiac output.

[6.4] **D.** It is important to systematically check for bleeding sources in the chest, abdomen, pelvic girdle, soft-tissue compartments (long-bone fractures), and external bleeding. Intracranial bleeding, although a significant injury, is usually not the cause of hypotension. The exception to this is the patient who is moribund secondary to a head injury.

CLINICAL PEARLS

❖ The ABCs are always the first steps in the evaluation of the trauma patient.

❖ The most common cause of hypotension in a trauma patient is hemorrhage.

❖ In the acute setting, the hemoglobin or hematocrit does not help to assess blood loss.

❖ The three stages of shock are compensated, progressive, and irreversible.

❖ Serum lactate and/or base-deficit levels are not accurate prognostic signs in hemorrhagic shock, but their trend may have prognostic value.

REFERENCES

Holcroft JW. Shock—approach to the treatment of shock. In: Wilmore DW, Cheung LY, Harken AH, Holcroft JW, Meakins JL, Soper NJ, eds. ACS surgery. New York: Webmed Professional Publishers, 2003:61–74.

Mullins RJ. Management of shock. In: Mattox KL, Feliciano DV, Moore EE, eds. Trauma. New York: McGraw-Hill, 1999:195–234.

Wilson M, Davis DP, Coimbra R. Diagnosis and monitoring of hemorrhagic shock during the initial resuscitation of multiple trauma patients: a review. J Emerg Med 2003;24(4):413–22.

An intoxicated 25-year-old man was brought to the emergency department (ED) by paramedics after he was involved in an altercation at an acquaintance's house and sustained several stab wounds to the torso and upper extremities. His initial vital signs in the ED showed a pulse rate of 100 beats per minute, blood pressure of 112/80 mmHg, respiratory rate of 20 breaths per minute, and Glasgow Coma Scale score of 13. A 2-cm stab wound is noted over the left anterior chest just below the left nipple. Additionally, a 2-cm wound is identified next to the umbilicus, and several 1- to 2-cm stab wounds are noted in right arm and forearm, near the antecubital fossa. The abdominal and chest wounds are not actively bleeding and there is no apparent hematoma associated with these wounds; however, one of the wounds in the right arm is associated with a 10-cm hematoma that is actively oozing.

◆ **What are the next steps in the evaluation of this patient?**

◆ **What are the complications associated with the injuries?**

ANSWERS TO CASE 7: Penetrating Trauma to the Chest, Abdomen, and Extremities

Summary: A 25-year-old hemodynamically stable, intoxicated man presents with stab wounds to the chest, abdomen, and upper extremities.

◆ **Next steps:** Assess ABCDE: airway, breathing, circulation, disability, and exposure. After completing this survey, consider probing the knife wounds to see whether they are superficial or deep.

◆ **Potential complications from injuries:** Chest wound: Heart/pericardium, pneumothorax, hemothorax, diaphragm.

◆ Abdominal wound: Bowel, vascular, urinary solid organs (spleen, liver).

◆ Extremities: Vascular, nerve, tendon.

◆ Prioritization of evaluation and treatment of these wounds is based on the physiological changes induced by the injuries and not the injury location or type.

Analysis

Objectives

1. Be able to classify penetrating injuries by location, including chest, thoracoabdominal region, abdomen, flank, back, and "cardiac box."
2. Learn the priorities involved in the initial management of penetrating injuries.
3. Become familiar with the treatments of penetrating truncal and extremity injuries.

Considerations

This 25-year-old man arrives to the ED with slight tachycardia, but stab wounds to the chest, abdomen, and upper extremity. A systematic approach must be undertaken, and **the clinician must guard against being distracted by "peripheral" findings**. Likewise, young healthy individuals, particularly those intoxicated, may have significant injuries and not manifest many findings. Advanced trauma life support (ATLS) guidelines stress the initial primary survey to identify and address the potentially life-threatening issues: the **ABCDEs: airway, breathing, circulation, disability, and exposure.** Exposure (removing all of the patient's clothing and rolling the patient to examine the patient's backside) is particularly important in a patient with penetrating trauma because puncture wounds may be hidden in skin fold areas including, axillary and inguinal creases, and gluteal folds.

Radiographic adjuncts include upright chest x-ray (CXR) (preferably at end expiration) and a focused abdominal sonogram for trauma (FAST) examination to look for intraperitoneal free fluid. For this patient, who is hemodynamically stable and who possesses minimal abdominal findings, a very reasonable strategy is to perform a local exploration of the abdominal wound to determine the depth of penetration. A wound that does not penetrate the abdominal fascia may be irrigated and closed, without further diagnostic requirement. Notably, this patient is intoxicated, and the physical examination may not be very sensitive for this reason.

APPROACH TO PENETRATING TRAUMA

Anatomical Regions

Chest: Clavicles to costal margins, 360 degrees around.

Thoracoabdominal: From the inframammary crease (women) or nipples (men), down to the costal margins, 360 degrees around. The significance of penetrating wounds to this region is that intrathoracic, intraabdominal contents, and diaphragm are all at risk for injury.

"Cardiac box": Represents the anatomical region bordered by imaginary lines drawn along the clavicles superiorly, and midclavicular lines bilaterally down to the costal margins inferiorly. This box would also include the epigastric region between the costal margins. The clinical significance of the "box" is that roughly 85 percent of penetrating cardiac stab wounds originate from punctures to the "box."

Anterior abdomen: From the costal margins, down to the inguinal ligaments, and anterior to the mid-axillary line bilaterally.

Flank: The costal margin down to the iliac crest, and between the anterior and posterior axillary lines.

Back: Area between the posterior axillary lines. Because of the thick musculature over the back, only approximately 5 percent of stab wounds to the back actually cause significant injuries. Stable patients with penetrating injury and no abnormalities on abdominal examination can be evaluated with CT scans to identify wound tracks and depth of penetration of wounds.

Initial Management

The primary survey, or ABCs should be addressed first (see Table I-2 in section I). The clinician should not be distracted by eye-catching, but not immediately life-threatening injuries. In an unstable patient, treatment decisions often need to be made before obtaining diagnostic tests. For example, a patient with a stab wound to the chest and rapidly dropping oxygen saturations will require tube thoracostomy ("B" breathing) prior to confirmatory CXR. Bleeding, even if profuse, is usually most effectively controlled by direct application of hand pressure to the bleeding site, whereas gauze and pressure dressings are generally far less effective. All patients should have immediate placement of large-bore IV access at two sites, where warm IV fluid may be initiated. After completion of the primary survey, a detailed examination for potential injuries (secondary survey), as well as diagnostic tests should be performed in an expeditious fashion (see Table 7-1).

In general, gunshot wounds possess much greater injury potential than stab wounds because of the higher kinetic energy transfer to the tissue from bullets. When managing a patient with gunshot wounds, it is important to bear in mind

Table 7-1

IDENTIFICATION OF INJURIES

ANATOMICAL REGION	PHYSICAL EXAMINATION	FURTHER TESTING
Chest	Auscultation for symmetry of breath sounds to identify hemo- or pneumothorax. Auscultate heart for muffled heart sounds, presence of distended neck veins suggest pericardial tamponade. Assess for sucking chest wound	Ultrasound evaluation of the heart is a reliable diagnostic study for cardiac tamponade. A CXR may detect hemo- or pneumothorax, or free air under the diaphragm.
Abdomen	Palpate abdomen for distension, the "doughy" feel of hemoperitoneum, peritoneal signs, or tenderness beyond the immediate site of the laceration may identify significant intra-abdominal injuries.	CXR and plain abdominal films not usually helpful. FAST examination for free fluid fairly specific, but may not be sensitive. Options include observation with serial physical examinations; computed tomography; local wound exploration; diagnostic peritoneal lavage (DPL); laparoscopy; and laparotomy.
Extremity	Assess the 6 Ps of arterial insufficiency: pain, paresthesias, paralysis, pulselessness, pallor, and poikilothermia (or polar for cold). Assess pulsatile bleeding, expanding hematoma, pulse deficit, bruit or thrill; evaluate skin temperature, capillary refill, and pulses distal to the injury, and a complete motor and sensory examination.	CT angiography or angiographic examination if vascular injury suspected.

Source: Townsend, CM, Beauchamp RD, Evers BM, and Mattox KL, eds. Sabiston textbook of Surgery, 16th ed. Philadelphia: W.B. Saunders, 2001.

that the bullet path and tissue destruction can be quite unpredictable, and it may not be assumed that the projectile has taken a direct path between the entrance and exit wounds.

The management of patients with penetrating injuries has undergone significant evolution over the past two decades. During the 1980s and 1990s, most patients underwent invasive diagnostic evaluations, including exploratory laparotomy and angiography on the basis of the injury mechanism and location. Currently, selective management of penetrating injuries is acceptable, which has led to a significant reduction in unnecessary operations and invasive diagnostic studies in these patients. The application of selective management must be individualized based on the clinical presentation, available personnel, and resource available, and as always, the conservative approach must be balanced against the risk of delay in the diagnosis and treatment of injuries. Options may involve close observation, with or without additional minimally-invasive diagnostic studies such as ultrasonography, laparoscopy, and thoracoscopy. The decision to proceed with nonoperative treatment is most appropriately determined by qualified surgeons, after the initial evaluation.

Specific Anatomical Regions

Chest Injuries   Generally, only 10 to 15 percent of patients with penetrating chest trauma require urgent operative intervention, while the remaining patients may require only observation, diagnostic imaging, with or without tube thoracostomy. Fortunately, the majority of the patients requiring an operation can be identified within the first few minutes by initial hemodynamic instability, the presence of a large hemothorax on CXR, or high chest tube output. The **chest x-ray** has adequate sensitivity to evaluate for pneumothorax and hemothorax. Roughly 15 percent of pneumothoraces may present in a delayed fashion; therefore the absence of either should be confirmed by repeat CXR in 4 to 6 hours. Obtaining an end-expiratory film may increase the likelihood of detecting a small pneumothorax. Computed tomography (CT) of the chest is highly sensitive for the detection of pneumothorax. A small pneumothorax visualized by CT and missed by CXR is referred to as an "occult pneumothorax". These are reevaluated by CXR in 3 to 6 hours for progression.

Local wound exploration of chest injury is not recommended because the procedure itself can penetrate the pleura and cause a pneumothorax. Pneumo- or hemothorax found by CXR is treated by placement of a 36- or 40-French chest tube. **The best treatment** of a **tension pneumothorax** is often **needle thoracostomy** for faster relief of the pleural pressure. Smaller tubes clot easily with blood and are not indicated in the setting of trauma. If the pneumo- or hemothorax does not resolve on the postplacement CXR, a second tube should be inserted. Considerations for thoracotomy in the operating room include initial output of 1500 mL of blood, or > 200 mL/h over the next 5 hours.

Any patient with an injury within the cardiac box should undergo prompt **FAST** examination of the heart by an experienced emergency medicine physician or surgeon. The subxiphoid view may be complemented by a parasternal view and can detect pericardial blood with up to 100 percent sensitivity (Fig. 7-1). Hemopericardium is an indication for pericardial exploration in the operating room.

Resuscitative (or so-called emergency department) thoracotomy is reserved for those patients who are *in extremis* **or who have lost vital signs within a few minutes prior to arrival.** Both discussions and performance of this procedure can be associated with a great deal of controversy, drama, and emotion. It must be borne in mind that in these situations, mortality exceeds 97 percent, and these interventions may expose the health care providers to unnecessary accidental injury and infectious exposure. The best opportunity for successful outcome is associated with procedures performed in a properly selected patient by an experienced surgeon, with the capabilities to provide definitive treatment in the operating room.

Thoracoabdominal   Thoracoabdominal wounds are of particular interest because injuries to the diaphragm are difficult to detect, and in the presence of negative intrathoracic pressure, herniation of intraabdominal contents may eventually occur. Unless the diaphragmatic defect is large, herniation of

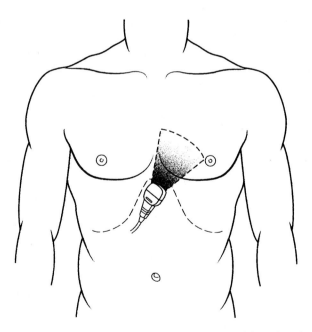

Figure 7-1. FAST examination imaging the subxiphoid region for pericardial fluid.

stomach or intestines are rarely visualized by CXR in the ED. Consultation from a surgeon should be obtained when diaphragmatic injury is suspected, because the definitive diagnostic study is surgical evaluation by **laparoscopy or thoracoscopy**.

Anterior Abdomen   Immediate indication for **laparotomy** includes clinical evidence of **shock** (hypotension, tachycardia, cold and clammy skin, or diaphoresis), **peritonitis**, **gun-shot wound** with probable course through the abdominal cavity, or **evisceration** of abdominal contents. In the absence of these findings, further evaluation or observation is indicated.

Local Wound Exploration   This is probably the best initial evaluation for a stable patient with an abdominal stab wound. This procedure is performed after preparing the skin with an antiseptic agent and creating a sterile field and anesthetizing the skin and soft tissues with lidocaine. The skin laceration is enlarged, and the wound tract is gently followed until either its termination or its violation of the anterior abdominal fascia. An intact fascia connotes the unlikelihood of an intraabdominal injury, and therefore the wound may be irrigated and closed. If the anterior abdominal fascia has been penetrated, then several options are available at that point. One of these options is the **diagnostic peritoneal lavage (DPL)**. The bladder should be decompressed with a Foley catheter and the stomach decompressed with a nasogastric tube prior to the procedure. The periumbilical skin is cleansed, draped, and anesthetized. A small incision is made and the peritoneum is entered either by open dissection or an over-guidewire Seldinger-type technique to insert the lavage catheter (Fig. 7-2). After intraperitoneal placement of the catheter, aspiration with a syringe is attempted. A grossly positive test is defined as aspiration of 10 mL of blood, or any bowel contents.

When the initial evaluation is negative, the test proceeds with instillation of 1 L of warmed saline, which is then drained by gravity and submitted for microscopic analysis. There is no clear consensus on the accepted criteria of a "microscopic positive" result in penetrating trauma, and the criterion may vary from center to center, ranging from 1000 red blood cells (RBC)/mm^3 to 100,000 RBC/mm^3, or 500 WBC/mm^3. If the DPL is positive, the patient should proceed to the operating room for exploratory laparotomy. If the DPL is negative, the patient should be **observed** for 24 to 48 hours, during which time antipyretics, antibiotics, and narcotic analgesics are withheld. DPL use has been abandoned in many centers, because "positive" DPLs in hemodynamically stable patients may lead to a high rate of nontherapeutic laparotomies. It is critical that a surgeon becomes involved in the patient's care prior to a DPL, because other options, including observation, laparoscopy, or laparotomy, are possible in these patients.

Microscopic hematuria in penetrating abdominal, flank, or back trauma necessitates evaluation of the kidneys, ureters, and possibly the bladder by CT, intravenous pyelogram (**IVP**), and perhaps retrograde cystography. Recent lit-

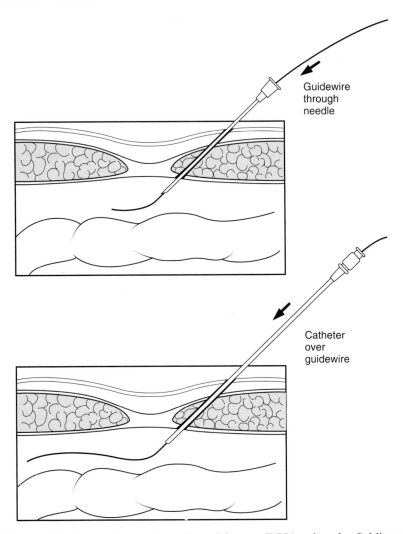

Figure 7-2. Closed diagnostic peritoneal lavage (DPL) using the Seldinger technique.

erature suggests that most renal injuries without associated hemodynamic compromise or urinary collection system leaks do not mandate exploration.

The use of CT imaging to evaluate patients with penetrating abdominal, back, and thoracoabdominal injuries has become more acceptable recently. In these settings, CT may help to identify the wound tract and assess for possible intraabdominal and retroperitoneal injuries. Good sensitivity of this test occurs when thin (3-mm) cuts are performed and read by an experienced radiologist. Specificity of CT is excellent in identifying free air or free fluid in the abdomen; however, the study may lack sensitivity in identifying actual injuries to hollow viscera.

Back   Physical exam, FAST, and DPL are all quite insensitive when it comes to injuries to the retroperitoneum (including colon, kidneys, ureters). Patients may indicate a desire to flex their hips and this may be the only clue to a retroperitoneal process irritating the psoas muscles. Here, CT may be used to evaluate a wound tract, but still thin cuts and interpretation by an experienced radiologist are critical.

Extremities   As outlined above, the six Ps of arterial insufficiency and the hard signs of vascular injury (such as pulsatile bleeding) should be sought. These are indications for immediate operative or angiographic evaluation. A careful pulse exam should be performed, to look for a deficit. A site of injury can be auscultated to identify a bruit that could represent a traumatic arteriovenous fistula. Similarly, Doppler examination of the brachial artery at the antecubital fossa and the palmar arches can confirm flow or identify a bruit. Additionally, a motor or sensory deficit can represent nerve (or tendon) injury that is best evaluated and treated in the operating room.

Comprehension Questions

[7.1]   A 23-year-old man is involved in an altercation in the parking lot after a baseball game. He suffers a single stab wound 2-cm medial and superior to the left nipple. His blood pressure is 110/80 mmHg and heart rate is 80 beats per minute. Which of the following management options is most appropriate for this patient?

A.   CXR, wound exploration, and EKG
B.   CXR and CT scan of the chest and abdomen
C.   CXR and echocardiography
D.   CXR, echocardiography, and laparoscopy

[7.2]   For which of the following patients is CT imaging an appropriate diagnostic option?

A.   A 38-year-old man with diffuse abdominal pain and a 6-inch knife impaled just below the umbilicus
B.   A 22-year-old man with a single stab wound to the back, pulse rate of 118 beats per minute, blood pressure of 94/80, and gross hematuria
C.   A 16-year-old boy with a single stab wound 2 cm above the left inguinal crease, with heart rate of 120 beats per minute and blood pressure of 90/78 mmHg
D.   A hemodynamically stable, 34-year-old woman, who is 26 weeks pregnant and has a single stab wound to the back and no other abnormalities on physical examination

[7.3]   A 34-year-old man is brought into the emergency room after a motor vehicle accident. He complains of dyspnea and initially had an oxygen saturation of 88 percent. On examination, he has decreased breath sounds of the right chest and now has an oxygen saturation of 70 percent on room air. Which of the following is the most appropriate next step?

A. Chest radiograph
B. CT of the chest
C. Tube thoracostomy
D. Heparin anticoagulation

Answers

[7.1]   **C.** CXR is sensitive in identifying hemothorax and pneumothorax, while echocardiography is useful in identifying pericardial fluid. Wound exploration of the chest wound is not recommended because the information gained is limited and the procedure is associated with the potential of producing a pneumothorax. An EKG provides limited information regarding cardiac injury and is generally not done. A stab wound above the nipple line is rarely associated with intraabdominal injury, therefore CT scan of the abdomen or diagnostic laparoscopy are unnecessary.

[7.2]   **D.** CT of the abdomen may be useful in identifying injuries to the retroperitoneal structures in a patient with a stab wound to the back. That the patient is 26-week pregnant does not contraindicate CT scan. Further diagnostic study would not be beneficial in patients listed in choices A, B, and C because these patients are exhibiting signs of significant injury that would necessitate urgent exploratory laparotomy.

[7.3]   **C.** The constellation of clinical signs points toward a pneumothorax. With the dropping oxygen saturations, tube thoracostomy (chest tube) should be placed even before chest radiograph confirmation, because the patient may progress to cardiovascular collapse.

CLINICAL PEARLS

❖   The systematic approach to the trauma patient is ABCDE (airway, breathing, circulation, disability, exposure).

❖   A wound that does not penetrate the abdominal fascia may be irrigated and closed without further diagnostic studies.

❖   Penetrating trauma to the chest below the nipple line may cause intraabdominal injury as well as chest injury.

❖   The FAST (focused abdominal sonogram for trauma) is fairly accurate in assessing intraperitoneal free fluid.

❖   Approximately 85 percent of penetrating cardiac stab wounds originate from a puncture to the "cardiac box."

REFERENCES

Alameda County Medical Center/Highland General Hospital. Protocols and guide-
    lines for the division of trauma. Available at: www.eastbaytrauma.org.
Cameron JL, ed. Current surgical therapy, 7th ed. St. Louis: Mosby, 2001.
Townsend CM, Beauchamp RD, Evers BM, Mattox KL, eds. Sabiston textbook of
    surgery, 16th ed. Philadelphia: W.B. Saunders, 2001.
Trunkey DD, Lewis FR, eds. Current therapy of trauma, 4th ed. St. Louis: Mosby,
    1999.

A 22-year-old student is brought in by paramedics from the campus health center. The nurse called 911 after the patient collapsed. On further questioning, the nurse states that the patient had been complaining of some itching and tongue swelling shortly after receiving an injection of penicillin for presumed "strep throat." When paramedics arrive, the patient has perioral cyanosis, stridor, and wheezing, and was tachycardic and hypotensive. On arrival to the emergency department, the patient is confused and diaphoretic with labored breathing. His blood pressure is 80 mmHg on palpation heart rate 150 beats per minute, respiratory rate 30 breaths per minute, and his pulse oximetry is 82 percent on 15 L/min of oxygen by face mask. Physical exam reveals significant perioral and laryngeal edema with near obstruction of the posterior oropharynx. Auscultation of the neck and lungs confirms stridor and severe wheezing. His skin has diffuse flushing and multiple large urticarial lesions on the trunk and extremities.

◆ **What are the next steps?**

◆ **What treatments should be instituted?**

ANSWERS TO CASE 8: Anaphylaxis

Summary: This is a patient with a systemic allergic reaction, likely to penicillin. The patient's cardiovascular instability categorizes him at the most extreme end of the spectrum of allergic responses, better known as anaphylaxis.

◆ **Next steps:** Resuscitation and stabilization should be the focus. Airway, breathing, and circulation should be managed appropriately and in that order, which will mean both procedural and pharmacological intervention. A **definitive airway** will need to be immediately established in the face of impending airway obstruction (see Case 1), and the patient's cardiovascular compromise must be supported with epinephrine.

◆ **Further treatments to be instituted:** In addition to airway management and early administration of epinephrine, pharmacological therapy is tailored to the other widespread manifestations of the anaphylactic response. These include volume resuscitation with crystalloid, nebulized beta agonists for wheezing, nebulized racemic epinephrine to decrease laryngeal edema, systemic steroids, antihistamines (including H_2 blockers), and removal of any remaining antigen.

Analysis

Objectives

1. Recognize the characteristic clinical features of anaphylaxis and anaphylactoid reactions.
2. Understand the underlying pathophysiology of anaphylaxis.
3. Become familiar with the available treatment options and how to implement them.

Considerations

This young man is brought into the ED with swelling of the tongue and itching. The perioral cyanosis, diffuse wheezing, stridor, and struggle to breathe all indicate **impending respiratory failure**. A delay of even a minute may be life-threatening. The most important intervention for this individual is **securing an airway.** This patient likely has edema of the pharynx and larynx, and his life likely depends on successful airway management, most likely **cricothyroidotomy** in the ED setting. Intubation or tracheostomy may be technically very difficult in this patient. Intravenous access with administration of **epinephrine** is likewise important, but not before securing the airway. This patient's clinical presentation is classic for anaphylaxis, and indeed penicillin is one of the most common pharmacological agents to be implicated. Identification of the inciting agent is not essential for treatment of anaphylaxis, but is helpful in preventing further exposures and recurrence of symptoms.

Treatment of anaphylaxis is supportive, and requires knowledge of general resuscitative techniques, airway management, and some basic pharmacology.

APPROACH TO ANAPHYLAXIS

Millions of people present to emergency departments every year complaining of allergic symptoms ranging from the minor dermatologic to the multisystem anaphylactoid reactions. Much of the time, it is difficult if not impossible to identify the trigger. Indeed many of these reactions may occur in response to medical therapies such as antibiotics and radiologic contrast agents. The broad spectrum of allergic responses makes it difficult to calculate a precise incidence of this disease. There are an estimated 30,000 ED visits every year for adverse food reactions. However, there are far more visits for more vague complaints and unknown exposures that at first glance may be difficult to identify as anaphylaxis. In the emergency department the goal is symptomatic treatment and prevention of further episodes.

True anaphylaxis is a **type 1 hypersensitivity** reaction occurring after a previous sensitizing exposure. In its purest form, this means an immune-mediated **activation of basophils and mast cells with subsequent release of prostaglandins, leukotrienes,** and **histamine**. From a clinical standpoint, an anaphylactoid reaction also includes release of these compounds but through non–immune-mediated pathways. The only clinical significance of this difference is that anaphylactoid reactions can occur without prior sensitization. Regardless of the underlying mechanism, their effects are similar, and early recognition will determine successful clinical management of these patients.

Pathophysiology

While the biochemical interactions involved in anaphylaxis are complicated, they boil down to good things gone bad. When first exposed to a substance, binding antibodies trigger class switching and regulatory changes in gene expression, effectively priming the immune system for its next encounter with the offending agent. In certain cases, this leads to **immunoglobulin (Ig) E binding mast cells and basophils**. In the classically defined anaphylactic reaction, the antigen again encounters the immune system, binds to the IgE on the mast cells and basophils, and releases a flood of cytokines that sets the clinical response in motion. In an anaphylactoid reaction, the antigen causes direct release of cytokines by mast cells and basophils, without need for prior sensitization. In both cases, the end result is the same, and clinically indistinguishable.

The early stages of some anaphylactic reactions involve increased secretion by mucous membranes. In addition to **watery eyes and rhinorrhea, increased bronchial secretions and increased smooth muscle tone cause wheezing** and increase the work of breathing. Decreased vascular tone and **increased capillary permeability** lead to **cardiovascular compromise and hypotension**. Other cytokines, specifically histamine, can cause **urticaria and**

angioedema. There are numerous cytokines involved in the immunologic cascade following exposure, but no one major substance is felt to be primarily responsible. Leukotriene C_4, prostaglandin D_2, histamine, and tryptase are known key components in the reaction.

Some of the most common causes of anaphylaxis are medications, most notoriously penicillin and sulfa agents. Some studies suggest as many as 1 in 500 exposures to penicillin will result in anaphylaxis. Because the use of penicillin is so widespread, it leads to far more cases of anaphylaxis than even radiographic intravenous contrast agents, even though the incidence is higher in the contrast group, approximately 1 to 2 percent of all patients. The later reaction is not IgE mediated, and is more common in patients receiving the less-expensive hyperosmolar agents. Overall, there are an estimated 0.9 fatal reactions per 100,000 patients exposed to IV contrast. This number skyrockets to 60 percent in patients who have had a prior exposure and reaction.

Hymenoptera, or bees and wasps stings, are another cause of anaphylaxis. Anaphylaxis from stings result in an average of 50 deaths per year in the United States. Overall, the number of cases of arthropod anaphylaxis seen by physicians is small compared to the number of iatrogenic cases, but because exposures often occur miles from medical treatment, they can have serious outcomes.

Food sources round out the major causes of serious allergic reactions. **Peanuts** are easily the **most common cause of serious allergies**, but any food can be responsible. Other common food allergens include eggs and shellfish. Anyone with a known shellfish allergy should be treated as if (s)he has a potential radiographic contrast allergy, because iodine in both may be the offending component.

Diagnosis

There are no specific tests for anaphylaxis, so **the diagnosis is made clinically**. The most commonly affected system is the skin, which manifests with **angioedema, urticaria, erythema, and pruritus** in greater than 90 percent of patients with anaphylaxis. The cardiovascular system is also affected, primarily as a result of decreased vasomotor tone and capillary leakage. This leads to **hypotension and tachycardia**, and resultant altered mental status. The most clinically significant system to be compromised by anaphylaxis is the respiratory tract. **Bronchospasm and bronchorrhea** in the lower respiratory tract in combination with edema of the upper respiratory tract are the most feared and difficult to manage aspects of anaphylaxis. Control of the airway and maintaining oxygenation and ventilation become the most important therapeutic interventions, as **nearly all deaths caused by anaphylaxis are a result of airway compromise.** Thus early and aggressive airway management—surgical if needed—is indicated in these patients. Although less common, patients may also complain of abdominal cramping, nausea, vomiting, and diarrhea.

The severity of any given reaction is impossible to predict; however, rapid onset of symptoms tends to indicate a more severe and diffuse response. While reactions are almost always temporally related to an exposure, patients can develop symptoms up to 4 days after exposure.

Treatment

Treatment of anaphylaxis begins with patient education and avoiding known precipitants. **Patients with known allergies should carry self-injectable epinephrine** (Epi-Pen and Epi-Pen Jr). However, this is not always possible. Once the medical system has been alerted and activated to a potential anaphylaxis case, treatment must center on resuscitation and supportive care. This begins with the **ABCs, large-bore IVs for volume resuscitation, oxygen, and hemodynamic monitoring**. The airway must be assessed immediately. It is imperative that providers have a *low* **threshold to secure the airway as laryngeal edema can increase to the point of occlusion quickly** making standard orotracheal intubation impossible (Table 8-1). **When attempting an orotracheal intubation, the provider should also be prepared to quickly switch to a surgical airway such as a cricothyroidotomy should the oral attempt fail.**

The primary medication to initiate is **epinephrine** (Table 8-2). Epinephrine will act as a pressor for hemodynamic support as well as to counteract released mediators and prevent their further release. It can be dosed subcutaneously or intravenously; however, in true anaphylaxis, IV administration is preferred. Epinephrine dosing can be confusing and potentially dangerous. In general, all **ampules of epinephrine have 1 mg of medication** (1 mL of 1:10,000 = 1 mg of medication; 10 mL of 1:100,000 = 1 mg of medication). **One method of administration is to place 1 mg (1 ampule) of epinephrine into 1 L of intravenous fluid (equivalent to 1 mcg/mL) and infuse to 1 to 4 cc/min (1-4 mcg/min).** This allows for precise titration of dosing to desired effect, and provides more rapid onset. Caution should be exercised in the elderly and in those with known cardiovascular disease. Inhaled beta agonists are indicated for wheezing, and nebulized racemic epinephrine has been hypothesized to decrease laryngeal edema. Intravenous **glucagon** is often useful for individuals on **beta blockers**, because they generally will not respond to epinephrine.

Other adjuvants include systemic **steroids**, specifically methylprednisolone (Solu-Medrol) and prednisone. Steroids will not take action for about 6 hours, but will blunt further immune responses and the so-called

Table 8-1
PITFALLS IN ANAPHYLAXIS

Failure to recognize the symptoms of anaphylaxis

Underestimating the severity of laryngeal edema and failure to secure the airway early

Reluctance to administer epinephrine early

Forgetting to remove the allergen; e.g., the IV drip of penicillin or bee stinger

Lack of appropriate patient education

Failure to prescribe an Epi-Pen prior to discharge

Table 8-2

TREATMENT FOR ANAPHYLAXIS

DRUG	ADULT DOSE	PEDIATRIC DOSE
Epinephrine	IV single dose: 100 mcg over 5–10 min; 1:100,000 dilution given as 0.1 mg in 10 mL at 1 mL per min IV infusion: 1–4 mcg per min IM: 0.3–0.5 mg (0.3–0.5 mL of 1:1000 dilution)	IV infusion: 0.1–0.3 mcg/kg per min; maximum 1.5 mcg/kg/min IM: 0.01 mg/kg (0.01 mL/kg of 1:1000 dilution)
IV fluids: NS or LR	1–2 L bolus	10–15 mL/kg bolus
Diphenhydramine	25–50 mg q6h IV, IM, or PO	1 mg/kg q6h IV, IM, or PO
Ranitidine	50 mg IV over 5 min	0.5 mg/kg IV over 5 min
Cimetidine	300 mg IV	4–8 mg/kg IV
Hydrocortisone	250–500 mg IV	5–10 mg/kg IV (max: 500 mg)
Methylprednisolone	125 mg IV	1–2 mg/kg IV (max: 125 mg)

Albuterol	Single treatment: 2.5–5.0 mg nebulized (0.5–1.0 mL of 0.5% solution) Continuous nebulization: 5–10 mg/h	Single treatment: 1.25–2.5 mg nebulized (0.25–0.5 mL of 0.5% solution) Continuous nebulization: 3–5 mg/h
Ipratropium bromide	Single treatment: 250–500 mcg nebulized	Single treatment: 125–250 mcg nebulized
Magnesium sulfate	2 g IV over 20 min	25–50 mg/kg IV over 20 min
Glucagon	1 mg IV q5min until hypotension resolves, followed by 5–15 mcg per min infusion	50 mcg/kg q5min
Prednisone	40–60 per day PO divided bid or qd (for outpatients: 3–5 days; tapering not required)	1–2 mg per day PO divided bid or qd (for outpatients: 3–5 days; tapering not required)

"biphasic anaphylaxis." Steroids should be continued for days after the reaction and gradually tapered. H_1 and H_2 blockers should also be administered. Again, the goal of therapy is to mitigate the effects of as many cytokines as possible. Diphenhydramine and ranitidine are the most commonly employed agents. It should be remembered that these other medications, while safe and easy to administer, are not first-line agents, and will not counteract respiratory and cardiovascular compromise.

Comprehension Questions

[8.1]   Which of the following most suggests anaphylaxis rather than a simple allergic reaction?

A. Hives
B. Watery eyes
C. Blood pressure of 80/40 mmHg
D. Swollen lips
E. Flushing

[8.2]   A patient with a peanut allergy is brought to the ED by ambulance after accidentally eating his friend's peanut butter sandwich. He is wheezing and anxious. Your first intervention should be:

A. Diphenhydramine 50 mg IV
B. Normal saline at 120 mL/h
C. Examine the skin
D. Epi-Pen 0.3 mg SQ
E. Assess the airway

[8.3]   Which of the following management options is the greatest determinant of patient outcome in anaphylaxis?

A. Timely administration of steroids
B. Immediate identification of the allergen
C. Early airway intervention and respiratory support
D. Correct dosing of epinephrine
E. Intravenous fluids

[8.4]   A 32-year-old man collapses in the emergency center after being brought in by paramedics. He was stung by a bee and is known to be highly allergic. He appears cyanotic and had extreme stridor in the ambulance. Severe laryngeal edema is notable. After securing the airway, which of the following is the best next step?

A. Immediate intravenous epinephrine
B. Immediate high-dose corticosteroids intravenously
C. Injection of lidocaine into the laryngeal region
D. Intravenous antihistamines

Answers

[8.1]   **C.** Hypotension indicates a systemic reaction and cardiovascular compromise, thereby classifying this allergic reaction as anaphylaxis. The other options may all be part of an anaphylactic response, but may also just be simple allergic reactions.

[8.2]   **E.** In any resuscitation, airway is always first. This is especially true in anaphylaxis where airway compromise is most likely to kill your patient. The other interventions are all appropriate to quickly institute, but not before the airway.

[8.3]   **C.** Again, airway is paramount. Once the airway is secure, the greatest pitfall of this disease has been contained, and other organ systems and symptoms can be appropriately managed.

[8.4]   **A.** Establishment of an airway is paramount. Because of the significant laryngeal edema, endotracheal intubation will be nearly impossible; hence, cricothyroidotomy is likely to be lifesaving. After securing an airway, epinephrine is the most important medication to administer in anaphylaxis.

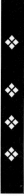

CLINICAL PEARLS

❖   The airway should be secured early and often. It is much easier to extubate a patient without severe laryngeal edema than to intubate a patient with an occluded posterior oropharynx.

❖   Epinephrine should be given at the first sign of cardiovascular compromise.

❖   Look for causes of anaphylaxis *after* you have started your initial resuscitation.

❖   Steroids, antihistamines, and beta agonists are all helpful pharmacological adjuvants for managing the many symptoms of anaphylaxis.

REFERENCES

Braunwald E, Fauci AS, Kasper DL, et al, eds. Harrison's principles of internal medicine, 15th ed. New York: McGraw-Hill, 2001.

Rowe BH, Carr S. Anaphylaxis and acute allergic reaction. In: Tintinalli JE, Kelen GD, Stapczynski JS, eds. Emergency Medicine, 6th ed., New York: McGraw-Hill: 2004:108-24.

At 3 AM the paramedics call to inform you that they are en route to the emergency department with a 33-year-old asthmatic. As she is brought in, you immediately notice that she is struggling to breathe. Sweat pours from her face and body as her neck and chest heave in an attempt to inhale another breath. Her efforts are ultimately futile as consciousness slips away and she becomes apneic.

◆ **What are your initial priorities in the management of this patient?**

◆ **What are your standard treatment options in managing her emergency medical condition?**

ANSWERS TO CASE 9: Acute Exacerbation of Asthma

Summary: This is a case of a 33-year-old female experiencing a severe asthma attack. Respiratory arrest is imminent.

◆ **Initial Priorities:** The first priority in this patient's management is addressing the ABCs (airway, breathing, circulation). Based on this presentation, immediate protection of her airway with rapid-sequence endotracheal intubation is indicated. Simultaneously, this patient should be placed on a cardiac monitor with automated blood pressure measurement, establishment of IV access, and continuous pulse oximetry.

◆ **Standard treatment options:** Basic treatment options include adrenergic agonists (e.g., albuterol [Proventil], terbutaline [Brethine]), anticholinergic agents, and corticosteroids. Intravenous magnesium sulfate is often given to patients with severe asthma exacerbations.

Analysis

Objectives

1. Understand the pathophysiology of respiratory distress caused by acute asthma exacerbation.
2. Describe the key historical and physical exam features.
3. Be able to discuss treatment options for the patient with acute bronchospasm caused by asthma.

Considerations

This 33-year-old asthmatic patient has progressive respiratory difficulty until she becomes apneic. Regardless of the underlying etiology, airway and breathing are the most important initial concerns in any patient. Attention to the airway is critical, and in this case, **rapid-sequence endotracheal intubation** is the best option. Because airway issues may arise at any given time, the emergency room physician must be skilled, rehearsed, and have equipment to perform endotracheal intubation at any given time. Protection of the airway, and mechanical ventilation is the best therapy in this instance. Administration of beta-agonist agents, corticosteroids, anticholinergic agents, and a search for the trigger are likewise important.

APPROACH TO ASTHMA

Epidemiology and Pathophysiology

In the United States, asthma accounts for more than 2 million emergency department (ED) visits, 470,000 hospitalizations and 5000 deaths each year. Overall, between 4 and 8 percent of all adults carry a diagnosis of asthma, with a higher prevalence reported in children and the elderly. It is the most common chronic disease in children and adolescents and the third leading cause of preventable hospitalizations in the United States. Asthma results in more than 10 million lost school and workdays per year, and results in $14.5 billion dollars of medical expenses per year.

Asthma is considered a **chronic inflammatory disorder of the airways** in which inflammatory cells and cellular elements play a key role. In susceptible individuals, precipitating allergens incite an acute inflammatory reaction that results in recurrent episodes of wheezing, breathlessness, chest tightness, and cough. These episodes are usually associated with widespread but variable **airflow obstruction** from acute **bronchospasm, mucous plugging, and airway inflammation, and edema**. Although patients appear to completely recover following an asthma attack, some recent evidence suggests that asthmatic patients develop chronic airflow limitation as a result of sub-basement membrane fibrosis of the pulmonary epithelium.

Two distinct phases of asthma have been described. The **early** (or immediate) phase of asthma consists of acute **bronchoconstriction**. Following allergen challenge, the lungs begin to constrict within 10 minutes. Peak bronchoconstriction occurs at 30 minutes and either, spontaneously or with treatment, resolves within 1 to 3 hours. With continued allergen challenge or with refractory bronchoconstriction, this initial phase can progress onto the late phase of asthma. This **late (or delayed) phase** of asthma begins **3 to 4 hours after the allergen challenge** and constitutes the **inflammatory component** seen with acute asthma. Inflammatory cell recruitment, bronchial edema, mucoserous secretion, and further bronchoconstriction all play key roles in the development and propagation of late-phase asthma. Whereas beta$_2$ agonists target the immediate phase of asthma, **corticosteroids target the delayed phase**.

Diagnosis

The typical asthma exacerbation is characterized by cough, chest tightness, dyspnea, and wheezing in a patient with a known asthma history. Although wheezing is often thought of as the hallmark finding in asthma, it is not specific to asthma (Table 9-1) and can be absent during severe asthma exacerbations. The history and physical examination should focus on excluding other diagnoses while evaluating the extent of the current asthma exacerbation. Key features to elicit are the nature and time course of the symptoms, precipitating events, use of medication prior to arrival, and any high-risk historical features (Table 9-2).

The evaluation of an asthmatic patient begins with the general appearance of the patient. Patients who are **extremely anxious or drowsy, unable to speak in full sentences secondary to respiratory distress**, or are using **accessory muscles** of inspiration are at significant risk for rapid decompensation. Additional worrisome features are signs of **central cyanosis, hypoxia** (pulse oximetry <90 percent), significant **tachypnea** (>30 breaths per minute), **diaphoresis, diffuse or absent wheezing**, and **poor air entry** on pulmonary examination.

Table 9-1
DIFFERENTIAL DIAGNOSIS OF WHEEZING

Asthma

Congestive heart failure

Chronic obstructive pulmonary disease

Allergic reaction

Foreign-body aspiration

Pneumonia

Pulmonary embolism

Upper airway obstruction

Toxic inhalation

Tumor

Table 9-2
HIGH-RISK HISTORICAL ASTHMA FEATURES

At any time
  History of previous sudden life-threatening asthma exacerbation
  History of prior intubation
  History of prior ICU admission

In the past year
  ≥2 hospital admissions
  ≥3 ED visits

In the past month
  Hospital admission
  ED visit
  ≥2 canisters of short-acting bronchodilator used

Other
  Current or recent use of oral steroids
  Complicating health (e.g., cardiovascular, COPD) or psychiatric (e.g., depression)
  condition
  Poor patient perception of severity of asthma
  Severe allergen hypersensitivity
  Low SES and urban residence
  Illicit drug use

Abbreviations: COPD, chronic obstructive pulmonary disease; SES, socioeconomic status

The pulmonary exam is the most helpful in the evaluation of asthma. The chest should be inspected for respiratory rate and degree of accessory muscle use. **Intercostal (best seen in the flank and back) and supraclavicular retractions indicate significant respiratory distress.** Following inspection, the lungs should be auscultated to determine the loudness and duration of wheezing. An exacerbation can be graded as mild, moderate, or severe based on the duration and quality of wheezing and air entry. Wheezing only during forced active breathing or only during the expiratory phase in a patient that has good air entry and a near normal expiratory phase indicates a mild exacerbation. A moderate exacerbation is characterized by wheezing that occurs during inspiration and expiration in a patient with diminished air entry and a prolonged expiratory phase. And finally, marked wheezing with obviously decreased or near-absent breath sounds in a patient with poor air entry indicates severe asthma. Routine laboratory investigations (e.g., complete blood count, basic metabolic panel), arterial blood gas analysis, chest radiography, and cardiac monitoring are not required in the uncomplicated asthmatic. Table 9-3 suggests indications for each of these modalities. Bedside testing that measures **peak expiratory flow rate** (PEFR) or **fractional expiratory volume at 1 second** (FEV_1) is commonly used to monitor response to treatment in the ED. These measurements are often compared to the patient's personal best measurement to gauge improvement.

Management

Immediate priorities in the management of all asthma patients include an initial assessment of the patient's airway, breathing, and circulation status.

Table 9-3
SUGGESTED INDICATIONS FOR FURTHER TESTING IN ASTHMA

Complete blood count—suspected pneumonia

Metabolic panel—patient on diuretic therapy

Theophylline level—patient on theophylline therapy

BNP—suspicion of CHF

Arterial blood gas—patient with suspected hypoventilation, severe respiratory distress, or PEFR or FEV_1 <30% predicted after treatment

Chest radiography—patient with asthma requiring admission, severe respiratory distress, failure to improve in the ED, immunocompromised host, unexplained fever, or clinical suspicion for alternative diagnosis (e.g., pneumonia, pneumothorax, CHF)

Cardiac monitoring—patient with severe respiratory distress, coexisting cardiac morbidity, or clinical suspicion of tension pneumothorax, CHF, or pulmonary embolus

Abbreviations: BNP, brain natriuretic peptide; CHF, congestive heart failure; FEV_1, fractional expiratory volume at 1 second; PEFR, peak expiratory flow rate.

Patients *in extremis* **require placement of peripheral intravenous lines, continuous supplemental oxygen therapy, and cardiac monitoring.** While these interventions are underway, the physician should ascertain a history, perform a physical exam, and initiate appropriate therapy.

Oxygen, Compressed Air, and Heliox **Oxygen should be provided to maintain a pulse oximetry reading of at least 90 percent in adults and at least 95 percent in infants, pregnant women,** and **patients with coexisting heart disease.** Oxygen is often used as the delivery vehicle for nebulized medications, although compressed air and **helium:oxygen mixtures** (Heliox) can also be used. Although Heliox mixtures produce more laminar air flow and potentially deliver nebulized particles to more distal airways, they have not been shown to consistently lead to improved ED outcomes for asthmatics.

Adrenergic Agents Inhaled albuterol, through nebulization or metered dose inhaler (MDI) with spacer device, is the mainstay of treatment for acute asthma. **Typically 2.5 to 5 mg of albuterol is intermittently nebulized every 20 minutes for the first hour of therapy** and then repeated every 30 minutes thereafter for 1 to 2 more hours. Continuous nebulization with higher doses of albuterol benefits severe asthmatics. Beta$_2$ agonists bind pulmonary receptors and activate adenyl cyclase which results in an **increase in intracellular cyclic adenosine monophosphate (cAMP).** This results in a drop in myoplasmic calcium and subsequent bronchial smooth-muscle relaxation. In addition, Beta$_2$ agonists are thought to have some antiinflammatory properties by inhibiting inflammatory mediator release. **Side effects** of these agents are generally mild and include **tachycardia, nervousness, and shakiness or jitteriness.**

Alternatively, albuterol can be administered with an **MDI** and spacer device. In the ED, patients can receive 4 to 8 puffs every 20 minutes for the first hour of therapy and then every 30 minutes thereafter for 1 to 2 more hours. MDI with spacer device therapy is therapeutically equivalent to nebulizer therapy in adults and may be more efficacious than nebulizer therapy in children. Implementation of MDI with spacer device therapy for asthmatics in the ED is associated with decreased health care cost.

Although inhalation therapy is optimal, occasionally patients with severe obstruction or who cannot tolerate inhalation therapy are given subcutaneous administration of epinephrine or terbutaline. **Epinephrine is given in a dose of 0.3 to 0.5 mg subcutaneously every 20 minutes to a maximal dose of 1 mg. Terbutaline** is given 0.25 to 0.5 mg subcutaneously every 30 minutes to a maximal dose of 0.5 mg over 4 hours. Generally, terbutaline is preferable because of its Beta$_2$ selectivity and fewer cardiac side effects.

Levalbuterol, the L isomer of racemic albuterol, has received considerable attention recently and has a role in patients that develop dose-limiting side effects on traditional albuterol therapy. Currently, levalbuterol is not approved for the treatment of acute asthma.

Anticholinergic Agents When added to albuterol, **anticholinergic agents** lead to a modest improvement in pulmonary function and decrease the admission rate in patients with moderate to severe asthma exacerbations. **Anticholinergics decrease intracellular cyclic guanosine monophosphate (cGMP)** concentrations, which reduce vagal nerve-mediated bronchoconstriction on medium- and larger-sized airways. Additionally, anticholinergic agents may have some minor antiinflammatory properties that help to stabilize capillary permeability and inhibit mucous secretion. The typical dose for **ipratropium bromide is 2 puffs from a MDI with spacer device, or 0.5 mL of the 0.02% solution**. Practitioners often combine the first dose of albuterol with ipratropium in the medication holding chamber of hand-held nebulization devices. Side effects are typical of other anticholinergic medications.

Corticosteroids Corticosteroids have been used to treat chronic asthma since 1950 and acute exacerbations of the disease since 1956. Although a tremendous amount of research has been done on the value of corticosteroids in asthma, many fundamental issues have yet to be resolved, such as the optimal dose, route, and timing of steroids. It is generally agreed that **corticosteroids should be initiated early in the treatment of acute asthma in patients with moderate/severe asthma attack**, worsening asthma over many days (>3 days), and mild asthma not responding to initial bronchodilator therapy. Some authors believe that more liberal use of corticosteroids is warranted and advocate steroids for any patient whose symptoms fail to resolve with a single albuterol treatment. Even more liberal asthmatologists prefer that steroids be given for every asthma patient who is sick enough to warrant ED evaluation.

Steroids act on the delayed phase of asthma and modulate the inflammatory response. They have been shown to improve pulmonary function, decrease the rate of hospital admission, and decrease the rate of relapse in patients that receive them early in their ED treatment course. Oral administration of prednisone (dose 40 to 60 mg) is usually preferred to intravenous methylprednisolone (dose 125 mg) because it is less invasive and the effects are equivalent. Intravenous steroids, however, should be administered to patients with severe respiratory distress who are too dyspneic to swallow, patients who are vomiting, or patients who are agitated or drowsy.

Leukotriene Antagonists The development of **leukotriene antagonists** represents an important advancement in the treatment of **chronic asthma**. Studies involving **zileuton (Zyflo Filmtab), zafirlukast (Accolate), and montelukast (Singulair)** demonstrate that their daily use over the course of several months can lead to improvement in pulmonary function and decrease in asthma symptomatology. Recent trials in the ED with montelukast and zafirlukast have shown that these agents may have a role in the acute setting.

Magnesium Although no benefit has been shown in mild to moderate asthmatics, **magnesium sulfate given intravenously at dosages of 2 to 4 g benefits asthmatics with severe airway obstruction**. Magnesium is thought to compete with calcium for entry into smooth muscle, inhibits the release of calcium from the sarcoplasmic reticulum, prevents acetylcholine release from nerve endings, and inhibits mast cell release of histamine. Additionally, there is some evidence that magnesium may directly inhibit smooth muscle contraction, but this is controversial. The onset of magnesium is quick and effects can be seen 2 to 5 minutes after initiation of therapy. The effects are short-lived and diminish quickly when the infusion is stopped. The dose of magnesium is 2 to 4 g IV in adults and 30 to 70 mg/kg IV in children given over 10 to 15 minutes. Magnesium has minimal side effects. The most commonly reported are hypotension, a flushing sensation, and malaise.

Other Agents The marginal benefit, significant side effects, and difficulty achieving a therapeutic level of theophylline argue against its routine use in acute asthma. Despite these concerns, some intensivists recommend loading with aminophylline for severe asthmatics. The routine administration of antibiotics has not been shown to decrease symptomatology in asthma in patients without concurrent bacterial lower respiratory infection or sinusitis.

Positive Pressure Ventilation Positive pressure ventilation (PPV), with either invasive or noninvasive methods, is indicated for patients with respiratory failure or impending failure who are not responsive to therapy. **Noninvasive ventilation with bilevel positive airway pressure (BiPAP) is an appropriate choice for cooperative patients with normal mentation and normal facial anatomy.** The BiPAP machine should be set at inspiratory pressure 8 to 10 cm H_2O and expiratory pressure 3 to 5 cm H_2O. Patients who fail to improve over 30 to 60 minutes may require intubation. **Immediate rapid-sequence endotracheal intubation should be reserved for unconscious or near-comatose patients with respiratory failure.** With an **awake patient**, an appropriate **induction agent** (e.g., ketamine) and **paralytic agent** (e.g., succinylcholine) should be used prior to intubation. Suggested initial settings are Assist Control mode at a respiratory rate of 8 to 10 breaths per minute, tidal volume 6 to 8 mL/kg, no extrinsic peak end-expiratory pressure (PEEP), and an inspiratory flow rate of 80 to 100 L/min. These ventilator settings promote the goal of permissive hypercapnia while limiting plateau pressures. Following initiation of PPV, blood gas analysis can be used to modify ventilator or BiPAP settings.

Admission/Discharge Criteria Acute asthma is a heterogeneous condition and as such patients should be individualized when it comes to disposition decisions. Patients who respond well to therapy by improved subjective and objective criteria (e.g., symptoms resolved, normal or near-normal pulmonary exam) are suitable candidates for discharge. **An improvement of PEFR or FEV$_1$ to greater than 70 percent predicted or personal best can also be used as a sign of objective improvement.**

Asthmatics that are discharged should receive **albuterol, a MDI spacer device, and a 3- to 10-day course of oral steroids**. This duration of oral steroids does not require tapering as long as the patient has not recently been on steroid therapy. Inhaled steroids or oral leukotriene antagonists can be added to the treatment plan of patients who meet specific criteria. While awaiting discharge, MDI with spacer device technique should be reviewed with the patient, and the patient should be instructed on how to monitor peak flow readings at home. Additionally, patients should be educated about the common asthma precipitants and how to avoid them, as well as receive written and verbal instructions on when to return to the ED. Finally, patients should be referred for a followup medical appointment in a timely manner. Patients who are unable to followup with their primary physician can be instructed to return to the ED for a recheck of their symptoms.

Hospital admission should be considered in patients that fail to respond to therapy (i.e., PEFR or FEV$_1$ <50 percent predicted) or patients with partial response to therapy (i.e., PEFR or FEV$_1$ between 50 and 70 percent predicted) that also have significant medical or social issues that impair access to health care, personal judgment, or understanding of their disease.

Comprehension Questions

[9.1] A 24-year-old male is brought into the ED complaining of an exacerbation of his asthma. Which of the following is the most appropriate method of assessing the severity of his disease?

A. Spirometry
B. Measurement of the diffusion capacity of the lungs
C. Measurement of the peak expiratory flow
D. Measurement of the alveoli oxygen tension

[9.2] A 19-year-old female is admitted to the hospital for an exacerbation of asthma likely precipitated by pollen and colder weather. Her inpatient regimen includes both intravenous and inhalant medications. Which of the following medications is most likely to be used as part of discharge plan?

A. Theophylline
B. Antibiotics
C. Magnesium
D. Histamines
E. Corticosteroids

[9.3]   Which initial ventilator setting is appropriate for intubated asthmatics?

   A. IMV mode, rate 16, tidal volume 6 to 8 mL/kg
   B. IMV mode, rate 16, tidal volume 10 to 12 mL/kg
   C. AC mode, rate 8 to 10, tidal volume 6 to 8 mL/kg
   D. AC mode, rate 8 to 10, tidal volume 10 to 12 mL/kg
   E. AC mode, rate 16, tidal volume 6 to 8 mL/kg

Answers

[9.1]   **C.** The peak expiratory flow is a reliable and fairly accurate method of assessing asthma. Spirometry, although providing important information, is rarely available in the ED.

[9.2]   **E.** Corticosteroids are often used after a hospitalization. None of the other medications are used routinely for discharged asthma patients.

[9.3]   **C.** The initial settings for patients with obstructive lung disease should be AC mode, rate 8 to 10, tidal volume 6 to 8 mL/kg. Low volumes and small tidal volumes are used to prevent air stacking and barotrauma.

CLINICAL PEARLS

❖ Initiate therapy with albuterol while obtaining history and performing physical for patients with significant asthma.

❖ Corticosteroids should be administered early for asthmatic exacerbations.

❖ Use lower than traditional ventilator settings to prevent barotrauma in the intubated asthmatic.

❖ The individual who presents with an initial episode of "wheezing" may have etiologies other than asthma, for example, foreign body, pneumonia, or congestive heart failure.

❖ Absence of wheezing can sometimes be misleading in the individual *in extremis* because of very little air movement.

REFERENCES

Cydulka RK, Jarvis HE. New medications for asthma. Emerg Med Clin North Am 2000;18(4):789–801.

Jain S, Hanania NA, Guntupalli KK. Ventilation of patients with asthma and obstructive lung disease. Crit Care Clin 1998;14(4):685–705.

National Institutes of Health, National Heart, Lung, and Blood Institute. *Guidelines for the diagnosis and management of asthma.* NIH publication, Washington, D.C., No. 97-4051. April 1997.

A 32-year-old man is involved in a motor vehicle accident (MVA) and brought into the emergency department (ED). He was the driver of a sports car that hit the freeway barricade at a high speed. He was thrown against the windshield of the car and hit his face and forehead against the windshield, but denies a loss of consciousness. On examination, he has a 7-cm laceration of his right face coursing from the front of his right ear to just below the lower lip. He appears alert and has normal papillary reflexes. When he is asked to smile, the right side of his mouth droops.

◆ **What is the most likely diagnosis?**

◆ **What is the likely therapy?**

ANSWERS TO CASE 10: Facial Laceration

Summary: A 32-year-old man presents to the ED after an MVA in which he was the driver of a sports car that hit the freeway barricade at a high speed. He was thrown against the windshield but did not lose consciousness. On examination, he has a 7-cm laceration of his right face coursing from the front of his right ear across the cheek to just below the right lower lip. His neurological examination is normal except for inability to smile on the right.

◆ **Most likely diagnosis:** Right facial nerve laceration

◆ **Likely therapy**: Microsurgical repair of right facial nerve

Analysis

Objectives
1. Understand the critical structures that may be injured in facial lacerations.
2. Understand the need for tetanus immunization in trauma.
3. Know the basic principles of repair of facial injuries.

Considerations

This patient suffered a laceration across his right cheek from a motor vehicle accident. The **first steps in management of trauma include the ABCs** (airway/cervical spine, breathing, circulation), and then the **secondary survey**, assessment of nonhemorrhaging lacerations. **Any trauma to the head, face, or neck should raise concern about a cervical spine injury.** Also, bony injuries such as orbital fractures or mandibular fractures are possibilities. Injury to cranial nerves V or VII are common. The facial nerve leaves the stylomastoid foramen and gives motor and sensory branches to the temporal, zygomatic, buccal, and mental regions. Laceration to the buccal branch may also be associated with injury to the parotid duct (Fig. 10-1). Identification of a facial nerve injury is critical, because results are best when repaired as soon as possible. Microsurgical techniques give fairly good results. After repair of the injury, the patient needs a tetanus immunization, if the last time the patient received a tetanus vaccine was longer than 5 years ago (Table 10-1). (See Case 7 for discussion of systematic trauma survey.)

APPROACH TO FACIAL LACERATIONS

Basic approach to wound care includes assessment for other injuries, probing the depth of the wound, irrigation, a neurovascular examination, and deciding on whether primary closure is advisable (leave open if infection is likely such as contamination or delay in time). The length of time the suture stays in place depends on the body location (Table 10-2). Finally, the time of the last tetanus vaccination should be assessed.

Table 10-1
TETANUS PROPHYLAXIS IN WOUND MANAGEMENT

IMMUNIZATION HISTORY	DT (0.5 ML) IM	TIG*
Fully immunized, <10 years since booster	No	No
Fully immunized, >10 years since booster	Yes	No
Incomplete series (<3 injections) or unknown immunization record	Yes	Yes†

* TIG dose is 75 units in patients younger than 5 years of age; 125 units in patients 5–10 years of age, and 250 units in patients older than 10 years of age.

†Some experts would not administer TIG in conditions of low risk for tetanus and, minor, clean wounds that are less than 6 hours old in an immunocompetent host.

Source: Adapted from Tintinalli JE, Kelen DG, Stapczynski JS, eds. Emergency Medicine, 6th ed. New York: McGraw-Hill, 2004:943–946.

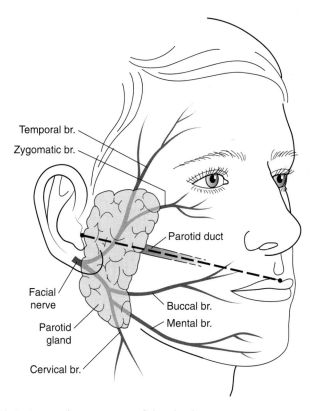

Figure 10-1. Anatomic structures of the cheek.

Table 10-2

TIME FROM WOUND CLOSURE TO SUTURE REMOVAL

LOCATION	NUMBER OF DAYS
Face	3–5
Scalp	7
Chest	8–10
Back	10–14
Arm	10–14
Fingers	7–10
Hand	7–10
Leg or foot	8–12

Source: Tintinalli JE, Kelen GD, Stapczynski JS, eds. Emergency medicine, 6th ed. New York: McGraw-Hill, 2004:331.

Scalp and Forehead

These lacerations are usually caused by a combination of blunt and sharp trauma. Careful inspection of the wound is critical, with care to palpate for depressed skull fractures, and assess the integrity of the galea, which covers the periosteum. Repair usually follows the skin lines for the best cosmetic result. The **scalp** should be closed with a **4-0 monofilament suture of different color than the patient's hair** (or **staples** can be used) and **removed after 7 to 10 days**. Because scalp lacerations may be associated with significant hemorrhage, rapid closure with staples may decrease the blood loss. If the galea is involved, this should be closed with buried nonabsorbable suture. **Forehead** lacerations should be likewise closed in layers, with the skin approximated with **6-0 nonabsorbable continuous running or interrupted suture, removed after 5 days**. Care should be taken to precisely approximate hair lines.

Eyelids

The eyelid is thin and delicate and is functionally and cosmetically important. Because of the risk of periorbital trauma, the emergency room physician should have a low threshold to refer to an oculoplastic specialist or ophthalmologist for evaluation and repair. Findings especially concerning include injuries involving the inner aspect of the lid, affecting the lid margin, the lacrimal duct, extending into the tarsal plate, or associated with ptosis. Repair is generally undertaken **with 6-0 interrupted suture, with care to stay super-ficial; the suture is removed after 3 to 5 days.**

Nose

The nose is commonly injured, and is the most common fracture in victims of domestic violence. Inspection for the depth of injury is important. Infection can occur when all layers are penetrated or when cartilage is visible. **Septal trauma may lead to hematoma formation, which can lead to necrosis of the septum** or chronic obstruction of the nasal passageway. Anesthesia in this area is difficult because of the tightness of skin over the cartilage. Epinephrine must be avoided in this area. Topical lidocaine is generally helpful. Septal hematomas must be drained. Cartilage lacerations should be repaired, and the skin closed with 6-0 nonabsorbable suture for 3 to 5 days. Lacerations to the nasal alae are usually complex and difficult to anesthetize; these wounds often require consultation of a plastic or ear, nose, and throat (ENT) surgeon.

Lips

The junction between the skin and the red portion of the lip, called the ver-million border, is of vital cosmetic importance. Additionally, the orbicularis oris muscle that surrounds the mouth is critical for retention of saliva and facial expression and for producing speech. Inspection of the teeth, tongue, gums, and mandible is paramount. Lacerations involving the lip but not cross-ing the vermillion border can be closed in layers with **6-0 nonabsorbable suture, left in place for 5 days. Wounds involving the vermillion border need to be repaired precisely, because even a 1-mm discrepancy will be noticeable** (Fig. 10-2). Regional anesthesia may be helpful, because local anesthetic infiltration may obscure the anatomy. A plastic surgeon may be con-sulted for these circumstances. When intraoral lacerations are present, peni-cillin prophylactic antibiotics may be useful.

Ears

Basilar skull fracture (particularly with **raccoon-eyes**) or tympanic mem-brane rupture should be suspected. After inspection, cotton may be placed into the ear canal during irrigation. Regional auricular block is effective, and again, epinephrine should be avoided. Superficial lacerations may be repaired with 6-0 nonabsorbable suture for 5 days. Any cartilage that is showing should be covered to reduce the infection risk. Meticulous hemostasis is important to pre-vent hematoma formation. Auricular hematoma, or avulsed tissue, or crushed cartilage is probably best handled by a plastic or ENT surgeon.

Cheeks and Face

Lacerations of the **cheek and face** should be repaired after investigating the vital structures in the region such as the facial nerve and parotid duct.

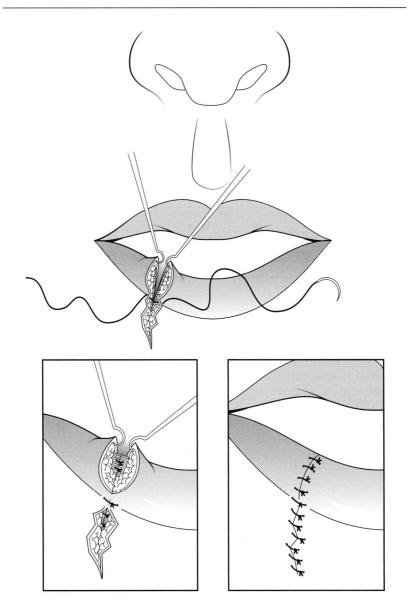

Figure 10-2. Lip laceration crossing the vermillion border. The first step is to approximate the vermillion-skin junction, the orbicularis muscle is then reapproximated, and, finally, the skin is repaired.

Generally, a **6-0 monofilament interrupted suture technique is used and removed after 5 days.**

Tetanus Immunization

Tetanus is an acute, often fatal, but preventable disease caused by the gram-positive bacterium *Clostridium tetani*. The **spores are ubiquitous in soil** and animal manure. Contamination of a wound (puncture) with *C. tetani*, particularly in **devitalized, crushed, or infected tissue,** can lead to its proliferation and expression of the neuroexotoxin **tetanospasmin.** This powerful exotoxin acts on the motor endplates of skeletal muscle, the spinal cord, the sympathetic nervous system, and the brain, leading to generalized muscle rigidity, autonomic nervous system instability, and severe muscle contractions. **The most common presentation of tetanus is muscle spasm of the masseter muscles,** "lockjaw," but the back, arms, diaphragm, and lower extremities can also be affected. The diagnosis is made clinically. In up to 10 percent of tetanus cases, the patient does not recall a wound. The usual incubation period varies from 7 to 21 days, but can extend from 3 to 56 days.

Patients with tetanus should be **admitted to the intensive care unit.** Wound debridement, respiratory support as needed, and muscle relaxants or neuromuscular blockade may be helpful. **Patients with tetanus should receive passive immunization with tetanus immunoglobulin (TIG) 3000 to 6000 units IM on the side opposite of the tetanus toxoid injection.** It clearly reduces morbidity and mortality. Penicillin is usually given, but is of questionable value.

Prevention of tetanus is accomplished with regular active immunization of all individuals. The dose of tetanus toxoid (t) or diphtheria/tetanus toxoid (dT) is 0.5 mL IM regardless of age. **TIG is given when incomplete tetanus immunization** (<3 injections) is encountered, the dosage varying with age (see Table 10-1). Again, the TIG and tetanus toxoid should be given in different body sites with different syringes.

Comprehension Questions

[10.1] An 18-year-old man was involved in an altercation at a local bar. He suffered lacerations of the scalp, neck, forehead, and upper lip. Which of the following is likely to be most challenging to repair from a cosmetic perspective?

A. Scalp
B. Neck
C. Forehead
D. Cheek
E. Upper lip

[10.2] A 24-year-old woman was the victim of domestic violence and received treatment at the local emergency room for multiple contusions and lacerations of the face. Six months after treatment, she notices a defect of the nasal septum with communication between the right and left nasal passageways. Which of the following is the most likely diagnosis?

A. Physician use of epinephrine on the nasal septum
B. Patient use of cocaine
C. Hematoma of the nasal septum
D. Posttraumatic stress syndrome

[10.3] The emergency physician is preparing a 4-cm deep scalp laceration for repair and notices a step-off of the underlying skull. Which of the following is the best next step?

A. Traction on the bone to take pressure off the underlying brain
B. CT imaging of the head
C. Ultrasound imaging of the head
D. If no neurological complaints, repair of the scalp and advise wearing a helmet for 4 weeks

[10.4] A 48-year-old man was rock climbing when he slipped and suffered a laceration to his right lower leg. He put pressure on it, wrapped the area, and made his way to the ED, and is seen about 10 hours after the injury. He recalls getting "all his shots" when he was a child, but doesn't recall the last tetanus booster. Which of the following is the best choice regarding tetanus prevention?

A. dT 0.5 mL IM
B. dT 0.5 mL IM and TIG 250 units IM
C. dT 0.5 mL IM, TIG 250 units IM, and intravenous penicillin 600,000 units every 6 hours
D. Admit to the ICU, observe for muscle spasm, 2500 units TIG IM, and 0.5 mL tetanus toxoid IM in the opposite deltoid muscles

Answers

[10.1] **E.** Lining up the vermillion border is by far the most challenging to repair because of the demands of precise approximation.

[10.2] **C.** The patient likely developed a nasal septal hematoma that caused necrosis to the septum and the subsequent communication between the nasal passageways.

[10.3] **B.** A depressed skull fracture is an emergency and may be associated with injury to the underlying brain. A CT scan of the head is critical.

[10.4] **A.** Because he has likely received a full series of immunizations, but does not remember the last booster, he should receive the tetanus toxoid 0.5 mL IM.

CLINICAL PEARLS

❖ The vermillion border must be exactly approximated because of its important cosmetic characteristics.

❖ The facial nerve has a course from the mastoid region across the cheek area.

❖ Meticulous hemostasis is important in repairing ear lacerations.

❖ Tetanus is an acute disease of wound contamination, which is largely preventable with immunization.

REFERENCES

Tintinalli JE, Kelen GD, Stapczynski JS, eds. Emergency medicine, 6th ed. New York: McGraw-Hill, 2004:302–304.

After lunch, a 15-year-old boy was cleaning some items in the shed in his backyard, when he saw a bat making a strange noise in the middle of the shed. The bat flew into a table and furniture, and flopped onto the floor. Wanting to show his new "pet" to friends, the boy attempted to catch the bat by placing it into a fishing net. The bat bit the boy on his dominant hand, after which the teenager ran into the house. The boy was brought to the emergency department (ED) by his parents. Inspection of the wound shows deep bite marks with a laceration close to the index finger joint. The bat escaped after the boy was bitten and has not been found.

◆ **What is the most likely diagnosis?**

◆ **What is the next step in treatment?**

ANSWERS TO CASE 11: Rabies/Animal Bite

Summary: A teenager complains of a deep bite to his dominant hand by a bat acting strangely. The bite is fresh and the bat cannot be located.

◆ **Most likely diagnosis:** Unprovoked attack by a rabies-infected bat.

◆ **Next step in treatment:** Notify animal control to locate the animal, then clean the wound and administer both passive and active rabies immunization to the patient. Administer tetanus toxoid if not received within the last 5 years.

Analysis

Objectives
1. Recognize that bat bites are a common vector for rabies.
2. Know that unprovoked attacks by wild animals such as raccoons, skunks, coyotes, or dogs should raise the concern for rabies.
3. Know the clinical presentation of rabies.
4. Know the treatments for rabies and common bite injuries.

Considerations

This 15-year-old teenager encountered a bat exhibiting very abnormal behavior. The bat, which is usually a nocturnal animal, is active in the afternoon, is in a peculiar location, and making strange sounds. Furthermore, it is having difficulty flying. These findings are suspicious for a rabies-infected bat. In the United States, bats comprise 15 percent of animals found to have rabies; wild raccoons and skunks have a higher incidence. However, 90 percent of human rabies is caused by bat bites, suggesting a higher virulence of strains of insectivorous bat rabies virus. Importantly, worldwide, particularly in geographical locations with incomplete animal vaccination, dogs are the most frequent vector for rabies transmission to humans.

As in any **bite injury, appropriate authorities should be notified to find, test, or observe the animal for abnormal behavior**. In the field, any open wound or bite should be thoroughly washed with soap, water and an antiseptic such as povidone-iodine. In the ED, irrigation with **sterile saline** is important; there is no added benefit to the addition of hydrogen peroxide or povidone-iodine to the irrigant. **Removal of any foreign body, and debridement of devitalized tissue** is the next step. Primary closure of the wound is the most commonly used technique; however, in a wound at risk for infection, delayed primary closure (leaving it open for 4 to 5 days and closing if no infection is seen), or secondary healing (spontaneous closure) may be used. Prophylactic antibiotics may have a role.

In this patient's case, a thorough **evaluation for neurovascular integrity** of the finger, and a **delayed primary closure** to observe for infection would be reasonable. **Prophylaxis for rabies** should include a combination of immediate passive (rabies immunoglobulin [RIG]) and active immunization (human diploid cell vaccine [HDCV]). Tetanus vaccine should be administered if the patient has not received it within the last 5 years.

APPROACH TO ANIMAL BITES

A bite is the most common means of transmission of rabies. Immunization of animals has decreased the incidence of rabies, but all animal bites should be suspect. Risk factors for transmission include unprovoked attacks, unknown or unobserved animals, or animals displaying unusual behavior. Animals with increased lacrimation, salivation, dilated irregular pupils, unusual behavior, or hydrophobia are particularly suspect. **Bites to the face or hands confer the highest risk of rabies transmission**, but a breakage of the skin anywhere can be causative. Dogs or cats that are vaccinated are unlikely to harbor rabies, although rarely, animals having only received one vaccine have been infected. **No cases have been recorded in animals having received two injections.** Healthy dogs, cats, or ferrets should be confined and **observed for at least 10 days for signs of illness**; with any sign of illness, the animal should be euthanized and its head shipped refrigerated to a laboratory qualified to assess for rabies.

Rabies is a single-stranded ribonucleic acid (RNA) rhabdovirus that attacks the central nervous system. It has a variable incubation period, averaging 1 to 2 months, but may be as short as 7 days or as long as 1 year. Bite location is an important factor determining transmission with face bites highest, lower extremity lowest, and upper extremity intermediate. Classic pathological finding **are *Negri bodies* found in neurons approximately 80 percent of the time**. Clinical presentation begins with a 1- to 4-day prodrome with fever, headache, malaise, nausea, emesis, and a productive cough. An encephalopathic stage follows with hyperactivity, excitation, agitation and confusion. Brainstem dysfunction follows with cranial nerve involvement, excessive salivation, hydrophobia, followed by coma and respiratory failure.

Rabies Prophylaxis

Preexposure prophylaxis with active vaccination may be given to individuals at risk (animal trainers, animal control field workers, etc.). This does not obviate the need for postexposure prophylaxis. **Prophylaxis is indicated for any person possibly exposed to a rabid animal. Passive immunization** with human rabies immunoglobulin (HRIG) 20 IU/kg should be injected around the wound site as soon as feasible. Any residual vaccine should be injected in the deltoid intramuscularly. **Active immunization should then be given intramuscularly with a different syringe and at a different site. The active vaccines include** HDCV, purified chick embryo cell vaccine (PCEC), or rabies vaccine adsorbed (RVA), and should be administered on days 0, 3, 7, 14, and 28. **Species identification and/or capture of the animal** will permit definitive pathological diagnosis and identify probable pathogens as well as toxin/venom. **Hydrophobia** is the **violent contraction of respiratory, diaphragmatic, laryngeal, and pharyngeal muscles initiated by consumption of liquids**. Additional signs of rabies include excessive lacrimation/salivation.

A thorough history and physical examination in the context of the geographical location will give important clues for treatment. Identification of the animal and observation will aid treatment. Although all mammals can harbor rabies, dogs, bats, and cats are of highest suspicion while rabbits and rodents are low. Snake bites require species identification to administer the correct antivenin because cross-reactivity is poor (Table 11-1 has additional information on animal bites and stings).

Important clues for high-risk cases demanding immunization for rabies include unprovoked attacks, wild dogs, areas endemic for rabies, and abnormal animal behavior. If the animal cannot be found or observation of the animal identifies abnormal/sick behavior within 10 days of the bite, then postexposure prophylaxis should be started and pathological examination should be performed.

Regardless of risks, all bites should be thoroughly cleaned both mechanically with soap and water as well as chemically with an antiseptic. Simple bites of the trunk and extremities (except for hand and feet) less than 6 hours old can generally be closed primarily. Simple bites of the head and neck area less than 12 hours old also can usually be reapproximated primarily. However, **puncture wounds, bites of the hand or foot, wounds more than 12 hours old, or those obviously infected or involving crushed tissue, are usually left open**.

Bacterial Infections

Dogs account for about 80 to 90 percent of mammalian bite injuries to people, followed by cats (7 to 10 percent) and humans (2 to 3 percent). **Cats** most often lead to a bacterial infection of the wound with *Pasteurella multocida* being the most commonly isolated bacteria. **Human bites are also prone to become infected, with multiple organisms responsible**. Bacterial infections result from 20 percent of dog bites, 50 percent of cat bites, and, most often, from human bites. Dogs and cats harbor *Staphylococcus aureus*, *Pasteurella* spp., *Capnocytophaga canimorsus*, streptococcus, and oral anaerobes. Humans usually have mixed flora, including *S. aureus*, *Haemophilus influenzae*, and beta-lactamase–positive oral anaerobes. Good initial-choice antibiotics include **amoxicillin–clavulanic acid, ticarcillin–clavulanic acid**, ampicillin–sulfate, or a second-generation cephalosporin. Duration of administration for established infections is 10 to 14 days and 3 to 5 days for prophylaxis. Cultures of wounds will usually dictate subsequent antibiotic choices. Tetanus boosters should be administered if more than 5 years has elapsed since the last administration (see Case 10).

The clenched-fist injury is especially important to assess, because a small bite injury may **deeply imbed bacteria into the metacarpophalangeal (MCP) joint of the hand,** leading to serious infection. A polymicrobial infection

Table 11-1

COMMON BITE OR STING INJURIES

ANIMAL	APPEARANCE	INFECTION & CLINICAL COURSE	TREATMENT
Human		50–60% infection rate Staphylococcus, streptococcus, Eikenella corrodens	If high risk, leave wound open Irrigation, tetanus, amoxicillin–clavulanate
Cat		Pasteurella multocida	Wound care as above Penicillin or amoxicillin
Dog		Pasteurella multocida, streptococcus, staphylococcus	Wound care as above Amoxicillin–clavulanate
Black Widow spider	1-cm–long body, classic "red hourglass" on abdomen	Neurotoxin injected leading to target lesion, muscle cramps	Clean wound, give antivenin
Brown Recluse spider	Violin- or fiddle-shaped marking on cephalothorax	Initially painless bite, becomes erythematous, and 3–4 days later, eschar and necrotic area forms	Support, analgesia
Scorpion sting		Southwestern United States Neurotoxin with paresthesias, sometimes cranial and motor nerve dysfunction, seizures	Supportive measures

Table 11-1 (*Continued*)
COMMON BITE OR STING INJURIES

ANIMAL	APPEARANCE	INFECTION & CLINICAL COURSE	TREATMENT
Hymenoptera (bees and wasps)		Venom contains histamines, melittin protein that causes degranulation of mast cells Erythema, edema, pruritus	Remove bee stinger, wash wound, ice NSAIDs and oral antihistamines If anaphylaxis, give epinephrine, antihistamines, steroids (see Table 8-2)
Crotalid (rattlesnake, water moccasin, copperhead)		Fang marks, localized pain, and progressive edema Nausea, weakness, oral numbness, tachycardia, muscle fasciculations	Avoid snake bite kits O_2, immobilize limb, IV line Take patient to medical facility for antivenin Use constriction band instead of tourniquet (allow arterial supply but inhibit lymph and venous drainage)
Elapid (coral snake)		Fang marks, nausea, headache, diplopia, muscle weakness, discolored urine, seizures	See above (wrap over the wound) Immobilize and transfer to medical facility for antivenin

Source: Schwab RA, Powers RA. Puncture wounds and mammalian bites. In: Tintinalli JE, Kelen GD, Stapczynski JS, eds. Emergency medicine, 6th ed. New York, McGraw-Hill: 2004:324–328.

including **staphylococcal and streptococcal** organisms is common. A **radiograph** to assess for **fracture or foreign body** is commonly performed. The wound should be irrigated, the tendons examined, and depending on the circumstances, either oral or intravenous antibiotics should be administered.

Comprehension Questions

Match the single best therapy (A to D) to the clinical scenario [11.1 to 11.4].

  A. Identify the species, clean and immobilize the site, apply suction to the entry wound, and administer antivenin.
  B. Clean bite site, treat with presumptive antibiotics, and notify social services.
  C. Clean site, observe animal, and watch for signs of secondary infection.
  D. Clean the site and begin rabies prophylaxis with active and passive immunization.
  E. Admit for radical surgical debridement in the operating room.

[11.1] A neighbor is bitten by your house dog who has received rabies immunization within the last year.

[11.2] A woman arrives in your ED with a bite wound to her breast which she says occurred during sexual activity.

[11.3] A boy scout is brought in by his scoutmaster with a snakebite to his left foot. He says he heard the snake's rattle just before it bit him. His entire foot is purple, swollen to his mid-calf, and very painful to the touch.

[11.4] While raking leaves under his fruit tree at dusk, a man says a bird flew into his face. When he checked his face in the mirror he saw a bite mark under blood streaks.

Answers

[11.1] **C.** This is a low-risk bite. The dog is your house dog with a low risk of ever contracting rabies. You have it immunized every year and can observe it for 10 days. As always, clean the bite thoroughly, consider radiographs to be sure no broken teeth are in the wound or that the bone has been penetrated. Administer tetanus if indicated and watch for secondary bacterial infection. If the bite had been from a human or cat, you would give prophylactic antibiotics.

[11.2] **B.** Human bites have high rates of infectivity. Clean the wound and administer prophylactic antibiotics. Tetanus toxoid, if indicated, should be given. Question the woman very carefully to determine if any abuse is present and consider a social services consult to address any related issues. Human immunodeficiency virus (HIV) and hepatitis can be transmitted by bites, so consider immediate and interval screening for these illnesses as well.

[11.3] **A.** This is a high-risk snake bite. The authorities should immediately be notified to search for the snake. Although 20 percent of venomous snakebites fail to inject venom, this bite is clearly injected. The rapid swelling, pain, and discoloration demands immediate attention. First responders should immobilize the site, place constriction bands that *do not* obstruct arterial flow, and suction the existing bite marks without incising for at least 30 minutes. Avoid incisions, packing in ice, or placing tourniquets. Immediate antivenin injection in and around the site should be a priority. Remember that species-specific antivenin is important and that administration time is critical. Best results are obtained within 4 hours. Mark the swelling every 15 minutes, evaluate coagulation profiles, electrocardiogram (EKG), renal function, and liver function, and consider ICU admission to insure adequate perfusion and to avoid disseminated intravascular coagulation (DIC). The University of Arizona Poison and Drug Information Center maintains a 24-hour hotline to assist with locating antivenin (520-626-6016).

[11.4] **D.** This injury is at high risk for rabies transmission. Dusk is the usual time for bat activity, and although this man did not feel a bite, he has discovered bite marks under his injury site. Bats carry high rates of rabies and this man was bitten on the face. Because the animal cannot be examined, immediate passive and active immunization should be initiated and tetanus administered, if indicated. As always, watch for secondary bacterial infection.

CLINICAL PEARLS

Dogs bites are the most common mammalian animal bites, and the most common vector for rabies.

Cat bites most commonly lead to infection, usually caused by *Pasteurella multocida*.

Bites that are more than 6 hours old are, in general, left open, because of the risk of infection.

Black widow spider bites usually cause muscle cramps and systemic neurotoxic effects, whereas brown recluse spider bites usually cause a necrotic center of the wound.

REFERENCES

Corey L. Rabies virus and other rhabdoviruses. In: Braunwald E, Fauci AS, et al., eds. Harrison's principles of internal medicine, 15th ed. New York: McGraw-Hill, 2001:1149–1151.

Disorders caused by reptile bites and marine animal exposures. In: Braunwald E, Fauci AS, et al., eds. Harrison's principles of internal medicine, 15th ed. New York: McGraw-Hill, 2001:2617–2618.

Madoff LC. Infectious complications of bites and burns. In: Braunwald E, Fauci AS, et al., eds. Harrison's principles of internal medicine, 15th ed. New York: McGraw-Hill, 2001:817–820.

A 59-year-old man with a history of hypertension presents to the emergency department (ED) with right-sided paralysis and aphasia. Per the patient's wife, he was in his usual state of health when he went to the bathroom about 1 hour prior to arrival in the ED. A few minutes later, his wife heard a thud in the bathroom and found her husband collapsed on the floor. She then called emergency medical services, who transported the patient to your ED. En route, his fingerstick blood sugar was 108 mg/dL.

On arrival in the ED, the patient is placed on monitors and an IV is established. His temperature is 36.8°C (98.2°F), blood pressure is 156/93 mmHg, heart rate 86 beats per minute, and respiratory rate is 20 breaths per minute. The patient has a noticeable left-gaze preference and is verbally unresponsive, although he will follow simple commands such as raising his left thumb. He has a facial droop, no motor activity, decreased deep tendon reflexes (DTRs), and no light-touch sensation on the right, although a normal exam on the left.

 What is the most likely diagnosis?

 What is the most appropriate next step?

 What is the best therapy?

ANSWERS TO CASE 12: Stroke

Summary: This is a 59-year-old man with acute onset of left-sided paralysis.

◆ **Most likely diagnosis:** Stroke

◆ **Most appropriate next step:** CT scan of the head

◆ **Best therapy:** Thrombolytics if the CT does not show hemorrhage

Analysis

Objectives
1. Recognize the clinical findings of an acute stroke.
2. Understand the diagnostic and therapeutic approach to suspected stroke patients.
3. Be familiar with the National Institutes of Health (NIH) Stroke Scoring system.

Considerations

This 59-year-old male has acute symptoms of involuntary motor deficits. The most common etiology by far is cerebrovascular accident. Other causes may include a conversion reaction, Todd paralysis, or hypoglycemia. The patient's presentation is typical for an acute stroke. Priorities include management of ABCs and determining whether this is an ischemic or hemorrhagic event. If ischemic, quick evaluation for thrombolytic administration is crucial. The **NIH Stroke Score (NIHSS)** is a standardized method of assessing the severity of stroke (see Table 12-1).

APPROACH TO SUSPECTED STROKE

More than 700,000 persons are affected each year by stroke. It remains the **third leading cause of death in the United States and the number one cause for disability.** Twenty percent of persons affected will die within 1 year. Many of the remaining population are left with severe neurological deficits and/or are unable to care for themselves.

Strokes can be divided into two categories: **ischemic and hemorrhagic.** Ischemic stroke is the result of impaired blood flow to the brain tissue. Cerebral arterial blood flow can be occluded by thrombus, emboli, or structural occlusion of the vessel. **Ischemic events account for approximately 80 percent of strokes** and occur most commonly in patients age 50 years and older. **Hemorrhagic strokes** occur when there is spontaneous bleeding from cerebral vessels and are more common in **younger patients**.

At the time of presentation, a complete history must be taken. Common medical conditions that predispose patients to having strokes include transient ischemic attack (TIA), hypertension, atherosclerosis, cardiac disease (e.g.,

Table 12-1

NATIONAL INSTITUTE OF HEALTH STROKE SCORE

CATEGORY	PATIENT RESPONSE	SCORE
Level of Consciousness Questions (Know month and age?)	Answers both questions correctly Answers one correctly Answers none correctly	0 1 2
Level of Consciousness Commands (Patient instructed to open & close eyes and then to grip and release nonparetic hand)	Obeys both correctly Obeys one correctly Obeys none correctly	0 1 2
Best Gaze (Horizontal gaze tested)	Normal gaze Partial gaze palsy Forced deviation, or total gaze paresis	0 1 2
Best Visual (Visual fields tested by confrontation)	No visual loss Partial hemianopsia Complete hemianopsia Bilateral hemianopsia (blind including cortical blindness)	0 1 2 3
Facial Palsy (Patient instructed to show teeth or raise eye brows or close eyes)	Normal symmetric movement Minor paralysis Partial paralysis Complete paralysis of one or both sides	0 1 2 3

Best motor arm
   Right _____
   Left _____
	No drift
	Drift < 10 seconds
	Falls < 10 seconds
	No effort against gravity
	No movement	

Best motor leg
   Right _____
   Left _____
	No drift
	Drift < 10 seconds
	Falls < 10 seconds
	No effort against gravity
	No movement	

Limb ataxia (finger-nose-finger and heel-toe bilaterally)	Absent Ataxia in one limb Ataxia in two limbs	0 1 2
Sensory (sensation or grimace to pinprick)	No sensory loss Mild sensory loss Severe sensory loss	0 1 2
Best Language (describe picture, name items on sheet)	No aphasia, normal Mild to moderate aphasia Severe aphasia Mute, global aphasia	0 1 2 3
Dysarthria (Read or repeat words from a sheet)	Normal Mild to moderate Severe	0 1 2
Extinction and Inattention	No abnormality Visual, tactile, spatial or personal inattention or extinction to bilaeral simultaneous stimulation Profound hemi-attention or hemi-attention to more than one modality	0 1 2

National Institute of Health, 2000.

atrial fibrillation, myocardial infarction, valvular disease), diabetes, dyslipidemia, and hypercoagulable states. Cigarette smoking and alcohol use are also risk factors. The onset of symptoms and sequence of events prior to presentation is helpful in the differential diagnosis. Symptoms will vary greatly depending on the type of infarct, the location, and the amount of brain involved (Tables 12-2 and 12-3).

A complete and thorough physical examination is very important. For example, carotid bruits suggest atherosclerotic disease while an irregularly irregular cardiac rhythm is consistent with atrial fibrillation. In addition, a detailed neurologic exam must be performed, including level of consciousness, visual assessment, motor and cerebellar function, deep tendon reflexes, sensation, language, and cranial nerves.

Table 12-2
ISCHEMIC STROKE SYNDROMES

SYNDROME	SYMPTOMS
Transient ischemic attack (TIA)	Neurological deficit resolving within 24 hours; highly correlated with future thrombotic stroke
Dominant hemisphere	Contralateral numbness and weakness, contralateral visual field cut, gaze preference, dysarthria, aphasia
Nondominant hemisphere	Contralateral numbness and weakness, visual field cut, contalateral neglect, dysarthria
Anterior cerebral artery	Contralateral weakness (leg > arm); mild sensory deficits; dyspraxia
Middle cerebral artery	Contralateral numbness and weakness (face, arm > leg); aphasia (if dominant hemisphere)
Posterior cerebral artery	Lack of visual recognition; altered mental status with impaired memory; cortical blindness
Vertebrobasilar syndrome	Dizziness, vertigo; diplopia; dysphagia; ataxia; ipsilateral cranial nerve palsies, contralateral weakness (crossed deficits)
Basilar artery occlusion	Quadriplegia; coma; locked-in syndrome (paralysis except upward gaze)
Lacunar infarct	Pure motor or sensory deficit

Source: Tintinalli JE, Kelen GD, Stapczynski JS, eds. Emergency medicine, 6th ed. New York: McGraw-Hill, 2004:1382-85

Table 12-3
HEMORRHAGIC STROKE SYNDROMES

SYNDROME	SYMPTOMS
Intracerebral hemorrhage	May be clinically indistinguishable from infarction; contralateral numbness and weakness; aphasia, neglect (depending on hemisphere); headache, vomiting, lethargy, marked hypertension more common
Cerebellar hemorrhage	Sudden onset of dizziness, vomiting, truncal instability, gaze palsies, stupor

Source: Tintinalli JE, Kelen GD, Stapczynski JS, eds. Emergency medicine, 6th ed. New York, McGraw-Hill: 2004:1382-85

Table 12-4
CRITERIA FOR INTRAVENOUS THROMBOLYSIS* IN ISCHEMIC STROKE

Inclusions
    Age 18 years or older
    Clinical criteria of ischemic stroke
    Time of onset well-established, <3 hours

Exclusions
    Minor stroke symptoms
    Rapidly improving neurological signs
    Prior intracranial hemorrhage or intracranial neoplasm
    Arteriovenous malformation or aneurysm
    Blood glucose <50 mg/dL or >400 mg/dL
    Seizure at onset of stroke
    Gastrointestinal or genitourinary bleeding within preceding 21 days
    Arterial puncture at a noncompressible site or lumbar puncture within 1 week
    Recent myocardial infarction
    Major surgery within preceding 14 days
    Sustained pretreatment severe hypertension (systolic blood pressure >185 mmHg, diastolic blood pressure >110 mmHg)
    Previous stroke within past 90 days
    Previous head injury within past 90 days
    Current use of oral anticoagulant or prothrombin time >15s or INR >1.7
    Use of heparin within preceding 48h or prolonged partial thromboplastin time
    Platelet count <100,000/mm^3

* Recombinant tissue plasminogen activator (rt-PA) should be used with caution in individuals with severe stroke symptoms, NIHSS > 22.
Source: Adams HP, Brott TG, Furlon AJ, et al. Guidelines for thrombolytic therapy for acute stroke, Circulation 1996;94:1167.

Differential Diagnoses

Other diseases that can be confused with stroke include Todd paralysis, complicated migraine headaches, nonconvulsive status epilepticus, spinal cord disorders, subdural hematoma, cerebral vasculitis, hypo- or hyperglycemia, hypo- or hypernatremia, hepatic encephalopathy, Bell palsy, hypertensive encephalopathy, meningitis/encephalitis, brain abscess, Rocky Mountain spotted fever, tumor, drug overdose, botulism, carotid/aortic/vertebral artery dissection, heat stroke, sickle cell cerebral crisis, and multiple sclerosis.

The **most urgent diagnostic studies** are (a) a bedside blood **glucose** to rule out hypo- or hyperglycemia and (b) **computed tomography (CT) imaging of the head** to detect any intracranial hemorrhage or ischemic changes. The stroke workup also includes electrolytes, blood urea nitrogen (BUN)/creatinine, complete blood count, coagulation studies, liver function tests, chest x-ray, cardiac enzymes, and an electrocardiogram (EKG). Other tests to consider are a lumbar puncture, angiography, magnetic resonance imaging (MRI), transcranial Doppler, and echocardiography.

Treatment

The **goals of treatment** include stabilizing the **ABCs**, evaluating for administration of **thrombolytics**, if appropriate, and addressing **comorbid conditions** such as hypertension. **Thrombolytic therapy** may be indicated if the symptoms began **less than 3 hours** prior to presentation and the patient does not meet any exclusion criteria (e.g., coagulopathy, recent major surgeries, etc.). The NIH/National Institute of Neurological Disorders and Stroke (NINDS) study found that intravenous recombinant tissue-type plasminogen activator (rt-PA) reduced disability as compared to placebo. **Strict criteria were used for study enrollment**, including **time of symptoms less than 3 hours**. Other studies have produced conflicting results, but allowed for a longer time window of symptoms. Thus, most practitioners use strict criteria (Table 12-4) and **lower rt-PA dosages**, such as 0.9 mg/kg with a maximum dose of 90 mg, with 10 percent of the dose administered as an IV bolus and the remainder infused over 60 minutes. Also, no heparin or aspirin is used during the initial 24 hours. Caution should be exercised when the NIHSS score is >22, because in these circumstances rt-PA may convert the ischemic strokes into hemorrhagic strokes. Elevated blood pressures are generally left untreated to maintain cerebral perfusion pressure. However, systolic blood pressures >220 mmHg and diastolic blood pressures >120 mmHg are best treated with easily titratable agents such as IV labetalol or nitroprusside. In these circumstances, the target blood pressure should not be "normal" and the blood pressure should not be lowered more than 25 percent of the presenting blood pressure. rt-PA is contraindicated with systolic blood pressures exceeding 185 mmHg. In addition, hemorrhagic strokes warrant a neurosurgical consultation.

Comprehension Questions

[12.1] A 58-year-old man experienced a neurological deficit and is diagnosed as having a stroke. Which of the following is the most likely etiology?

A. Ischemic
B. Hemorrhagic
C. Drug-induced
D. Trauma-induced
E. Metabolic-related

[12.2] A 59-year-old man is being evaluated for possible thrombolytic therapy after presenting with 4 hours of right arm weakness and aphasia. Which of the following is a contraindication to thrombolytic therapy?

A. Bilateral cerebral infarct
B. Hemorrhagic stroke
C. Hypertension-related stroke
D. Cocaine-induced stroke

[12.3] A 45-year-old woman is taken to the ED with probable stroke. Which of the following are the most urgent diagnostic studies?

A. Coagulation studies
B. EKG and cardiac enzymes
C. Bedside blood glucose and CT scan of the head
D. MRI of the head with and without contrast

[12.4] A 67-year-old woman is seen in the emergency room with left arm weakness and right facial droop. Her blood pressure is 160/100 mmHg. Which of the following is the best management for the hypertension?

A. Lower the blood pressure to below 140/90 mmHg
B. Lower the blood pressure to below 120/80 mmHg
C. Observe the patient
D. Use a beta-blocker to lower the blood pressure if she complains of a headache

Answers

[12.1] **A.** Ischemic strokes are more common than hemorrhagic.

[12.2] **B.** In general, a hemorrhagic stroke is the most significant contraindication to thrombolytic therapy.

[12.3] **C.** Bedside blood glucose and CT scan of the head are the most urgent diagnostic studies in evaluating possible stroke patients.

[12.4] **C.** Elevated blood pressures are generally left untreated unless there is severe hypertension (systolic blood pressures >220 mmHg and diastolic blood pressures >120 mmHg). Lowering the blood pressure may lead to cerebral ischemia and worsen the stroke.

CLINICAL PEARLS

❖ Strokes can present in many different ways. Besides asking about actual symptomatology, the clinician must take a careful history of the time of onset of symptoms and sequence of events prior to presentation.

❖ The most urgent diagnostic studies are a bedside blood glucose and CT scan of the head.

❖ Treatment is aimed at stabilizing the ABCs, evaluating for administration of thrombolytics, if appropriate, and addressing comorbid conditions such as hypertension.

❖ Unless the blood pressure is markedly elevated, hypertension should not be lowered in stroke patients.

REFERENCES

Asimos AW. Code stroke: a state-of-the-art strategy for rapid assessment and treatment. Emerg Med Prac 1999;1(2):1–24.

Lewandowski C, Barsan W. Treatment of acute ischemic stroke. Ann Emerg Med 2001;37(2):202–16.

The National Institute of Neurological Disorders and Stroke rt-PA Stroke Study Generalized efficacy or tPA for acute stroke. Stroke 1997;28:2119–25.

The National Institute of Neurological Disorders and Stroke rt-PA Stroke Study Tissue plasminogen activator for acute ischemic stroke. N Engl J Med 1995;333(24):1581–7.

Tintinalli JE, Kelen GD, Stapczynski JS, eds. Emergency medicine, 5th ed. New York: McGraw-Hill, 2000:1430–9.

A 64-year-old man is brought into the emergency department (ED) by his family after fainting at home. He had been standing, dusting a bookshelf, when he fell backward onto the couch. He was noted to be pale and clammy during the incident, and recovered spontaneously in approximately 30 seconds. He did remember the moments just prior to and after the incident. He felt lightheaded and had palpitations just prior to falling, but did not describe any shortness of breath, chest pain, headache, nausea, diplopia, or loss of bowel or bladder control. His history included a myocardial infarction 2 years prior. The patient has been taking his regular medicines as directed, which include aspirin, a beta-blocker, and a cholesterol-lowering agent. His primary medical doctor had not recently started any new medicines or changed his doses. On presentation to the emergency department, the patient's vitals were blood pressure 143/93 mmHg, heart rate of 75 beats per minute, respiratory rate of 18 breaths per minute, temperature of 37.1°C (98.8°F), and oxygen saturation of 97 percent on room air. His exam was significant for a cardiac gallop. No carotid bruits, neurological abnormalities, rectal bleeding, or orthostatic changes were noted. A 12-lead electrocardiogram (EKG) demonstrated a normal sinus rhythm at 75 beats per minute with no significant changes from a prior study 6 months earlier; the EKG reveals Q waves in leads II, III, and aVF.

 What is the most likely diagnosis?

 What is your next step?

ANSWERS TO CASE 13: Syncope

Summary: This is a 64-year-old male with a history of a previous myocardial infarction who presents with an episode of syncope. The patient has an EKG with inferior Q waves but no acute changes at the time of presentation.

 Most likely diagnosis: Syncope most likely as a result of cardiac dysrhythmia with spontaneous resolution.

 Next step: Management of ABCs, intravenous access, and initiation of continuous cardiac monitoring.

Analysis

Objectives

1. Recognize the worrisome historical and physical features of syncope.
2. Understand the emergency physician's role in the evaluation of patients with syncope.
3. Recognize which patients need to be admitted to the hospital.

Considerations

Syncope is a temporary loss of consciousness and has many different etiologies. It is often difficult to determine the cause of the syncopal episode in the emergency department. The emergency physician's role is largely to ensure that syncope is the accurate clinical problem, and to rule out severe causes for the event.

APPROACH TO SYNCOPE

Syncope is defined as a **transient loss of consciousness** with a corresponding **loss of postural tone**. It is an extremely common presenting symptom to the emergency department, accounting for approximately 5 percent of all visits in this country. One to 6 percent of hospitalized patients will have been admitted for an evaluation of syncope. The list of potential causes for syncope is extensive, and includes cardiac, reflex mediated, orthostatic, medication related, psychiatric, hormonal, neurological, and idiopathic. Inappropriately used ancillary testing can consume thousands of health care dollars per patient and increase emergency department length of stay. With a carefully taken history and physical exam, clinicians can more easily tailor their secondary evaluation of the patient, and more efficiently use consultants and specific test modalities.

Etiologies

Cardiac syncope is loss of postural tone secondary to a sudden and dramatic fall in cardiac output. **Bradydysrhythmias, tachydysrhythmias**, and mechanisms that **disrupt outflow or preload** are the functional physiological abnormalities that cause these sudden changes in blood flow and ultimately inadequate perfusion of the brain. Patients with various forms of organic heart disease (aortic stenosis and hypertrophic cardiomyopathy), and those with coronary artery disease, congestive heart failure, ventricular hypertrophy, and myocarditis are at highest risk. Causes of bradydysrhythmias include sinus node disease, second/third-degree heart block, long-QT syndrome, and pacemaker malfunction. Causes of some of the tachydysrhythmias include ventricular tachycardia, ventricular fibrillation, Wolfe-Parkinson-White syndrome, torsade de pointes, and supraventricular tachycardia. When syncope is precipitated by tachydysrhythmias, patients will often complain of palpitations. Pericardial tamponade and aortic dissection should be considered in causes of cardiac syncope as both entities will result in a significant fall in functional cardiac output. Massive pulmonary embolism also is included in this category because syncope can arise from dysrhythmia or from severe pulmonary hypertension and a fall in left-sided filling pressure.

Reflex-mediated syncope (also known as situational syncope) includes **vasovagal, cough, micturition, defecation, emesis, swallow, Valsalva, and emotionally** (fear, surprise, disgust) related syncope. Loss of consciousness and loss of motor tone is caused by stimulation of the **vagal reflex**, resulting in transient bradycardia and hypotension. Warmth, nausea, lightheadedness, and the impending sense that often precedes loss of consciousness are common complaints of those affected by vagal syncope. Carotid sinus disease, or stimulation of overly sensitive baroreceptors in the neck (a tight collar) is another cause of sudden reflex-related syncope. These patients will often note a specific activity that is temporally related to their syncopal episodes (turning the head in a certain direction).

Orthostasis, or fall in blood pressure resulting from a **rapid change in body position**, usually from a supine to more upright posture, is another common cause of syncope. Orthostatic hypotension can be related to physiological changes (especially in the elderly), volume depletion, medications, and autonomic instability commonly seen in diabetics. Diaphoresis, lightheadedness, and graying of vision may suggest orthostatic syncope. Volume depletion secondary to sudden blood loss needs to be considered in all patients with syncope. Patients of all ages can develop a sudden gastrointestinal (GI) bleed and the initial blood flow can be occult because it is confined to the lower GI tract. Elderly patients, usually with abdominal and/or back pain, can loose massive amounts of blood from a leaking or ruptured abdominal aortic aneurysm.

Medication, especially polypharmacy, commonly seen in the elderly, is another important cause of syncope. **Antihypertensives, antidepressants, antianginals, analgesics, central nervous system depressants**, medications that can **prolong the QT interval** (erythromycin, clarithromycin, haloperidol, amiodarone, and droperidol are some of the more common medications), **insulin, oral hypoglycemics, and recreational polypharmacy** are common culprits. Geriatric patients with complicated medical histories are particularly at risk, although a detailed ingestion history should be obtained from all patients presenting with syncope. One should look closely for recent additions or changes to a medication regimen, including over-the-counter medications.

Neurological causes of **syncope** are **rare**, unless seizure is included in the differential diagnosis. Seizure can usually be quickly identified by history, witnessed seizure activity, and physical exam findings (tongue biting, loss of bowel/bladder control) and especially observation of a postictal state, which invariably resolves slowly over time. The onset of a severe headache associated with sudden loss of consciousness suggests a subarachnoid hemorrhage as the cause of syncope. Although uncommon, other neurological causes of syncope include migraines, subclavian steal, and transient ischemic attack or stroke of the vertebrobasilar distribution. Other neurological symptoms may accompany or persist past the sudden loss of consciousness.

Not uncommonly, patients with **psychiatric disease** will present with the complaint of sudden loss of consciousness. The history of these patients may include several prior episodes of syncope. Typically, these incidents will present with **minimal physical trauma** and none of the signs or symptoms that are commonly associated with cardiac syncope. Anxiety (with or without hyperventilation), conversion disorder, somatization, panic attacks, and breath holding spells can all cause syncope. Psychiatric/emotional causes, however, are a diagnosis of exclusion that should be considered seriously only after appropriate laboratory or ancillary testing has ruled out other more serious etiologies.

Diagnosis

Much to the disappointment of patients and providers, the **underlying cause is not elucidated in approximately 50 percent of patients who present to the emergency department with syncope.** Most of the young and otherwise healthy patients will be discharged home without a clearly defined cause for their loss of consciousness. Many of the elderly patients will be admitted for additional testing and observation. Of all the diagnostic tools available to physicians, the most useful is a good, thorough history and physical exam. The information gathered from the history and physical exam alone will identify the cause of syncope in 45 percent of cases.

Clinical Approach

The **initial history and physical** (including a rectal exam), combined with the **electrocardiogram,** form the preliminary workup of patients with syncope. This approach is often diagnostic in cases of vasovagal, situational, orthostatic, polypharmacy, and some cardiac-related syncope. Although laboratory testing rarely elucidates the cause of the syncope, it can be helpful in a limited number of situations. Inexpensive laboratory tests include hemogram for blood loss, glucometer for hypoglycemia, and electrolytes and blood urea nitrogen (BUN)/creatinine levels for dehydration/adrenal insufficiency or evidence of a recent seizure (anion gap). Rarely, toxicology screening for drug-related syncope can be helpful. A urinalysis is an inexpensive useful screening test that can provide information about glucose, infection, the patient's state of hydration, and the presence or absence of ketones. A urine pregnancy test should always be obtained in women of childbearing age, because early pregnancy and ectopic pregnancy can present as syncope.

In patients with a more complex history, consideration can be given to continuous cardiac monitoring, echocardiography, Doppler vascular studies, or contrast computed tomography (CT) imaging of the chest. Those patients with unexplained syncope and worrisome clinical features (advanced age, abnormal electrocardiogram [EKG], previous cardiac history, exertional syncope) often require further investigation such as treadmill testing, tilt-table testing, CT imaging of the head, cardiac enzymes, cardiac catheterization, and electrophysiological studies.

While the diagnosis and treatment are the usual goals in the evaluation of syncope, the decision tree for emergency medicine physicians is more focused than that of the specialist or outpatient physician (see algorithm in

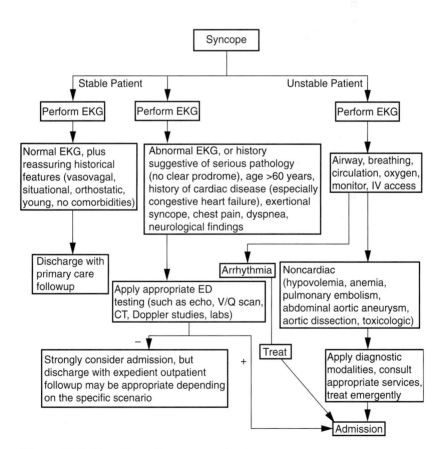

Figure 13-1. Algorithm of syncope evaluation.

Fig. 13-1). Unstable patients with syncope, including those with persistent hypotension, malignant arrhythmias, active blood loss, acute coronary syndromes, hemodynamically significant pulmonary emboli, and cardiac tamponade must be managed emergently. Patients with worrisome clinical features indicating a potentially life-threatening cause of syncope (organic heart disease, dysrhythmias, uncommon neurological causes, persistent medication effects) may not require vigorous stabilization in the emergency department, but should be admitted to the hospital for observation and further testing. Patients older than age 60 years, those with known cardiovascular disease, and those without a reassuring prodrome or situational cause should also be considered for admission.

The younger patient with no comorbidities, reassuring first-time symptoms, and a normal electrocardiogram can usually be discharged from the emergency department to home. Referral to a primary medical doctor should be made for coordination of any outpatient studies that may be warranted in the evaluation of recurring syncope. Patients with specific job-related concerns, such as heavy machine operators, pilots, or physicians, may require more expeditious referral and notification of the appropriate authorities. **Even benign causes of syncope, such as vasovagal syncope, can be fatal when the patient is driving**, and **driving restrictions may need to be recommended** by the emergency physician. **Presyncopal patients or those with a clear inciting event should be allowed to drive.** Those with true loss of consciousness without a clear prodrome, or those with frequent syncope, can drive a private automobile only after seeking treatment and documenting control for 3 months. In severe untreated syncope, driving is strictly prohibited. While the onus is not on the emergency physician to permanently remove driving privileges, driving concerns should be made clear to the patient and, when possible, the patient's family.

Comprehension Questions

[13.1] A 43-year-old man is brought into the ED because he passed out at work for no apparent reason. Currently, he is lucid and has no neurological abnormalities. What is the most common etiology after investigation?

    A. Arrhythmia
    B. Orthostasis
    C. Idiopathic
    D. Iatrogenic

[13.2] A 35-year-old female presents to the emergency department complaining of feeling lightheaded since she started spotting vaginally several hours earlier. Her blood pressure is 85/53 mmHg and her heart rate is 130 beats per minute. The most important next step is:

A. Obtain a urine pregnancy test
B. Obtain a serum quantitative beta human chorionic gonadotropin (beta-hCG) level
C. Obtain IV access and fluid resuscitate the patient
D. Obtain a formal pelvic ultrasound

[13.3] A 76-year-old man with a pacemaker presents to the emergency department after having an episode of syncope, followed by persistent lightheadedness. The patient's family mentions that he looks a little ashen. The patient is mentating, with a blood pressure of 110/60 mmHg, heart rate of 40 beats per minute. The most likely cause of this patient's symptoms is:

A. Myocardial infarction
B. Gastrointestinal bleed
C. Pacemaker malfunction
D. Micturition syncope
E. Sick sinus syndrome

Answers

[13.1] **C.** Idiopathic. Approximately 50 percent of all patients with a presenting complaint of syncope will not have a diagnosis.

[13.2] **C.** Obtain IV access and fluid resuscitate the patient. Investigating the possibility of pregnancy, specifically ectopic pregnancy, is incredibly important. However, initial stabilization of the patient takes precedence. Hypovolemia and hypotension must be treated emergently.

[13.3] **C.** Pacemaker malfunction. The patient's persistent symptoms, vitals, and history of pacemaker placement make pacemaker malfunction the most likely diagnosis. The other diagnoses must also be entertained in an elderly patient, with a more complete history, hemoglobin/hematocrit, stool Hemoccult test, cardiac enzymes, and an EKG.

CLINICAL PEARLS

❖ The causes of syncope are varied, and a successful diagnosis hinges on diligent history collection and appropriate use of diagnostic tools.

❖ Even the most experienced clinician will be unable to determine the cause of syncope in up to 50 percent of patients.

❖ Reassuring clinical signs in syncope are youth, a clear prodrome, no comorbidities, and reassuring historical features.

❖ Unstable patients should be treated emergently and stabilized, first addressing the ABCs.

REFERENCES

Linzer M, Yang EH, Estes NA, et al. Diagnosing syncope part 1: value of history, physical examination, and electrocardiography. Ann Intern Med 1997;126(12):989–96.

Linzer M, Yang EH, Estes NA, et al. Diagnosing syncope part 2: unexplained syncope. Ann Intern Med 1997;127(1):76–84.

Schipper JL, Kapoor WN. Cardiac arrhythmias: diagnostic evaluation and management of patients with   syncope. Med Clin North Am 2001;85(2):423-56

Syncope. In: Marx, ed. Rosen's emergency medicine: concepts and clinical Practice, 5th ed. Mosby, 2002.

A 63-year-old woman presents to the emergency department complaining of dyspnea and chest discomfort that she describes as tightness and difficulty in catching her breath. The patient has a history of breast carcinoma (stage IIB) for which she underwent left mastectomy 4 weeks ago and is currently undergoing chemotherapy with doxorubicin (Adriamycin) and fluorouracil (5-FU). In addition, she is taking tamoxifen. The patient describes her respiratory complaints and states that they are recent and sudden in onset. On physical examination, she appears uncomfortable and slightly anxious. Her pulse is 106 beats per minute and regular, blood pressure is 130/85 mmHg, and respiratory rate is 28 breaths per minute. The pulse oximetry indicates 97 percent on 2 L of O_2 by nasal canula. The lungs are clear to auscultation with occasional wheezing in the right lung field. Swelling of the lower extremities and minimal left calf tenderness are noted. Her laboratory studies reveal white blood cell count (WBC) of 8000/mm³, normal hemoglobin and hematocrit. The chest radiographs reveal no infiltrates or effusions, and a 12-lead electrocardiogram (EKG) reveals sinus tachycardia.

◆ **What is the most likely diagnosis?**

◆ **What is your next diagnostic step?**

ANSWERS TO CASE 14: Pulmonary Embolism

Summary: A 63-year-old woman with a history of breast cancer presents with dyspnea, chest discomfort, wheezes, leg swelling and tenderness, and a normal chest x-ray (CXR).

◆ **Most likely diagnosis:** Pulmonary embolism (PE) secondary to deep venous thrombosis (DVT) in the left lower extremity.

◆ **Next diagnostic step:** D-dimer level, arterial blood gas, venous duplex ultrasonography, ventilation–perfusion scan (V/Q scan), CT angiography, and pulmonary angiography are available and may be applied on a selective basis.

Analysis

Objectives

1. Learn the clinical presentations of PE.
2. Learn to formulate a reasonable diagnostic strategy for the diagnosis of pulmonary embolism in the emergency department setting.
3. Learn the sensitivity, specificity, and limitations of the D-dimer test for the diagnosis of DVT and PE.

Considerations

This 63-year-old patient has numerous risk factors for venous thromboembolism including age (>60 years), recent operation, and malignancy. The presentation of acute dyspnea, chest pain, tachycardia, and lower extremity swelling and pain in the absence of identifiable alternative cardiopulmonary disease place her in the high probability category for PE diagnosis. EKG for patients with suspected PE is generally helpful for identifying ischemic heart disease as a source of chest pain and respiratory complaints, and in some instances, the EKG may reveal right-heart strain patterns that are more specific for the diagnosis of PE. In this case, the EKG revealed sinus tachycardia, which although nonspecific, is nevertheless the most frequent presenting EKG finding among patients with PE. The relatively normal CXR is valuable in eliminating alternative diagnoses, such as pneumonia, pneumothorax, and congestive heart failure. Taking into consideration the clinical, radiographic, and EKG data, a presumptive diagnosis of PE can be made. The next steps in management thus include maintenance of cardiopulmonary stability, consideration of empiric anticoagulation therapy, and confirmation of the diagnosis.

APPROACH TO DVT AND PE

Definitions

Pulmonary embolism: Blockages of the pulmonary arteries, most often caused by blood clots originating from deep veins in the legs or pelvis.

In rare circumstances, air bubbles, fat droplets, amniotic fluid, clumps of parasites, or tumor cells may also cause PE.

Deep venous thrombosis: Formation of clot (thrombus) in a deep vein (a vein that accompanies an artery). DVT should be distinguished from thrombosis of superficial veins. Thromboses of deep veins in the calf (tibial veins) generally are clinically silent, do not lead to PE, and may not require specific treatment.

D-dimer assay: D-dimer is released into the circulation following degradation of cross-linked fibrin by plasmin. Elevated levels may indicate the presence of concurrent thrombus formation and degradation. Other conditions in which D-dimer elevation occur include sepsis, recent myocardial infarction or stroke (<10 days), recent surgery or trauma, disseminated intravascular coagulation, collagen vascular disease, metastatic cancer, and liver disease.

Venous duplex ultrasonography: Ultrasound imaging modality combining direct visualization of veins with Doppler flow signal to assess lumenal patency and compressibility of the deep venous system in the extremities and the presence of thrombosis. This imaging modality is most accurate for assessment of the iliac, femoral, and popliteal veins.

Ventilation-perfusion (V/Q) scan: Radioisotope used to identify ventilation–perfusion mismatches. Results are categorized into probability-ranked groups after taking into account the coexisting pulmonary pathology and the patient's overall clinical picture.

Computed tomography (CT) pulmonary angiography: Magnified CT imaging of the pulmonary vasculature obtained during the arterial phases of venous contrast injection. While highly specific for PE, the reported sensitivity is variable and ranges from 50 to 90 percent. The diagnostic sensitivity is higher for centrally located PE but reduced for subsegmental clots. The diagnostic accuracy is also related to observer experience/expertise.

Pulmonary angiography: Imaging involving intravascular contrast injection and fluoroscopy to determine patency of the pulmonary arterial vasculature. Offers >96 percent accuracy and is therefore considered the "gold standard" in the diagnosis of PE. It is an invasive technique that requires a trained interventionalist, and its application is associated with a 1 to 2 percent procedural complication rate, and 0.5 percent mortality.

Clinical Approach

Deep Venous Thrombosis   Up to **60 percent of patients with untreated proximal DVT will develop PE**; consequently, accurate diagnosis of this condition is critical for emergency physicians. **Unfortunately, the clinical features of DVT are frequently nonspecific**, and may include pain, tenderness, swelling/edema, and erythema. The physical examination and thromboembolic

Table 14-1
RISK FACTORS FOR DEEP VENOUS THROMBOSIS

Factor V Leiden mutation

Antithrombin III, protein C or S deficiency

Age > 60 y

Obesity

Pregnancy and postpartum

Previous thromboembolism

Smoking

Antiphospholipid syndrome

Immobilization

Malignancy

Medical illness (congestive heart failure, myocardial infarction)

Surgery (pelvic, orthopedic)

Trauma

Reference: Tintinalli, Kelen, Stapczynski, Emergency Medicine, 6th ed., New York: McGraw-Hill, 2004:410

risk factors (Table 14-1) are important in assessing the clinical suspicion (pretest probability), and based on the pretest probability, clinical algorithm for the diagnosis of lower extremity DVT may be formulated (Fig. 14-1). **All patients with DVT at or above the popliteal level should be treated**, with the treatment goals directed toward the prevention of thrombus propagation and prevention of thrombus embolization. In patients with extensive DVT involvement of the iliac and femoral veins, the use of thrombolytic therapy should be considered to help minimize the postphlebitic sequelae. For most patients the acute management consists of anticoagulation with unfractionated heparin (UFH) or low-molecular-weight heparin (LMWH). When UFH therapy is selected, it is vital to achieve therapeutic levels rapidly (activated partial thromboplastin time 1.5 to 2.5 times the control), and when this is accomplished within 24 hours, the DVT recurrence rate is 4 to 6 percent, compared to 23 percent when therapeutic levels are delayed. LMWH can be administered for the treatment of DVT with or without PE. **Enoxaparin is the most commonly used LMWH,** and the recommended dose is either **1 mg/kg/bid or 1.5 mg/kg/qd**. Patients developing recurrent DVT during optimal anticoagulation therapy should undergo evaluation for hypercoagulability and be considered for inferior venal caval filter placement. **Vena cava filters can also be useful for individuals for whom anticoagulation is contraindicated.**

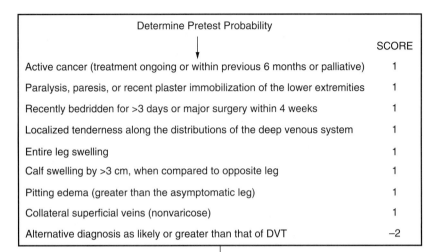

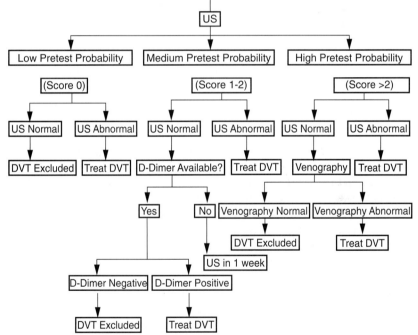

Figure 14-1. Algorithm for diagnosis of suspected lower extremity DVT. Modified, with permission, from Anand SS, Wells PS, Hunt D, et al. Does this patient have deep vein thrombosis? JAMA 1998; 279:1094–99.

Pulmonary Embolism Few common medical conditions are as difficult to diagnose as PE. The majority of patients have dyspnea and/or chest pain at presentation, whereas cardiovascular collapse is observed in 10 percent of the patients. Symptoms of PE include sudden onset **cough** (3 to 55 percent), blood-streaked sputum (3 to 40 percent), sudden onset of **dyspnea at rest or with exertion** (75 percent), splinting of ribs with breathing, **chest pain** (50 to 85 percent), and **diaphoresis** (25 to 40 percent). Nonspecific signs of PE include **tachypnea** (50 to 60 percent), **tachycardia** (25 to 70 percent), **rales/crackles** (50 percent), and **low-grade fever** (7 to 50 percent). Chest pains associated with PE may be pleuritic or nonpleuritic in nature, with pleuritic chest pains occurring most frequently with nonfatal peripheral pulmonary infarcts. The "classic triad" for PE (hemoptysis, dyspnea, and chest pain) occurs in fewer than 20 percent of patients in whom PE is diagnosed. PE can be proven in 20 percent of young, active patients presenting to the emergency department complaining only of pleuritic chest pain. Such patients are often dismissed inappropriately with inadequate workup and nonspecific diagnoses such as musculoskeletal chest pain or pleurisy. Spontaneous onset of chest wall tenderness without a history of trauma is worrisome, because this may be the only physical finding of PE. Unusual clinical presentations of PE also include seizure, syncope, abdominal pain, high fever, productive cough, adult-onset asthma, new-onset supraventricular arrhythmias, or hiccups.

Diagnosis Based on findings from the PIOPED (Prospective Investigation of Pulmonary Embolism Diagnosis) study, clinicians correctly excluded pulmonary embolism 91 percent of the time in low-clinical-probability patients; however, in the intermediate- and high-probability patients, clinicians correctly diagnosed PE only 64 to 68 percent of the time. Because **clinical variables alone lack power to permit treatment decisions**, patients with intermediate to high probability must undergo further testing until the diagnosis is proven, ruled out, or an alternative diagnosis is identified.

The initial CXR in a patient with PE is nearly always normal. Occasionally, the **Hampton's hump** (wedge-shaped pleural-based density caused by pulmonary infarction) can be seen. Serial CXRs obtained in a patient with PE are frequently associated with progression suggestive of atelectasis, pleural effusion, and elevated hemidiaphragm. After 2 to 3 days, the CXR in one-third of patients with PE demonstrates focal infiltrates mimicking pneumonia.

Interpretation of nuclear scintigraphic **ventilation–perfusion scanning (V/Q scan) may group patients into four result types: normal, low probability, indeterminate, and high probability.** Similar to the diagnosis of DVT, the clinical suspicion determines the pretest probability and the accuracy of V/Q scans, therefore the subsequent management following V/Q scans should be formulated on the basis of clinical impression and V/Q scan interpretations.

High-resolution computed tomographic angiography (CTA) is sensitive in identifying **most large and centrally located PEs, but may miss central clots in the middle (right) and lingular (left) pulmonary arteries** because of their nearly horizontal take-off from the hila. A negative CTA in a "high-probability" patient is not adequate to "rule out" PE diagnosis. **Pulmonary angiography remains the gold standard for the diagnosis of PE**, providing 100 percent certainty that obstruction to pulmonary blood flow exists. A negative pulmonary angiogram can rule out PE with 90 percent certainty. A complete negative study, however, requires the visualization of the entire pulmonary tree bilaterally. This can only be accomplished by selective injection of contrast in each branch of the pulmonary arterial system with multiple views of each area.

Laboratory Studies   **Pulse oximetry and arterial blood gas measurements are insensitive** in identifying PE and should never be used to direct diagnostic workup. Many recent investigations have focused on the use of the D-dimer assay for PE and DVT diagnosis. **D-dimers are cleavage products created by the degradation of cross-linked fibrin strands** by the fibrinolytic system. **The power of the D-dimer test is in its negative predictive value rather than its positive predictive value, provided a highly sensitive assay is chosen**. A normal D-dimer value is helpful for the exclusion of PE in patients with low pretest probability; however, because intravascular thrombosis may occur in conditions other than PE and DVT, the specificity of elevated D-dimer is limited. It is important to bear in mind that a combination of clinical history, physical exam findings, laboratory studies, and diagnostic investigations are frequently needed for the evaluation of high-risk patients. **In high-risk individuals, negative D-dimer assay alone cannot effectively rule out PE**, therefore additional imaging studies, such as V/Q scan, CTA, or pulmonary angiogram, may be needed to exclude the diagnosis.

Clinical Decision Making   Ultimately, it is the clinician's burden to combine the imaging and laboratory test results with clinical impression to determine whether treatment for DVT/PE is indicated. Figure 14-2 is an algorithm based on this approach. The treatment for pulmonary embolism is generally intravenous heparin therapy followed by Coumadin. **Thrombolytic therapy** has been advocated for those individuals with a serious PE, such as those with **hypotension**. To date, no studies have proven a survival advantage for thrombolytic therapy in PE.

Clinical Characteristics	Score
Signs of DVT (leg swelling, pain, tenderness with palpation of deep veins)	3
Heart rate >100	1.5
Immobilization or surgery in previous 4 weeks	1.5
Previous DVT/PE	1.5
Hemoptysis	1
Malignancy	1
An alternative diagnosis less likely than PE	3
(Total Score: Low clinical suspicion<2; Moderate clinical suspicion 2-6; High suspicion≥6	

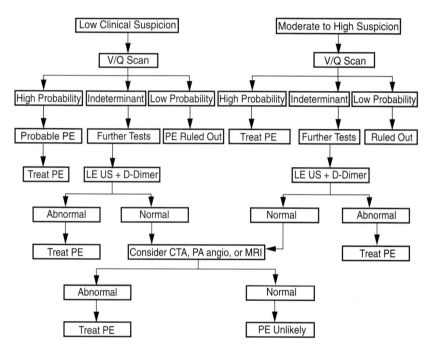

Figure 14-2. Diagnostic strategy for patients with suspected PE. Modified, with permission, from Wells PS, Ginsberg JS, Anderson DR, et al. Use of a clinical model for safe management of patients with suspected pulmonary embolism. Ann Intern Med 1998;129:997–1005.

Comprehension Questions

[14.1] Which of the following statements regarding DVT is *least* accurate?

A. A patient with thrombosis of the superficial femoral vein is not at risk for PE.

B. Venography is the definitive test for the diagnosis of DVT.

C. Thrombosis of the vena cava, subclavian veins, and right atrium are rare sources of PE.

D. Venous duplex ultrasonography is most useful in diagnosing DVT in veins easily compressible by the examiner.

E. The most likely source of a clinically devastating PE derives from the iliofemoral veins.

[14.2] A 60-year-old man has been diagnosed with a pulmonary embolism. Which of the following tests is most likely to be abnormal?

A. Electrocardiogram (EKG)

B. Chest x-ray

C. D-dimer level

D. Arterial blood gas (ABG)

E. Oxygen saturation

[14.3] Which of the following patients with shortness of breath has the lowest clinical probability for PE?

A. A 67-year-old man who underwent bilateral total knee replacements 2 weeks ago.

B. A 38-year-old man who underwent an uncomplicated open appendectomy 3 weeks ago.

C. A 35-year-old woman with a history of ovarian cancer.

D. A 35-year-old man with a history of a DVT 15 years ago, which occurred after an accident.

E. A 26-year-old woman who had an uncomplicated vaginal delivery 10 days ago.

[14.4] A 57-year-old man comes to the emergency room complaining of shortness of breath. The onset was sudden, and is associated with pleuritic chest pain. He was recently released from the hospital after being diagnosed with lymphoma. He had an indwelling catheter placed in his left subclavian vein the day before for chemotherapy administration. He was previously healthy without significant medical history. His vital signs are heart rate of 105 beats per minute, blood pressure 126/86 mmHg, respiratory rate of 28 breaths per minute, O_2 saturation 100 percent. Breath sounds are clear bilaterally without rubs or crackles. His heart sounds are normal without an S_3 or S_4 gallop. His left arm is mildly edematous, but otherwise painless, with a normal pulse exam. There is no swelling of his lower extremities and he has no pain with palpation of his calves. His catheter incision site is clean and intact. Of the following studies, which is inappropriate in the further workup of this patient?

A. Chest x-ray
B. EKG
C. Pulmonary angiography
D. D-dimer assay
E. Duplex ultrasonography of the deep veins of the upper and lower extremities

Answers

[14.1] **A.** Venography is the gold standard for diagnosing thromboses of the deep veins of the extremities and is useful when duplex studies are inconclusive. Duplex ultrasonography combines direct visualization of the vein with Doppler flow signals. Part of the study relies on the examiner's ability to visualize compression of the veins to rule out an occluding thrombus. Because intraabdominal and pelvic veins are difficult to compress, their evaluation by this method is limited. Most clinically significant PE's derive from the large veins of the lower extremity, especially the iliofemoral veins that can embolize large clots to the pulmonary vasculature with disastrous hemodynamic consequences. Infrequent sources of PE can be central veins of the upper extremity, the vena cava, or even the right atrium. Despite its name, the superficial femoral vein is considered a deep vein (it accompanies the superficial femoral artery), and can be the source of clinically significant thromboemboli.

[14.2] **C.** EKG findings are often normal or nonspecific in patients with PE. ST-segment and T-wave abnormalities are the most common, but occasionally signs of right-heart strain may be noted, including peaked P waves in lead II (P pulmonale), right bundle-branch block, supraventricular arrhythmias, and right axis deviation. The classic EKG findings of PE are S in lead I, Q in lead III, and inverted T in lead III (S1Q3T3). Chest radiographs are also usually normal. In severe PE, dilation of proximal pulmonary vessels with collapse of distal vasculature is noted (Westermark sign). Twenty-four to 72 hours after a PE, atelectasis and a focal infiltrate may be seen as a consequence of loss of surfactant. Pleural effusions may be noted, and, rarely, a triangular or rounded pleural-based infiltrate with its apex pointed to the hilum (Hampton hump) may be seen in the case of an infarction. ABG findings are often confusing, and abnormalities are usually a result of underlying pathology such as chronic obstructive pulmonary disease (COPD) or pneumonia. A low Po_2 in an otherwise healthy patient at risk for DVT/PE is more useful. O_2 saturation is rarely depressed and not very useful in the workup of PE. D-dimer levels are most useful in helping rule out PE. It is a very sensitive, but highly nonspecific, test, and when levels are normal, a PE is highly unlikely.

[14.3] **B.** Malignancy, acquired or inherited hypercoagulable states, previous DVT or PE, immobility, and pregnancy are all risk factors for DVT and PE. Although surgery is a known risk factor, the length of operation and postoperative immobility are factors that contribute to thrombosis.

[14.4] **C.** This patient may very well have a PE, but other sources of his chest pain and shortness of breath must also be considered. An EKG will aid in the diagnosis of cardiac etiologies including heart attacks or arrhythmias. A chest x-ray will show other possible pulmonary processes, including pneumonia or a pneumothorax from the central line placement (as well as confirm the position of the line). Duplex ultrasonography will help examine the venous system for thromboses and possible sources of PE, including the deep veins of the upper extremity, because this patient now has an indwelling catheter that can be a source of thrombus formation. A D-dimer assay, if negative, would be useful in excluding the diagnosis of DVT and PE, however this patient's results may be confused by his recent procedure. Pulmonary angiography is not yet indicated in this patient until further diagnostic workup leads one to suspect a PE as the source of his symptoms. Pulmonary angiography is invasive, costly, time-consuming, and not without its own complications, and should therefore be used judiciously.

CLINICAL PEARLS

❖ High clinical suspicion is the most important factor in determining the workup of PE.

❖ Negative D-dimer results are useful in excluding PE.

❖ V/Q scan and CT angiography are useful in risk-stratifying a patient with suspected PE.

❖ Pulmonary angiography is the gold standard for diagnosis but is expensive and not without its own inherent risks.

❖ Eighty percent of PEs develop from DVTs involving the iliac, femoral, or popliteal veins.

REFERENCES

Rosen CL, Tracy JA. The diagnosis of lower extremity deep venous thrombosis. Emerg Med Clin North Am 2001;19:895–912.

Sadosty AT, Boie ET, Stead LG. Pulmonary embolism. Emerg Med Clin North Am 2003;21(2):363–84.

Wells PS, Anderson DR, Rodger M, et al. Excluding pulmonary embolism at the bedside without diagnostic imaging: management of patients with suspected pulmonary embolism presenting to the emergency department by using a simple clinical model and D-dimer. Ann Intern Med 2001;135(2):98–107.

A 16-year-old nulliparous woman is brought into the emergency room complaining of severe headache and blurry vision. She is 28 weeks pregnant and has no complications with her pregnancy to date. On examination, her blood pressure is 180/120 mmHg, heart rate is 110 beats per minute, and respiratory rate is 18 breaths per minute. She is slightly lethargic. Her heart and lung examinations are normal. The abdomen reveals a fundal height of 28 cm and is nontender. The fetal heart tones are 120 beats per minute. Her reflexes are slightly brisk.

◆ **What is the most likely diagnosis?**

◆ **What is the best management?**

ANSWERS TO CASE 15: Preeclampsia/Malignant Hypertension

Summary: A 16-year-old nulliparous woman at 28 weeks' gestation has a severe headache and blurry vision. Her blood pressure is 180/120 mmHg and she is slightly lethargic. Her heart and lung examinations are normal. The fetal heart tones are 120 beats per minute. Reflexes are slightly brisk.

◆ **Most likely diagnosis:** Severe preeclampsia with malignant hypertension.

◆ **Best management:** Lower blood pressure with intravenous hydralazine or labetalol, initiate magnesium sulfate for seizure prophylaxis, and induce labor.

Analysis

Objectives

1. Be familiar with the diagnosis and treatment of preeclampsia.
2. Know how to diagnose and treat malignant hypertension.
3. Understand the complications of severe untreated hypertension.

Considerations

This 16-year-old woman at 28 weeks' gestation has severely elevated blood pressure, and is symptomatic. She has a severe headache and blurry vision. This is most likely **preeclampsia**, a hypertensive disease of unknown etiology unique to pregnancy. The underlying pathophysiology is **vasospasm and capillary leakage.** The clinical constellation is **hypertension, proteinuria, and peripheral or facial edema.** Table 15-1 lists the commonly affected end organs. This patient's headache and blurry vision are most likely caused by vasospastic effect on the brain. Lowering of the blood pressure and **magnesium sulfate** are important to initiate to prevent seizures (eclampsia). **Hydralazine 5 to 10 mg slow intravenous bolus over 5 to 10 minutes usually lowers the blood pressure to a safe range (diastolic blood pressure <115 mmHg);** the goal should not be to normalize the blood pressure because this can lead to placental insufficiency. Magnesium sulfate is more effective than phenytoin (Dilantin) or other anticonvulsant agents. A 4- to 6-g intravenous load of magnesium sulfate over 15 to 20 minutes is generally very effective. Thereafter, an intravenous infusion of 2 g/h is often used. Loss of deep tendon reflexes or hypoventilation must be monitored to assess for magnesium toxicity (which is treated with intravenous calcium gluconate).

APPROACH TO MALIGNANT HYPERTENSION

Definitions

Preeclampsia: hypertension with proteinuria greater than 300 mg in 24 hours at a gestational age greater than 20 weeks.

Table 15-1
END ORGANS AFFECTED BY PREECLAMPSIA

END ORGAN (BY SYSTEM)	SIGNS/SYMPTOMS OF PREECLAMPSIA
Neurologic	Headache Vision changes Seizures Blindness
Renal	Proteinuria Oliguria Elevated creatinine level
Pulmonary	Pulmonary edema
Hematologic/vascular	Thrombocytopenia Hemoconcentration Microangiopathic anemia Coagulopathy Severe hypertension (160/110 mmHg)
Fetal	Intrauterine Growth Restriction (IUGR) Oligohydramnios Decrease uterine perfusion (i.e. late decelerations)
Hepatic	Increased liver enzymes Subcapsular hematoma Hepatic rupture

Eclampsia: seizures associated with preeclampsia.

Malignant hypertension: severe hypertension characterized by an elevated diastolic blood pressure causing end-organ damage.

Clinical Approach

Hypertension is found in 20 to 30 percent of adults in developed countries. Hypertension is more common in men than in women, and blood pressure seems to increase with age. The incidence of hypertension is 1.5 to 2.0 times greater in African Americans than in whites. Hypertension is defined as two readings of greater than 140/90 mmHg on two different occasions. Treatment is usually successful, but uncontrolled hypertension can lead to hypertensive crises.

Hypertensive crises are critical elevations in blood pressure and are classified as **hypertensive urgencies or hypertensive emergencies** (malignant hypertension). Malignant hypertension occurs in less than 1 percent of hypertensive patients. More men than women are diagnosed with malignant hypertension and the average age of diagnosis is 40 years.

Now with the availability of effective medication, the life expectancy after diagnosis is greater than 5 years.

Hypertensive urgencies are elevations in blood pressure **without** the signs or symptoms of end-organ damage. Blood pressure in this circumstance should be reduced over several hours and the patient may be followed up in 24 to 48 hours. **Malignant hypertension** occurs with elevations in blood pressure **causing end-organ damage**. These patients **require immediate reduction of blood pressure** and should receive intravenous antihypertensive medications and be monitored in the intensive care unit.

Malignant Hypertension **Marked blood pressure elevation** along with **end-organ manifestations** characterize malignant hypertension. The symptoms include severe headache, vomiting, visual disturbances, transient paralyses, convulsions, stupor and coma resulting from hypertensive encephalopathy. **Papilledema** (Fig. 15-1) and retinal hemorrhages and exudates may also be seen. Although the mechanism of pathogenesis of malignant hypertension is

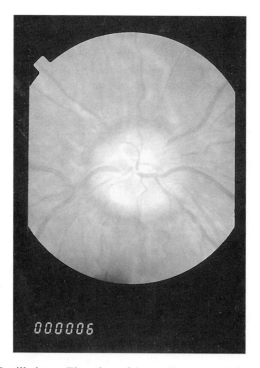

Figure 15-1. Papilledema. Elevation of the optic nerve and blurring of the disc margin are characteristic of papilledema. Reproduced with permission from Tintinalli JE, Kelen GD, Stapczynski JS, eds. Emergency Medicine, 6th ed. New York: McGraw-Hill, 2004:238.

unknown, these symptoms can be attributed to dilation of cerebral arteries and generalized arteriolar fibrinoid necrosis. Cardiac decompensation (e.g., Ml, pulmonary edema, aortic dissection) and declining renal function are also associated with malignant hypertension.

Malignant hypertension is a true medical emergency. Immediate evaluation is a necessity and the patient should be admitted to the hospital, preferably the intensive care unit. A detailed medical history must be obtained to determine if the patient has underlying renal, cardiac, or endocrine manifestations. Obvious etiologies of elevated blood pressure must be ruled out. The patient's current medications must be known and the possibility of ingestion of drugs or other substances must be considered. A thorough physical examination should be performed. Baseline laboratory studies such as a complete blood count (CBC), blood urea nitrogen (BUN), creatinine, and serum electrolytes should be obtained. For selective patients, calcium, phosphorus, thyroid function tests, lipid panel, erythrocyte sedimentation rate (ESR), catecholamines, plasma renin activity, aldosterone, and urinalysis with urine culture should be considered. A chest x-ray (CXR), renal ultrasound, echocardiogram, electrocardiogram (EKG), and possible head computed tomography (CT) scan should also be obtained. Depending on the severity of the hypertension, continuous intraarterial blood pressure monitoring may be considered. Appropriate therapy should then be initiated. This includes antihypertensive medications along with adequate control of pain or anxiety.

Treatment Antihypertensive medications must be used to prevent irreversible end-organ damage. The **initial goal in treating hypertensive crisis** is to rapidly lower the **diastolic** blood pressure to about **100 to 105 mmHg in 2 to 6 hours, but not by more than 25 percent of the presenting value**. More aggressive lowering of the blood pressure may lead to ischemia and hypotension. More normalization of the blood pressure may be contemplated over 24 to 48 hours. All of the commonly used drugs are vasodilators and therefore lower blood pressure by decreasing vascular resistance. Two categories of drugs are used: those that have an immediate onset and those that have a delayed onset. Those used for **immediate results include sodium nitroprusside, nitroglycerin, diazoxide, or trimethaphan**. Long-term control can be achieved with beta blockers, hydralazine, enalapril, or nifedipine.

Hypertensive disorders can also complicate pregnancies. These are responsible for a large number of maternal deaths each year. Pregnancy predisposes some women to a form of hypertension known as preeclampsia. Preeclampsia occurs in women at a gestational age greater than 20 weeks who present with hypertension and proteinuria.

Preeclampsia occurs as a consequence of vasospasm and leaky capillaries within the cardiovascular system. Various organ systems can be affected, especially with severe elevation in blood pressure, such as the kidney, liver, brain, and hematopoietic system. Proteinuria occurs secondary to damage to the renal glomerular system. Hepatic function is compromised and can lead to periportal hemorrhagic necrosis, subcapsular hematoma, or hepatic rupture. Vasospasm and impairment of the autoregulation system in the brain can cause cerebral edema, thrombosis, hemorrhage, blindness, seizure or coma.

Delivery is the only definitive treatment for preeclampsia. The gestational age and the severity of the disease must be considered so the risks and benefits of delivery versus expectant management can be assessed. Regardless of the decision, the blood pressure must be controlled, even if antihypertensive agents are needed. Persistently elevated blood pressures should be controlled with intravenous hydralazine or labetalol, the drugs of choice during pregnancy.

Comprehension Questions

[15.1] A 38-year-old male presents to the emergency department with complaints of a severe headache, diplopia, and vomiting. His blood pressure is 210/120 mmHg upon arrival. Which of the following is the best next step?

    A. Observe the blood pressure and recheck in 1 hour, and supportive measures for the headache and vomiting

    B. Give an antihypertensive such as sodium nitroprusside and admit to the intensive care unit

    C. Give intravenous furosemide (Lasix) to decrease the blood pressure

    D. Give lorazepam (Ativan) to help the patient relax

[15.2] A 54-year-old female is seen in the emergency department needing refills on her antihypertensive medications. She has been out of her medications for 2 weeks and cannot get an appointment with her private physician for 1 more week. She normally takes atenolol and hydrochlorothiazide. Her blood pressure is 190/100 mmHg. The patient has no complaints. She has been waiting for 4 hours and is in a hurry to get back to work. What is your next step?

    A. Change her medications to a calcium channel blocker

    B. Admit to the intensive care unit and initiate intravenous nitroprusside

    C. Give her a prescription for her medications, instruct her to take them immediately and have her followup in 48 hours

    D. Counsel the patient on the dangers of her noncompliance, admit to the hospital, and begin the patient on intravenous labetalol

[15.3] A 14-year-old female presents by ambulance in a postictal state. She is 35 weeks pregnant and was found by EMT personnel seizing at school. The patient is now unresponsive. Her blood pressure is 200/118 mmHg, heart rate is 125 beats per minute, and she is having difficulty breathing. Her heart and lung examinations are normal. The abdomen reveals a fundal height of 34 cm and is nontender. The fetal heart tones are 120 beats per minute. What is your best next step?

A. Emergent cesarean delivery followed by intravenous beta-blocker or hydralazine to lower blood pressure
B. Intubate, admit to the intensive care unit, and begin intravenous nitroprusside to lower the patient's blood pressure
C. Call a social worker and child protective services because the patient may have used cocaine
D. Assess ABCs of cardiovascular life support, begin intravenous beta-blocker or hydralazine to lower the blood pressure, begin magnesium sulfate for seizure prophylaxis, and induce labor

[15.4] A 38-year-old male presents to the emergency department after a motor vehicle accident with a broken right tibia. The patient has a history of hypertension for which he is on pharmacologic treatment. The patient is writhing on the gurney in pain. His blood pressure is 182/104 mmHg. After further evaluation the patient has no other evidence of injury. The patient has no complaints except for right leg pain. What is your next best step?

A. Pain control and monitor the patient's blood pressure
B. Start a beta-blocker and monitor the patient's blood pressure
C. Call a social worker because of suspected drug or alcohol abuse
D. Admit the patient to the hospital to get his blood pressure under control

Answers

[15.1] **B.** This man has malignant hypertension which is a medical emergency. He has symptomatic hypertension causing end-organ damage. The appropriate treatment is a fast-acting antihypertensive to decrease his diastolic blood pressure by one-fourth.

[15.2] **C.** This patient has hypertensive urgency. She has no symptoms related to her elevated blood pressure and no signs of end-organ damage. The patient should restart her medications and have her blood pressure reassessed in 48 hours.

[15.3] **D.** This patient has eclampsia and preeclampsia along with seizure activity. She needs immediate delivery along with intravenous medications to decrease her blood pressure and magnesium to prevent further seizure activity. Labetalol and hydralazine are the drugs of choice in pregnancy. A vaginal delivery should always be attempted if there is no previous history of cesarean delivery.

[15.4] **A.** Although this man has a history of hypertension, he is in excruciating pain, which could be causing his elevated blood pressure. The appropriate treatment is to control the pain, have the leg set back into place, and monitor his blood pressure. The blood pressure should decrease once his pain is controlled.

CLINICAL PEARLS

❖ Preeclampsia is defined as hypertension in pregnancy beyond 20 weeks' gestation and proteinuria.

❖ Malignant hypertension is defined as markedly elevated blood pressure in the face of end-organ symptoms, whereas hypertensive urgency is markedly elevated blood pressure without end-organ effects.

❖ One of the most common reasons for malignant hypertension is patient noncompliance with antihypertensive medication.

❖ Magnesium sulfate is the best medication to prevent and treat eclampsia.

REFERENCES

Cunningham FG, Gant NF, Leveno KJ, et al. Hypertensive disorders in pregnancy. In: Williams obstetrics, 21st ed. New York: McGraw-Hill:2001.

Fauci AS. Hypertensive vascular disease. In: Braunwald E, Fauci AS, Kasper DL, et al., eds. Harrison's principles of internal medicine, 14th ed. New York: McGraw-Hill, 1998:1380–94.

You are working in the emergency department of a 15-bed, rural hospital, and a 25-year-old, previously healthy woman presents for evaluation of abdominal pain. The patient describes her pain as having been present for the past 3 days. The pain is described as constant, exacerbated by movements, and associated with subjective fevers and chills. She denies any recent changes in bowel habits, urinary symptoms, or menses. Her last menstrual period was 6 days ago. The physical examination reveals temperature of 38.4°C (101.1°F), pulse rate of 110 beats per minute, blood pressure of 112/70 mmHg, and respiratory rate of 18 breaths per minute. Her skin is nonicteric. Cardiopulmonary examination is unremarkable. The abdomen is mildly distended and tender in both right and left lower quadrants. Involuntary guarding and localized rebound tenderness are noted in the right lower quadrant. The pelvic examination reveals no cervical discharge; cervical motion tenderness and right adnexal tenderness are present. The rectal examination reveals no masses or tenderness. Laboratory studies reveal white blood cell count (WBC) of 14,000 cells/mm³, a normal hemoglobin, and a normal hematocrit. The urinalysis reveals 3 to 5 WBC/high-power field (HPF), few bacteria, and trace ketones.

 What are the most likely diagnoses?

 How can you confirm the diagnosis?

ANSWERS TO CASE 16: Acute Abdomen

Summary: A 25-year-old, previously healthy woman presents with 3-day history of lower abdominal pain and fever. Her examination indicates the presence of fever, lower abdominal tenderness (right > left). The rectal examination is unremarkable. Her laboratory studies indicate leukocytosis.

 Most likely diagnoses: Likely diagnoses include perforated acute appendicitis, pelvic inflammatory disease (PID), ovarian torsion, or other pelvic pathology.

 Confirmatory studies: Begin with pregnancy test and pelvic ultrasonography to evaluate for possible ovarian and pelvic pathology. If these suggest pelvic source of pathology, then strong consideration should be given to exploratory laparoscopy or laparotomy.

Analysis

Objectives

1. Learn the relationships between symptoms, findings, and pathophysiology of the various types of disease processes capable of producing acute abdominal pain.
2. Learn to develop reasonable diagnostic and treatment strategies based on clinical diagnosis, resource availability, and patient characteristics.

Considerations

This is a healthy young woman, who presents with acute pain in the lower abdomen. Based on patient age and location of pain, acute appendicitis and gynecological pathology are the most likely sources of pathology, and additional history and diagnostic studies may help to differentiate these possibilities.

Pertinent gynecological history may include history of sexual contacts, menstrual pattern, previous gynecological problems, and the probability of pregnancy. A pregnancy test should be obtained early during the evaluation process to verify the presence or absence of pregnancy, and if the history and physical examination suggest the source of pathology to have originated from the pelvic organs, a pelvic ultrasound should be obtained.

In the event that the patient is pregnant, an ultrasound should be performed to verify intrauterine gestational sac and estimate the gestational age. If an intrauterine gestational sac is not visualized by ultrasound, the possibility of ectopic pregnancy should be considered and an immediate referral should be made for a gynecological evaluation and possible operative intervention. Whereas, if the pregnancy test is negative and pelvic pathology is strongly suspected, the initial priority would be to identify potential life-threatening and fertility reducing processes, including tuboovarian abscess, pelvic inflammatory disease, and ovarian torsion. **Pelvic ultrasonography** would be very valuable as the initial study to identify or rule out these processes. In the event that the pelvic ultrasound does not identify any pelvic pathology, a computed tomography (CT) scan of the abdomen and pelvis may be useful. The management approach for a patient with abdominal pain varies depending on resource availability. For this patient, if the 15-bed facility does not have CT capability, then the general surgeon should be consulted regarding possible transfer to another facility or further evaluation by laparoscopy or laparotomy.

APPROACH TO ABDOMINAL PAIN

Definitions

"Acute abdomen": describes the recent onset of abdominal pain. Patients with acute abdomen require urgent evaluation and not necessarily urgent operations.

Foregut: extends from oropharynx to mid-duodenum, including liver, biliary tract, pancreas, and spleen.

Hindgut: distal transverse colon to rectum.

Midgut: distal duodenum to mid-transverse colon.

Referred pain: this pain usually arises from a deep structure to a remote deep or superficial structure. The pattern of referred pain is based on the existence of shared central pathways between the afferent neurons of cutaneous dermatomes and intraabdominal structures. Frequently, referred pain is associated with skin hyperalgesia and increased muscle tone. (Classic example of referred pain occurs with irritation of the left hemidiaphragm from ruptured spleen that causes referred pain to the left shoulder because of shared innervation by the same cervical nerves.)

Somatic pain: arises from the irritation of the parietal peritoneum. This is mediated mainly by spinal nerve fibers supplying the abdominal wall. The pain is perceived as sharp, constant, and generally localized to one of four quadrants. Somatic pain may arise as a result of changes in pH and temperature (infection and inflammation) or pressure increase (surgical incision).

Visceral pain: generally characterized as dull, crampy, deep, or aching. Normal embryological development of abdominal viscera results in symmetrical bilateral autonomic innervation leading to visceral pain being perceived in the midline location. Visceral stimulation can be produced by stretching and torsion, chemical stimulation, ischemia, or inflammation. Visceral pain from gastrointestinal (GI) tract structures correlates with pain location based on their embryonic origins, where foregut pain is perceived in the epigastrium, midgut pain is perceived in the periumbilical region, and hindgut pain is perceived in the hypogastrium.

Clinical Approach

Abdominal pain is a common chief complaint of patients seen in the emergency department (ED), comprising approximately 5 to 8 percent of total visits. Overall, 18 to 25 percent of patients with abdominal pain evaluated in the ED have serious conditions requiring acute hospital care. In a recent series, the distribution of common diagnoses of adult ED patients with abdominal pain were listed as the following: 18 percent admitted, 25 percent undifferentiated abdominal pain (UDAP), 12 percent female pelvic, 12 percent urinary tract, and 9.3 percent surgical gastrointestinal. Approximately 10 percent of patients required urgent surgery, and most patients with UDAP were young women with epigastric symptoms who did not progress to develop significant medical problems.

Understanding of disease pathophysiology, epidemiology, clinical presentations, and the limitations of laboratory and imaging studies are important during evaluation of patients with abdominal pain in the ED. Patient evaluations should be directed toward identifying potentially serious medical conditions. Analgesia including narcotics should not be withheld in patients with pain. In the event that a diagnosis is not identified following a thorough evaluation, it may be appropriate to discharge the patient with the diagnosis of "abdominal pain of uncertain etiology." Usually, **individuals still under the effect of analgesia without a diagnosis should not be discharged.** For these patients, it is important to provide them with the reassurance that the pain most likely would improve and resolve; however because of the broad overlap in the early manifestation of serious disease, the patient should be instructed to seek early followup if symptoms do not resolve.

Abdominal Pain in Women Women make up approximately 75 percent of all patients evaluated in the ED with abdominal pain. Women of childbearing age represent a complex patient population from the diagnostic standpoint, because of a broader differential for pain. Acute appendicitis, biliary tract disease, urinary tract infection, and gynecological problems are the most common sources of abdominal pain in women of childbearing age. The history obtained from each patient should include details of menstrual history, sexual practices, gynecological and obstetrical history, and surgical history. For most individuals, the initial history and physical examination can help to direct the workup toward an organ system or body region. Laboratory evaluations, including CBC with differential, serum amylase, urinalysis, pregnancy test, and liver function test, may provide additional information to help rule in or rule out certain diagnoses. When indicated, imaging such as ultrasonography and CT scans can be helpful in assessing for biliary tract and pelvic pathology, and for acute appendicitis. **Because overreliance on laboratory and/or imaging can contribute to misdiagnoses, laboratory and imaging results should always be interpreted within the proper clinical context; clinical judgment should be exercised regarding the acquisition of consultation and/or observation.**

Abdominal Pain in Elderly Patients   Elderly patients account for approximately 15 percent of all ED visits, and about one-third of these visits result in inpatient admissions. In comparison to young adults, **elderly patients** with abdominal pain evaluated in the ED generally **have higher prevalence of serious diseases** causing abdominal pain, where the frequency of illnesses requiring surgical intervention has been estimated to be as high as 30 percent. Furthermore, the mortality rate associated with abdominal pain is increased in this population as a consequence of the increase in catastrophic illnesses (including mesenteric ischemia, leaking or ruptured aneurysm, and myocardial infarction). **Common diagnoses among elderly patients** include **biliary tract disease** (23 percent), **diverticular disease** (12 percent), **bowel obstruction** (11 percent), and undetermined (11 percent).

Because of a variety of reasons, including atypical clinical presentations and difficulty with communication, abdominal pain in the elderly is associated with high frequency of inaccurate diagnosis (up to 60 percent). Inability to accurately diagnose the cause of abdominal pain contributes to delayed treatment and increased mortality. Elderly patients whose abdominal pain were not accurately diagnosed in the ED were found to have a twofold increase in mortality when compared to elderly patients whose causes of abdominal pain were accurately diagnosed.

For most elderly patients, the evaluation should be broadened to help identify cardiac, pulmonary, vascular, and neurological causes of abdominal pain, as well as patient comorbidities. It is important to bear in mind that medications taken by many elderly patients may contribute to abdominal problems, as well as alter the clinical presentations (e.g., beta blockers may blunt pulse rate response to stress). When indicated, ancillary testing should be applied to assist in establishing the diagnosis; however it is important to remember that **the diagnostic accuracy of any test is dependent on the pretest probability, specificity, sensitivity, and disease prevalence of the test population.** Because abdominal pain in the elderly population is more frequently associated with serious pathology, appropriate consultations should be sought out and a liberal policy regarding inpatient or ED observation should be applied whenever causes cannot be clearly identified.

Patients with Chronic or Recurrent Abdominal Pain   Patients with chronic or recurrent abdominal pain represent one of the most difficult diagnostic and management challenges for emergency medicine physicians. The dilemma facing ED physicians during encounters with these patients include establishing the accurate diagnosis, determining appropriate use of diagnostic studies, determining the appropriateness of analgesic medications, and followup.

Similar to the approach taken toward patients with acute abdominal pain, the evaluation of chronic abdominal pain should begin with a thorough history. Events and activities that trigger or alleviate the symptoms may be helpful in identifying the organ systems of pain origin. Furthermore, detailed description of the patterns and location of pain are helpful for categorization of pain as visceral pain, somatic pain, or referred pain; based on these determinations, organ system and anatomical sources of abdominal pain also may be delineated.

The physical examinations in these patients should be focused to help sort out the differential diagnosis formulated on the basis of history, and not a search for pathology. Unfortunately, the physical examination findings are sometimes difficult to interpret because of psychological and personality changes, especially if the pain has been chronic, recurrent, and severe.

Unfortunately, no specific laboratory or imaging studies are completely sensitive or specific for the diagnosis of abdominal pain. As a general rule, diagnostic studies should be selected only if results of the studies will lead to specific additional evaluations or treatment. The CBC might be helpful in identifying leukocytosis, which may indicate an inflammatory or infectious condition, whereas the presence of anemia might help to verify the presence of ischemic colitis, GI tract malignancy, or inflammatory bowel disease. Abnormalities within the liver function panel may help identify choledocholithiasis, stenosing papillitis, and periampullary malignancy. Serum amylase elevation is generally seen in the setting of chronic or acute pancreatitis. Elevation in erythrocyte sedimentation rate may suggest the presence of autoimmune processes or collagen vascular disorders.

Frequently, even after the completion of extensive, appropriate evaluations the patient's condition may remain unrecognized. If possible, the results of the evaluation and diagnostic studies should be discussed with the patient's primary care physician, so that the patient may be provided with additional testing and followup. For those patients without primary care physicians, evaluation and consultation by an appropriate primary care physician or specialist should be obtained prior to discharge from the ED.

Comprehension Questions

[16.1] A 30-year-old woman presents with epigastric pain that developed following dinner. The patient describes having similar pain prior to the current episode, but previous episodes were less severe. The patient was diagnosed as having gastroesophageal reflux disease by her primary care physician and prescribed a proton pump inhibitor, which has been ineffective in resolving her pain. The current pain episode has been severe and persistent for 3 hours. The patient has a temperature of 38°C (100.4°F), heart rate of 100 beats per minute, respiratory rate of 20 breaths per minute, and blood pressure of 130/90 mmHg. The abdominal examination reveals no abdominal tenderness. The administration of 30 mL of antacids and 4 mg of morphine sulfate resulted in some relief of pain. Which of the following is the most appropriate next step?

A. Obtain CBC, amylase, liver functions test, and ultrasound of the gallbladder

B. Follow up with her primary care physician in 2 weeks

C. Admit the patient to the hospital for upper GI endoscopy

D. Prescribe antacids and discharge the patient from the ED, with followup by her primary care physician

[16.2] Which of the following features best characterize somatic pain?

A. Midline location

B. Sharp, persistent, and well-localized pain in the left lower quadrant

C. Intermittent pain

D. Pain is improved with body movement

[16.3] For which of the following patients is CT of the abdomen contraindicated?

A. A 60-year-old man with persistent left lower quadrant pain, fever, and a tender mass

B. A 45-year-old alcoholic man with diffuse abdominal pain, WBC 18,000 cells/mm³, and serum amylase of 2000 Iu/L

C. A nonpregnant 18-year-old woman with suprapubic and right lower quadrant pain, fever, and WBC of 15,000 cells/mm³

D. A 70-year-old man with abdominal pain and distension, a 10-cm pulsatile mass in the epigastrium, and blood pressure of 70/50 mmHg

[16.4] Which of the following factors *does not* influence the accuracy of diagnostic studies?

A. Disease prevalence in the testing population

B. Sensitivity of the study

C. Pretest probability

D. Availability of the test

Answers

[16.1] **A.** This patient has recurrent epigastric pain, which is attributed to gastroesophageal reflux disease. However, the fact that her symptoms have been poorly controlled with proton pump inhibitors in the past suggests that the diagnosis is probably inaccurate. Choice A represents testing for the evaluation of biliary tract disease, which is appropriate in this setting. Because of her fever, followup in 2 weeks is not appropriate.

[16.2] **B.** Somatic pain is generally associated with irritation of the parietal peritoneum, resulting in localized, sharp pain.

[16.3] **D.** This patient is hemodynamically unstable and possesses signs and symptoms suggestive of ruptured abdominal aneurysm. CT scan is contraindicated in this situation.

[16.4] **D.** Disease prevalence of the test population, sensitivity of the test, and pretest probability of the patient are all factors that can influence the accuracy of diagnostic studies.

CLINICAL PEARLS

❖ Most patients with the diagnosis of "undifferentiated abdominal pain" determined after thorough ED evaluation will have spontaneous resolution of pain.

❖ Narcotic medications will affect the characteristics and intensity of all abdominal pain, regardless of etiology.

❖ Up to one-third of elderly patients with abdominal pain evaluated in the ED have conditions that may require surgical intervention.

REFERENCES

Graff LG IV, Robinson D. Abdominal pain and emergency department evaluation. Emerg Med Clin N Am 2001;19:123–36.

Kamin RA, Nowicki TA, Courtney DS, Powers RD. Pearls and pitfalls in the emergency department evaluation of abdominal pain. Emerg Med Clin N Am 2003;21:61–72.

Liu CD, McFadden DW. Acute abdomen and appendix. In: Greenfiled LJ, Mulholland MW, Oldham KT, Zelenock GB, Liiemoe KD, eds. Surgery: scientific principles and practice, 2nd ed. Philadelphia: Lippincott-Raven Publishers, 1997.

Zackowski S. Chronic recurrent abdominal pain. Emerg Clin N Am 1998;16:877–94.

A 2-year-old boy is brought to the emergency department (ED) because of an episode of "choking." The patient was playing with marbles when his mother left the room for a few minutes. She ran back in when she heard the patient gagging and coughing. She denies seeing her son turn blue or any recent fever, cough, or other upper respiratory infectious symptoms. The patient was a term baby without any significant past medical history. He is not taking any medications, and his immunizations are all up to date. He attends daycare and has no recent sick contacts.

On exam, his temperature is 37.7°C (99.9°F), blood pressure is 80/50 mmHg, heart rate is 100 beats per minute, respiratory rate is 24 breaths per minute, and the O_2 saturation is 98 percent on room air. The patient is playful and alert. His exam is unremarkable except for moderate wheezes. He has no intercostal retractions nor use of any accessory muscles.

◆ **What are the potential complications in this patient?**

◆ **What is the most appropriate next step?**

ANSWERS TO CASE 17: Swallowed Foreign Body

Summary: This is a 2-year-old boy with probable ingestion of a foreign body (marble).

◆ **Potential complications:** Airway obstruction, esophageal stricture, perforation and mediastinitis, paraesophageal abscess, cardiac tamponade, and aortotracheoesophageal fistula.

◆ **Most appropriate next step:** Because the child is stable, x-ray to localize the foreign body.

Analysis

Objectives

1. Recognize the clinical scenario, signs, and symptoms of swallowed foreign bodies.
2. Learn the diagnostic and therapeutic approach to the various types of swallowed foreign bodies.

Considerations

Patients with swallowed foreign bodies may be asymptomatic or may present *in extremis.* Although most objects will pass through the gastrointestinal tract without problems, it is important to recognize which patients require observation and which will need some type of intervention (see Table 17-1). This 2-year-old boy appears to be in stable condition, but the astute ED physician will be prepared for respiratory decompensation at any time, because the foreign body may acutely obstruct the airway.

APPROACH TO SWALLOWED FOREIGN BODY

Foreign body ingestion is a relatively common presentation in the ED. Although children account for the vast majority of cases, edentulous adults, psychiatric patients, and prisoners also commonly swallow foreign objects. Children most commonly ingest things they can pick up and place in their mouths, such as coins, buttons, and small toys. Adults are more likely to have trouble swallowing meat, bones, and nuts. Although objects can be located anywhere throughout the alimentary tract, there are several areas where they lodge more frequently. In the pediatric patient, **most obstructions occur in the proximal esophagus** at **one of five places:** the **cricopharyngeal narrowing, thoracic inlet, aortic arch, tracheal bifurcation, and hiatal narrowing.** In contrast, most adult patients have distal esophageal obstructions caused by a structural or motor abnormality (e.g., stricture, malignancy, scleroderma, achalasia).

Most adult patients will be able to relate a history of ingesting a foreign object or of feeling food becoming lodged. They may complain of chest or epi-

Table 17-1
SPECIAL TYPES OF SWALLOWED FOREIGN BODIES

FOREIGN BODY	COMMENTS	TREATMENT
Food impaction	Barium swallow after treatment to confirm clearance of the impaction and to rule out esophageal pathology. Avoid proteolytic enzymes (e.g., papain) because of risk of esophageal perforation.	Expectant if handling secretions and impacted < 12 hours. Otherwise endoscopy preferred. Alternatives: IV glucagon, sublingual nifedipine, sublingual nitroglycerin, oral gas-forming agents.
Coin	Often asymptomatic. X-ray to confirm location (esophageal coins lie with flat side showing on anteroposterior x-ray).	Endoscopy preferred. Alternative: Foley catheter removal under fluoroscopy if lodged <24 hours.
Button battery	High risk of mucosal burns and esophageal perforation if lodged in esophagus. X-ray to confirm location.	Expectant management if past the esophagus and no symptoms. Endoscopy if in esophagus or has not passed through the pylorus after 48 hours. Alternative: Foley catheter removal if lodged in esophagus < 2 hours.
Sharp or pointed objects	X-ray to confirm location.	If >5 cm long or >2 cm wide or extremely pointed, remove before passing from stomach because of risk of intestinal perforation. If symptomatic or swallowed a sewing needle, surgical consult for endoscopy or laparotomy. Otherwise expectant management.
Cocaine (body packing)	Rupture of packet may be fatal. Avoid endoscopy because of risk of rupture.	If packet intact, may observe and use whole-bowel irrigation. Otherwise surgery.

Source: Tintinalli JE, Kelen GD, Stapczynski JS, eds. Emergency medicine, 6th ed. New York: McGraw-Hill: 2004:513–516.

gastric pain, retching, vomiting, wheezing, or difficulty swallowing. In children, the history may be less clear. Parents may have seen the child with an object in his or her mouth and suspect ingestion. Children can present with vomiting, gagging, choking, refusal to eat, or neck or chest pain. **Drooling or an inability to swallow suggests a complete obstruction.**

The physical **exam should focus on identifying patients with airway compromise**, inability to tolerate fluids, or **active bleeding**. It should include a careful evaluation of the oropharynx, neck, chest, and abdomen. Findings such as fever, subcutaneous air, or peritoneal signs suggest perforation. In patients with a suspected oropharyngeal foreign body, direct or indirect laryngoscopy can be useful. **Plain x-rays** may help locate radiopaque foreign bodies throughout the gastrointestinal (GI) tract and be used to follow their progression (if repeated every 2 to 4 hours). If plain films do not reveal the object, an esophagogram or endoscopy are other options. **Endoscopy is usually the study of choice because the object may be removed once it is visualized.** Some success has been reported using metal detectors to locate and follow metallic objects.

Most patients who are symptomatic require observation. In general, once a foreign object passes the pylorus, it will continue through the GI tract without incident. However, **if it cannot pass the esophagus or pylorus, it must be removed.** Again, endoscopy is usually the method of choice. However, surgery may be necessary if there is evidence of obstruction or perforation, if the object is too big to pass safely, or if it contains toxins.

There are several special considerations when dealing with certain types of swallowed foreign bodies such as **button batteries**, which generally need to be removed because of their toxic effects on mucosa.

Comprehension Questions

[17.1] The ED director embarks on a study to see the type of patient most likely to experience foreign-body ingestion. Which of the following groups of individuals is most likely to have foreign-body ingestion?

    A. Edentulous adults
    B. Children
    C. Psychiatric patients
    D. Prisoners

[17.2] A 21-year-old woman accidentally swallowed a penny. At which of the following locations is the coin most likely to be lodged in the esophagus?

    A. Cricopharyngeal narrowing
    B. Thoracic inlet
    C. Aortic arch
    D. Lower esophageal sphincter

[17.3] A 3-year-old girl accidentally swallowed a button battery from her mother's camera. She does not appear to be in respiratory distress. She has normal vital signs and is afebrile. What is the best management for this patient?

    A. Expectant management
    B. Recommend avoidance of citrus drinks
    C. Endoscopy
    D. Avoidance of magnets

[17.4] An 8-year-old girl presents to the ED having swallowed a penny as part of a bet with a friend. The abdominal radiograph reveals that the penny is in the stomach. Four hours later, it is still in the stomach. Which of the following is the best next step?

    A. Endoscopy
    B. Rigid bronchoscopy
    C. Laparotomy
    D. Lithotripsy
    E. Observation

Answers

[17.1] **B.** Foreign-body ingestion is most common in children.

[17.2] **D.** In adults, a swallowed object will most commonly lodge in the esophagus at the lower esophageal sphincter.

[17.3] **C.** Because of the high risk of mucosal burns and esophageal perforation, a button battery in the esophagus must be removed as soon as possible.

[17.4] **A.** In general, the preferred method of swallowed foreign-body removal is endoscopy (except in body packers because of rupture risk).

CLINICAL PEARLS

❖ Children account for the vast majority of cases of swallowed foreign bodies.

❖ In the pediatric patient, objects most commonly lodge in the proximal esophagus, whereas most adult patients have distal esophageal obstructions.

❖ Findings such as fever, subcutaneous air, or peritoneal signs suggest perforation and necessitate an emergent surgical consult.

❖ Button batteries in the esophagus must be removed as soon as possible, as well as sharp, pointed objects in the stomach. In general, the preferred method of swallowed foreign-body removal is endoscopy (except in body packers because of rupture risk).

REFERENCES

Gaasch WR, Barish RA. Swallowed foreign bodies. In: Tintinalli JE, Kelen GD, Stapczynski JS, eds. Emergency medicine, 5th ed. New York: McGraw-Hill, 2000:529–31.

Kuhns DW, Dire DJ. Button battery ingestions. Ann Emerg Med 1989;18:293.

McGuirt W. Use of Foley catheter for removal of esophageal foreign bodies. Ann Otol Rhinol Laryngol 1982;91:599–601.

Rosen P, Barkin R, ed. Emergency medicine: concepts and clinical practice, 4th ed. St. Louis: Mosby, 1998:869–74.

A 55-year-old man presents to the emergency department complaining of abdominal pain. The patient relates that he has been having intermittent pain throughout the abdomen for the past 8 to 10 hours, and since the onset of pain, he has vomited twice. His past medical history is significant for hypertension and colon cancer for which he underwent right colectomy 8 months ago. The patient indicates that he has not had any recent abdominal complaints. His last bowel movement was 1 day ago, and he denies any weight loss and hematochezia. On physical examination, the patient is afebrile. The pulse rate is 98 beats per minute, blood pressure is 132/84 mmHg, and respiratory rate is 22 breaths per minute. His cardiopulmonary examination is unremarkable. His abdomen is obese, mildly distended, with a well-healed midline scar. No tenderness, guarding, or hernias are noted. His bowel sounds are diminished, with occasional high-pitched sounds. The rectal examination reveals normal tone, empty rectal vault, and Hemoccult-negative stool.

◆ **What is the most likely cause of this patient's problems?**

◆ **What are the next steps in this patient's evaluation?**

ANSWERS TO CASE 18: Intestinal Obstruction

Summary: A 55-year-old man with history of previous abdominal operation for the resection of right colon carcinoma presents with intermittent abdominal pain and vomiting. The physical examination reveals no abdominal wall or groin hernias, no tenderness, and high-pitched bowel sounds.

   Most likely diagnosis: Bowel obstruction. It is unclear whether it is large or small bowel, or complete versus partial obstruction.

   Next steps in evaluation: An abdominal series of x-rays, comprised of a chest x-ray and a flat and upright view of the abdomen.

Analysis

Objectives

1. Learn to recognize the clinical presentations of intestinal obstruction (small bowel and colon).
2. Learn the common causes of bowel obstructions.
3. Learn the approach for selection of imaging modalities in the evaluation of patients with possible bowel obstruction.

Considerations

In this patient scenario, the differential diagnosis for obstruction includes intestinal ileus, adhesions, ischemia, and obstruction from recurrence of metastatic colon carcinoma. In this patient, the probability of ileus as the cause of his abdominal symptoms is unlikely, because the patient has a history of crampy abdominal pain and findings of high-pitched bowel sounds, which are clinical features compatible with mechanical obstruction and not functional obstruction. **The first imaging study to consider is the abdominal series**, because these x-rays will help to distinguish partial obstruction from high-grade, complete obstruction. The abdominal series would delineate the level of obstruction. **The presence of stool or air in the rectal vault may suggest a partial obstruction,** whereas the presence of air and fluid levels in the small intestine, with the absence of stool and air throughout the colon, indicate a high-grade, small-bowel obstruction. His past history of colon cancer points to the possibility that recurrent cancer may be the cause of his bowel obstruction; thus, a computed tomography (CT) scan of the abdomen may be helpful in identifying any obstructing tumor masses.

APPROACH TO BOWEL OBSTRUCTION

Definitions

Closed-loop obstruction: Blockage occurs both proximal and distal to the dilated segment preventing decompression. Examples include an isolated loop of small bowel caught in a tight hernia defect, a twisting of the bowel on itself causing a volvulus or a complete large-bowel obstruction in a patient with a competent ileocecal valve. These obstructions are unlikely to resolve with nonoperative therapy.

Complications of bowel obstruction: ischemia, necrosis, and perforation as a result of obstruction.

CT scan of the abdomen: This modality is increasingly used in the evaluation of patients with bowel obstruction. It can help to differentiate functional obstruction from mechanical obstruction. It is also useful in the evaluation of patients with previous abdominal malignancy to help determine if the obstruction is related to tumor recurrence.

Functional or neurogenic obstruction: Luminal contents cannot pass because of bowel motility disturbances preventing peristasis. Etiologies include neurogenic dysfunction, medication or metabolic related problems, bowel wall infiltrative processes such as collagen vascular diseases, or extraluminal infiltrative processes such as peritonitis or malignancy. Surgery generally does not improve the above conditions; however, complications related to the above conditions may require operative intervention.

Mechanical obstruction: Luminal contents cannot pass through the gastrointestinal (GI) tract because of a mechanical obstruction. The treatment can be operative or nonoperative.

Open-loop obstruction: Intestinal blockage is distal, allowing proximal bowel decompression of obstruction via nasogastric (NG) suction or emesis.

Simple (uncomplicated) bowel obstruction: partial or complete obstruction of the bowel lumen without compromise to the intestinal blood flow.

Upper GI–small-bowel follow through: This is contrast radiography done following the administration of oral contrast. The study accurately localizes obstruction site and caliber in the small bowel. The administration of contrast may be associated with worsening of obstruction and aspiration. This study is rarely indicated in the ED setting.

Clinical Approach

The causes of bowel obstruction in young children (<5 years of age) are quite different than those found in the adult population. The following discussion is limited to adult patients. **Adhesions** represent the most common cause of **small-bowel obstruction** whereas **colorectal carcinoma** is the most common cause of **large-bowel obstruction**. Table 18-1 lists the distribution and clinical features associated with obstructive causes.

Pathophysiology With mechanical obstruction, **air and fluid accumulate in the bowel lumen**. The net result is an **increase in the intestinal intraluminal pressure**, which further inhibits fluid absorption and stimulates the

Table 18-1

LARGE-VERSUS SMALL-BOWEL OBSTRUCTION

SMALL-BOWEL OBSTRUCTION	LARGE-BOWEL OBSTRUCTION
Causes	Causes
Adhesions (70–75%)	Carcinoma (65%)
Malignancy (8–10%)	Volvulus (15%)
Hernia (8–10%)	Diverticular disease (10%)
Volvulus (3%)	Hernias, peritoneal carcinomatosis, fecal impaction, ischemic colitis, foreign body, inflammatory bowel disease (total 10%)
Inflammatory bowel disease (1%)	
Intussusception, gallstone ileus, radiation enteritis, intraabdominal abscess, bezoar (all <1%)	
Symptoms	Symptoms
Vomiting (common)	Distension (common and usually significant)
Crampy pain (common, early)	Postprandial cramps and bloating
Distension (moderate)	Vomiting (unusual)
	Bowel habit changes (common)

influx of water and electrolytes into the lumen. Eighty percent of air found in bowel is from swallowed air (Fig. 18-1). Because of this, NG tube decompression may be useful in preventing progression of bowel distension. Initially following the onset of mechanical obstruction, there is an increase in peristaltic activity. However, as the obstructive process progresses (usually >24 hours), coordinated peristaltic activity diminishes along with the contractile function of obstructed bowel, giving rise to dilated and atonic bowel proximal to the point of obstruction. With this progression, the patient may actually appear to improve clinically with less frequent and less intense crampy abdominal pain. The effects of mechanical obstruction on intestinal blood flow include an initial increase in blood flow. **With unrelieved obstruction, blood flow diminishes leading to a breakdown of mucosal barriers and an increased susceptibility to bacterial invasion and ischemia.**

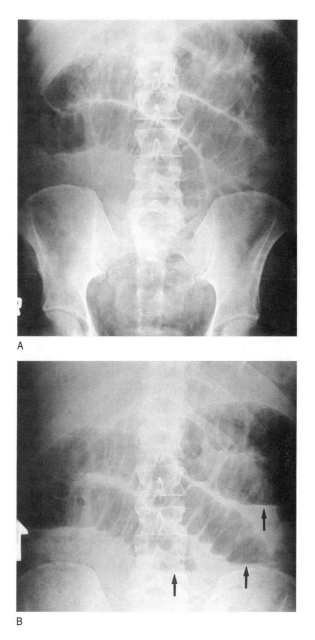

A

B

Figure 18-1. Abdominal radiographs in the supine (A) and upright (B) positions show a dilated small bowel with air-fluid levels. (Reproduced, with permission, from Kadell BM, Zimmerman P, Lu DSK. Radiology of the abdomen. In: Zinner MJ, Schwarz SI, Ellis H, et al, eds. Maingot's abdominal operations, 10 ed. New York: McGraw-Hill 1997:24)

Clinical Presentation   The **typical presentation of bowel obstruction involves pain, emesis, constipation, obstipation, distension, tenderness, visible peristalsis, and/or shock.** The presence or absence of these signs and symptoms are dependent on the severity of the obstruction. Pain associated with bowel obstruction is generally severe at the onset and is characterized as intermittent and poorly localized. With progression of a small-bowel obstruction, spastic pain decreases in intensity and frequency. However, continuous pain may develop as the result of ischemia or peritonitis.

In **large-bowel obstruction, pain frequently presents as postprandial crampy pain.** With chronic large-bowel obstruction, some patients may describe this pain as indigestion. Continuous pain may also develop with the progression of marked distension, ischemia, or perforation. Emesis is a symptom found commonly in patients with intestinal obstruction. In general, patients with proximal obstruction of the small bowel report the most dramatic episodes, whereas patients with distal obstructions do not experience as much emesis. The quality of the material vomited may help indicate the level of obstruction, as obstruction in the distal small bowel may produce feculent vomitus. Contrary to common beliefs, **obstruction of the large bowel often is not associated with vomiting**, because the presence of a competent ileocecal valve (found in 50 to 60 percent of individuals) may contribute to a closed-loop obstruction.

Absence of bowel movements and flatus are suggestive of a high-grade or complete obstruction. With the stimulation of peristalsis at the initiation of an obstructive episode, it is not unusual for a patient to describe having bowel movements. The presence of a recent bowel movement does not rule out the diagnosis of a bowel obstruction. The classic description of decreased stool caliber is not frequently reported by patients with large-bowel obstruction, and when reported, this finding is not specific for colonic obstruction. On the other hand, diarrhea is frequently reported by patients with progressive large-bowel obstruction. Presumably, with increased narrowing of the bowel lumen, passage of the solid and semisolid contents are blocked, therefore the stools become more liquid in character. Distension to some degree is generally found in most patients with intestinal obstruction; however, this finding may be absent in patients with obstruction of the proximal small bowel, therefore the absence of distension does not eliminate the possibility of intestinal obstruction.

Patients with uncomplicated obstruction usually have ill-defined nonlocalized abdominal tenderness. The tenderness results from compression of the distended bowel leading to the aggravation of visceral pain. In the case of open-loop obstruction, decompression by emesis or NG tube frequently results in the improvement or resolution of abdominal tenderness. **Localized tenderness is a finding that is infrequently encountered in patients with uncomplicated bowel obstruction**, and its presence **may be associated with complications involving an isolated bowel segment.** The presence of this finding may suggest the presence of a closed loop obstruction, necrosis or perforation, and in a patient without obvious need for urgent operative treatment, further evaluation with CT scan may be helpful.

Management of Small-Bowel Obstruction **When identified early, patients with uncomplicated small bowel obstruction should be managed by NPO, intravenous hydration, and NG tube decompression.** This therapy is directed at correcting the fluid and electrolyte deficits and reversing the cycle of inflammatory and metabolic events associated with an increased intestinal luminal pressure. Many patients with early, partial small-bowel obstruction can be successfully managed without further problems.

Typically, **patients who present late in the course of obstruction are less likely to resolve with nonoperative management**. Furthermore, in these patients with prolonged obstruction, the probability of **bowel ischemia and necrosis** is increased. The development of complicated small-bowel obstruction is associated with increased morbidity and mortality; therefore every effort should be made to identify and initiate early treatment in these patients. No clinical, laboratory, and radiographic criterion will reliably predict and identify patients with small-bowel obstruction who will go on to develop bowel necrosis. **The presence of fever, tachycardia, persistent abdominal pain, abdominal tenderness, leukocytosis, and high-grade obstruction are associated with the increased likelihood of bowel necrosis. These findings should prompt referral to a surgeon.**

The nonoperative approach does not address the source of the small-bowel obstruction. Therefore, prolonged nonoperative therapy would be considered inappropriate for patients with surgically correctable causes such as abdominal wall and groin hernias and obstructing neoplasms. Similarly, patients with no previous abdominal operations and no reason for intraabdominal adhesions should undergo resuscitation and prompt evaluation to identify a possibly treatable source of obstruction.

Management of Large-Bowel Obstruction Patients with **large-bowel obstruction are generally dehydrated** and should be managed with **nasogastric suction, intravenous fluid hydration, and monitored closely for the response to fluid** resuscitation. Patients with inappropriate response to fluid resuscitation should be admitted to an intensive care unit where invasive monitoring may be used to guide the resuscitation efforts.

The major diagnostic dilemma in patients with suspected large-bowel obstruction is differentiating mechanical obstruction from functional obstruction. In most patients, a **CT scan** will help make the differentiation. When mechanical and functional obstruction cannot be differentiated by CT imaging, a contrast enema without bowel preparation may be obtained.

Colorectal carcinoma is by far the most common cause of mechanical large-bowel obstruction. The site of obstruction of colon carcinoma correlates to the luminal diameter of the large bowel, rather than with the frequency of distribution of carcinoma. The generally reported frequency of distribution of obstructing colorectal carcinoma is **splenic flexure (40 percent), hepatic flexure (25 percent), descending and sigmoid colon (25 percent), transverse colon (10 percent), and ascending colon and cecum (10 percent)**. Less commonly, sigmoid volvulus, and diverticular disease may cause large-bowel obstruction. In these settings the plain radiographs generally will identify the sigmoid volvulus. When identified, the volvulus may be evaluated and resolved by proctosigmoidoscopy performed without bowel preparation. Because nearly all patients with large-bowel obstruction will require operative treatment, surgical consultations should be obtained early in these patients.

One of the most devastating complications associated with large-bowel obstruction is colonic perforation, which generally occurs in the cecum or right colon. **The risk for developing colonic perforation is increased among patients with severely dilated colon (>10 cm cecal diameter).** These patients may or may not present with frank peritonitis; however, most patients will have severe volume contraction as a consequence of the ongoing inflammatory changes. The diagnosis of colonic perforation should be entertained when patients fail to improve with aggressive fluid management.

Comprehension Questions

[18.1] A 44-year-old woman with a past history of appendicitis that was treated by appendectomy 2 years ago presents with abdominal pain of 4-days' duration. Her temperature is 38.5°C (101.3°F), pulse rate is 120 beats per minute, and blood pressure is 100/84 mmHg. Her abdomen is distended and diffusely tender, with guarding. An occasional, high-pitched bowel sound is present. A kidneys, ureters, bladder (KUB) x-ray reveals a markedly dilated small bowel without air or stool in the colon. Which of the following is the most appropriate course of management?

A. Place IV, NG tube, and Foley catheter, initiate broad-spectrum antibiotics, and obtain CT of abdomen

B. Place IV, NG tube, and Foley catheter, initiate broad-spectrum antibiotics, and prepare patient for operation

C. Place IV, NG tube, and Foley catheter, initiate broad-spectrum antibiotics, and attempt nonoperative treatment

D. Place IV, NG tube, and Foley catheter, initiate broad-spectrum antibiotics, obtain CT scan of abdomen, and prepare patient for an operation

[18.2] Which of the following is the most likely cause of small-bowel obstruction in 25-year-old woman with no previous abdominal operations?

A. Adhesions

B. Hernia

C. Crohn disease

D. Adenocarcinoma of the small bowel

[18.3] Which of the following approaches is *least likely* to help differentiate a functional obstruction from a mechanical obstruction in a 90-year-old female with Alzheimer disease, urinary tract infection, and abdominal distension?

A. CT scan of the abdomen
B. Four-view radiographs of the abdomen
C. Barium enema
D. History and physical examination

Answers

[18.1] B. This patient presents with signs and symptoms of high-grade small-bowel obstruction. The physical examination is highly suspicious for presence of intraabdominal complications associated with the obstruction, therefore CT scan is unlikely to contribute further in the diagnosis, and nonoperative therapy is inappropriate for a patient with suspected complicated small-bowel obstruction.

[18.2] B. Hernia would be the most likely cause of small bowel obstruction in a patient without previous abdominal operations or other causes of adhesions.

[18.3] D. History and physical examination is often inadequate in differentiating mechanical large-bowel obstruction from functional large bowel obstruction, and this would be especially true in a patient with Alzheimer disease and possible cause for functional large-bowel obstruction.

CLINICAL PEARLS

❖ Persistent pain in a patient with small-bowel obstruction is usually suggestive of bowel ischemia or impending bowel necrosis.

❖ Localized tenderness in a patient with small bowel obstruction may indicate an isolated segment of closed-loop obstruction, localized ischemic injury, or localized perforation.

❖ Because the symptoms and physical findings associated with large-bowel obstruction are nonspecific, they can be easily overlooked by both the patient and the physician.

❖ **Adhesions** represent the most common cause of **small-bowel obstruction,** whereas **colorectal carcinoma** is the most common cause of **large-bowel obstruction**.

REFERENCES

Drazan KE, Corman ML. Large bowel obstruction. In: Cameron JL, ed. Current surgical therapy, 6th ed. St Louis: Mosby-Year Book, 1998:186–90.

Hodin RA, Mathews JB. Small intestine. In: Norton JA, Bollinger RR, Chang AE, et al., eds. Surgery: basic science and clinical evidence. New York: Springer, 2001:617–46.

A 19-year-old female is brought into the emergency department (ED) complaining of abdominal pain and diarrhea of 3 days' duration. She has also been nauseous and has not been able to drink much liquids. Five days ago she returned from a camping trip in New Mexico, but did not drink from natural streams. She denies fever, but states that she has had some chills. Her stools have been watery, brown, and profuse. The patient denies health problems. On examination, the patient is thin and pale. Her mucous membranes are dry. Her temperature is 37.2°C (99°F), heart rate 110 beats per minute, and blood pressure 90/60 mmHg. The skin has no lesions. Her heart and lung examinations are unremarkable except for tachycardia. The abdominal examination reveals hyperactive bowel sounds and no masses. There is diffuse mild tenderness but no guarding or rebound. Rectal examination demonstrates no tenderness or masses, and is guaiac negative. The complete blood count reveals a leukocyte count of 16,000 cells/mm^3. The pregnancy test is negative.

◆ **What is your most likely diagnosis?**

◆ **What is your next diagnostic step?**

◆ **What is the next step in therapy?**

ANSWERS TO CASE 19: Acute Diarrhea

Summary: A 19-year-old healthy female presents to the ED with a 3-day history of abdominal pain, nausea, and nonbloody, watery, profuse diarrhea. Five days ago, she was on a camping trip in New Mexico but did not drink from natural streams. Her mucous membranes are dry. Her temperature is 37.2°C (99°F), heart rate 110 beats per minute, and blood pressure 90/60 mmHg. The abdominal examination reveals hyperactive bowel sounds, no masses, and diffuse mild tenderness without peritoneal signs. Rectal examination is occult blood negative. The leukocyte count is 16,000 cells/mm^3. The pregnancy test is negative.

◆ **Most likely diagnosis:** acute diarrhea with volume depletion and possible electrolyte abnormalities

◆ **Next diagnostic step:** Stool for fecal leukocytes

◆ **Next step in therapy:** Intravenous fluid hydration

Analysis

Objectives

1. Know a diagnostic approach to acute diarrhea including the role of fecal leukocytes and assessment for occult blood in the stools.
2. Understand that volume replacement and correction of electrolyte abnormalities are the first priorities in treatment of diarrhea.
3. Be familiar with a rational workup for acute diarrhea, and know the common etiologies of diarrhea, including *Escherichia coli, Shigella, Salmonella, Giardia,* and amebiasis.

Considerations

This 19-year-old woman developed severe diarrhea and nausea. Her most immediate problem is volume depletion as evidenced by her dry mucous membranes, tachycardia, and hypotension. The **first priority** should be **acute replacement of intravascular volume**, usually with **intravenous normal saline**. The electrolytes should be assessed and abnormalities such as hypokalemia should be corrected. After volume repletion, the next priority is to determine the etiology of the diarrhea. **Up to 90 percent of acute diarrhea is infectious in etiology**. This patient does not have a history consistent with inflammatory bowel disease or prior abdominal surgeries. She had been camping in New Mexico recently which predisposes her to several pathogens: *E. coli, Campylobacter, Shigella, Salmonella,* and *Giardia*. She does not have grossly bloody stools which would usually mandate an evaluation, and suggest invasive bacterial infections such as hemorrhagic or enteroinvasive *E. coli* species, *Yersinia* species, *Shigella,* and *Entamoeba histolytica*. Additionally, the stool for occult blood is negative. Fecal leukocyte examination is an inexpensive and good test to differentiate the various types of infectious diarrhea.

If the fecal leukocytes are present in the stool, the ED physician may have a higher suspicion for *Salmonella, Shigella, Campylobacter, Clostridium difficile, Yersinia,* enterohemorrhagic and enteroinvasive *E. coli,* and *E. histolytica.* Stool cultures may be helpful. In general, ova and parasite evaluation is unhelpful unless the history strongly points toward a parasitic source, or the diarrhea is prolonged. Most diarrhea is self-limited, and does not need evaluation. Table 19-1 summarizes the danger signs. Because of the severity of this patient's symptoms, empiric antibiotic therapy such as with ciprofloxacin (Cipro) might be indicated.

APPROACH TO ACUTE DIARRHEA

Definitions

Acute diarrhea: present for less than 2 weeks' duration.
Chronic diarrhea: diarrhea present for greater than 4 weeks' duration.
Diarrhea: passage of abnormally liquid or poorly formed stool in increased frequency.
Subacute (persistent) diarrhea: present for 2 to 4 weeks' duration.

Clinical Approach

Etiologies   Approximately 90 percent of acute diarrhea is caused by infectious etiologies, and the remainder is caused by medications, ischemia, or toxins. Infectious etiologies often depend on the patient population. For instance, **travelers to Mexico or Asia will frequently contract enterotoxigenic *E. coli* as a causative agent.** Those traveling to Russia and campers and backpackers will often be affected by *Giardia. Campylobacter, Shigella,* and *Salmonella* are also common causative agents.

Consumption of foods is also frequently a culprit. ***Salmonella* or *Shigella*** can be found in **undercooked chicken, enterohemorrhagic *E. coli* in undercooked hamburger**, and ***Staphylococcus aureus* or *Salmonella* in mayonnaise. Raw seafood may harbor *Vibrio*, *Salmonella*,** or hepatitis A, B, or C. Sometimes the timing of the diarrhea following food ingestion is helpful. For example, illness within **6 hours of eating a salad** (mayonnaise) suggests ***S. aureus*, 8 to 12 hours postingestion suggests *Clostridium perfringens*, and 12 to 14 hours postingestion suggests *E. coli*** (see Table 19-1).

Daycare settings are particularly common locales for *Shigella, Giardia,* and rotavirus transmission. Patients in nursing homes or who were recently in the hospital may develop *C. difficile* colitis from antibiotic use.

Clinical Presentation   Most patients with acute diarrhea have self-limited processes, and do not require much workup. Exceptions to this rule include **profuse diarrhea, dehydration, fever exceeding 38.5°C (101.3°F), grossly bloody diarrhea, an elderly patient, severe abdominal pain, duration exceeding 48 hours without improvement, and an immunocompromised patient.**

Table 19-1

ETIOLOGIES OF DIARRHEA

ETIOLOGIC AGENT	INCUBATION TIME	DIARRHEA	EMESIS	ABDOMINAL PAIN	FEVER	COMMENTS
Staphylococcus aureus, Clostridium perfringens	4–12 hours	Watery, profuse	Pronounced	Mild	Absent	Preforming toxin, may be in foods
Vibrio cholerae, entero-toxigenic *Escherichia coli*	8–72 hours	Watery, profuse	Moderate	Mild	Absent	Enterotoxin produced
E. Coli, Giardia	2–7 days	Variable, watery	Mild	Moderate	Variable	Enteroadherent or entero-pathogenic
Hemorrhagic *E. coli, Clostridium difficile*	1–3 days	Variable, often bloody	Mild	Severe	Mild	Cytotoxin producing, causing cell necrosis and inflammation
Salmonella, Campylobacter, Shigella, enteroinvasive *E. coli, Entamoeba histolytica*	1–4 days	Often bloody	Mild	Severe	Moderate to high	Invasive organisms leading to inflammation, abdominal pain and fever

Source: Ahlquist DA, Camilleri M. Diarrhea and constipation. In: Braunwald E, Faucis AS, Kaspar DL, et al. Harrison's principles of internal medicine, 15th ed. New York: McGraw Hill, 2001.

The history should be meticulous about trying to identify bowel processes that may be causative, exposures, including medications and foods, travel history, and other friends or family members with similar symptoms. A history of a viral illness may provide a clue to the etiology. Occupational history may be helpful. The clinician should determine what the patient can tolerate orally; in other words, if the patient is both vomiting and having profuse diarrhea, severe dehydration is likely. The amount and character of the stools may be helpful.

The physical examination should focus on the vital signs, clinical impression of the volume status, degree of sepsis, mental status, and abdominal examination. Volume status is determined by observing whether the mucous membranes are moist or dry, skin has good turgor or is tenting, jugular venous distention, and capillary refill. The principal laboratory test is the stool for microscopic and microbiological examination; usually it is sent for culture, but these results often require several days and are not useful in the ED setting. Ova and parasite evaluation is generally unhelpful except in selected circumstances of very high suspicion. Stool test for *C. difficile* **toxin** may yield the etiology in patients who develop symptoms after **antibiotic use**. Although classically associated with clindamycin, any antibiotic can cause pseudomembranous colitis. A complete blood count, electrolytes, and renal function tests are sometimes indicated.

If the etiology is still unclear and the patient is not improving while off oral intake, hospital admission and consultation with a gastroenterologist may be indicated. Radiological studies or endoscopy may be needed to find the cause. Diseases such as inflammatory bowel disease or ischemic bowel disease must be considered.

Treatment **Fluid and electrolyte replacement are fundamental to the treatment of acute diarrhea.** For mildly dehydrated individuals who can tolerate oral fluids, **sports drinks** such as Gatorade orally is often all that is needed. For those with more serious volume deficits, or elderly patients or infants, hospitalization and intravenous hydration is generally necessary. **Bismuth subsalicylate** may be used to alleviate the gastrointestinal symptoms, but should not be used in an immunocompromised individual because of the risk of bismuth encephalopathy. Many physicians choose to treat patients with moderately ill or severely ill appearance empirically with ciprofloxacin 500 mg twice daily for 5 days. Antimicrobial treatment may not alter the course of the disease.

Traveler's Prophylaxis The best method of preventing traveler's diarrhea, which is principally caused by enterotoxigenic *E. coli*, is avoidance of food and water in areas of high risk. Travelers should be advised to drink only bottled water, and avoid eating foods from street vendors or unhygienic locations. Peeled fruit should be avoided unless the traveler peels it himself/herself. The CDC endorses **bismuth subsalicylate, two 262-mg tablets chewed well four**

times a day (with meals and at bedtime), but does not advocate the use of antimicrobial agents because a false sense of security or the development of antibiotic resistance. Nevertheless, many practitioners prescribe **ciprofloxacin 500 mg once a day. Medical prophylaxis (either bismuth subsalicylate or antibiotic) should not be used for longer than 3 weeks**.

Comprehension Questions

Match the following etiologies (A to E) to the clinical situation in questions [19.1] to [19.4]:

A. *E. coli*
B. *Giardia*
C. Rotavirus
D. *S. aureus*
E. *Vibrio*
F. *Cryptosporidium*

[19.1] During the winter, a 24-year-old woman who works at a daycare center develops profuse watery diarrhea.

[19.2] A 22-year-old college student takes a trip during spring break to Cozumel and develops diarrhea.

[19.3] Several workers develop watery diarrhea and significant emesis within 4 hours after eating food at a potluck dinner.

[19.4] A 45-year-old man eats raw oysters and 2 days later develops abdominal cramping, fever to 38.3°C (101°F), and watery diarrhea

Answers

[19.1] **C.** Rotavirus usually causes a watery diarrhea, and is especially common in the winter.

[19.2] **A.** *E. coli* is the most common etiology for traveler's diarrhea.

[19.3] **D.** *S. aureus* usually causes prominent vomiting and diarrhea within a few hours of food ingestion as a consequence of the toxin produced.

[19.4] **E.** Raw seafood may harbor *Vibrio* species.

CLINICAL PEARLS

❖ The vast majority of acute diarrhea is caused by an infectious etiology.
❖ Most acute diarrheas are self-limited.
❖ One should be cautious when assessing acute diarrhea in immunosuppressed patients, very young, or elderly patients.

❖ Significant dehydration, grossly bloody diarrhea, high fever, and lack of improvement after 48 hours are warning signs of possible complicated diarrhea.

❖ In general, acute uncomplicated diarrhea can be treated with oral electrolyte-fluid solution with or without empiric ciprofloxacin.

REFERENCES

Ahlquist DA, Camilleri M. Diarrhea and constipation. In: Braunwald E, Fauci AS, et al., eds. Harrison's principles of internal medicine, 15th ed. New York: McGraw-Hill, 2001

Centers for Disease Control and Prevention. 2003. Available at: www.cdc.gov/travel/diarrhea.htm. Accessed 6/23/04.

A 30-year-old white male presents to the emergency department (ED) complaining of the sudden onset of abdominal bloating and back pain. The patient states that he was sleeping comfortably but the sudden onset of severe, constant pain that radiates from his back to his abdomen and down toward his scrotum caused him to awaken. He is unable to find a comfortable position and feels best when ambulating. He admits to having had occasional hematuria but denies ever having this type of pain before. He has no other significant medical problems. On physical exam the patient is diaphoretic and in moderate distress. His blood pressure is 128/76 mmHg, heart rate is 90 beats per minute, temperature is 37.4°C (99.4°F), and his respiratory rate is 28 breaths per minute. His cardiovascular exam reveals tachycardia without murmurs. Lung exam is clear to auscultation. Abdominal exam demonstrates good bowel sounds, no abdominal distension and costovertebral angle tenderness. A midstream voided urine specimen demonstrates gross hematuria.

◆ **What is the most likely diagnosis?**

◆ **How would you confirm the diagnosis?**

◆ **What is the next step in treatment?**

ANSWERS TO CASE 20: Nephrolithiasis

Summary: A 30-year-old healthy male complains of the acute onset of severe back pain and a history of gross hematuria. He appears to be in moderate distress and has not previously experienced these symptoms.

◆ **Most likely diagnosis:** Nephrolithiasis.

◆ **Confirmation of the diagnosis:** Perform a urinalysis, complete blood count (CBC), serum chemistries, kidneys, ureters, bladder (KUB) radiograph, intravenous pyelogram or computed tomography (CT) scan of the abdomen.

◆ **Next step:** Start IV fluids and provide adequate pain management for the patient before sending him for the appropriate imaging study. Strain all urine once the diagnosis of nephrolithiasis is suspected and perform stone analysis on any stone passed.

Analysis

Objectives

1. Recognize the history and typical presentation of a patient with nephrolithiasis.
2. Be able to order the appropriate laboratory and radiographic studies to diagnose nephrolithiasis.
3. Know how to treat and manage nephrolithiasis in an acute situation.

Considerations

This patient has a very typical presentation for nephrolithiasis; male (three times more common in men than in women) and the history of the sudden onset of pain that radiates from his back toward his abdomen. The emergency department physician must be careful to rule out any other acute abdominal etiologies that may mimic the same presentation (Table 20-1 lists the differential diagnosis). Patients with nephrolithiasis often have difficulty in finding a comfortable position. Patients with an acute abdomen often feel better when they remain supine without moving or with their knees bent toward their chest. The pain can be described as constant, colicky, or they may describe it as waxing and waning. A history of dark-brown tinged urine may represent old blood in the urine (i.e., from a stone high in the calyx) while a complaint of bright red blood in the urine, may be more consistent with a lower urinary tract stone. A family history of nephrolithiasis or a personal history of stones within the urinary tract may make the diagnosis easier. On physical exam, the patient is normotensive and afebrile, but tachycardic. The presence of fever would suggest urinary tract infection such as pyelonephritis or some other disease process (appendicitis). The increase in heart rate is most likely related to his pain. Furthermore, costovertebral angle tenderness and hematuria on urinalysis are highly suggestive of a urinary tract process.

APPROACH TO NEPHROLITHIASIS

Definitions

Calcium oxalate: the most common type of renal stone is radiopaque.

Extracorporeal Shock Wave Lithotripsy (ESWL): fluoroscopically focused shockwaves result in disintegration of the stone into fragments that are usually small enough to pass in the urine.

Nephrolithiasis: a condition in which stone formation has occurred within the urinary tract system.

Clinical Approach

Epidemiology   The incidence of stone formation within the United States depends on a multitude of extrinsic and intrinsic risk factors, such as socioeconomic status, diet, occupation, climate, medications, sex and age (Table 20-2). **Nephrolithiasis is more common in males** than in females (3:1) and has its peak incidence between the ages of 30 and 50 years. Individuals exposed to high temperature either by geographic location or through occupation are at an increased risk of dehydration, which can increase the risk of stone formation. Also, individuals with excessive sun exposure have increased calcium absorption because of increased vitamin D production. Medications can also predispose individuals to stone formation. **Calcium oxalate stones are the most**

Table 20-1

DIFFERENTIAL DIAGNOSIS OF NEPHROLITHIASIS

Appendicitis

Ectopic pregnancy

Salpingitis

Diverticulitis

Bowel obstruction

Renal artery embolism

Biliary stones

Ovarian torsion

Peptic ulcer disease

Abdominal aortic aneurysm

Gastroenteritis

common types and they account for greater that 75 percent of stones. The remainder of stones vary in type and include magnesium ammonium phosphate, calcium phosphate, uric acid, and cystine stones. **Magnesium ammonium phosphate stones are more common in women and are usually associated with urease-producing organisms.**

Clinical Presentation The vast majority of patients with renal stones will present to the emergency department complaining of **acute onset colicky or noncolicky renal pain**. Noncolicky pain is most likely caused by an upper urinary tract stone, whereas colicky pain is most likely caused by the stretching caused by the stone in the ureter. In addition, the presenting symptoms may be tachycardia, tachypnea, and hypertension all related to the severity of the pain. **Fever, pyuria, and severe costovertebral angle tenderness usually indicate a medical emergency, because pyelonephritis caused by obstruction often leads** to sepsis and rapid deterioration. Persistent nausea and vomiting because of stimulation of the celiac ganglion may require the patient to be hospitalized.

A dipstick and microscopic examination of the voided midstream urine is very helpful, but the **amount of hematuria does not correlate with the degree of obstruction**. Although microscopic hematuria is present in 90 percent of cases involving nephrolithiasis, a complete ureteral obstruction may present without hematuria. A careful analysis of urine sediment for crystals by an experienced individual should be performed promptly. In addition to the microscopic evaluation, a culture and sensitivity test should be performed.

A KUB radiograph is sometimes helpful in identifying a urinary tract stone (90 percent are radiopaque). Traditionally, the intravenous pyelogram (IVP)

Table 20-2
RISK FACTORS

Metabolic factors	Environmental factors
Hypercalciuria	Hot, dry, increased sunlight
Hyperuricosuria	Drugs
Hypocitraturia	Loop diuretics
Hyperoxaluria	Antacids
Primary hyperparathyroidism	Acetazolamide
Renal tubular acidosis	Glucocorticoids
Age	Theophylline
30-50 years	Allopurinol
Sex	Probenecid
Male 3:1	Triamterene
Diet	Acyclovir
Increased intake of calcium,	Indinavir
protein and oxalate	Vitamins D and C
Socioeconomic status	

has been the gold standard in evaluating a renal stone because it gives information about degree of obstruction as well as renal function. In many institutions, **newer-generation helical CT imaging without contrast is used as the imaging method of choice for acute renal colic**; its sensitivity and specificity seems to approach that of the IVP, but renal function is not assessed. CT imaging also has the advantage of assessing the appendix, aorta, and diverticulitis. Regardless of test, the clinician should interpret the clinical picture in conjunction with the imaging results. Before an IVP, the patient should be questioned about allergy to contrast dye or shellfish, the possibility of pregnancy, and preexisting renal disease. Pregnant women and children generally should have ultrasound imaging first to avoid the radiation exposure. Table 20-3 lists the risk factors of nephrotoxicity associated with contrast dye.

Management   **The critical issues surrounding nephrolithiasis are pain control, degree of obstruction, and presence of infection.** Adequate analgesia is critical in treating a patient with nephrolithiasis, and should not be delayed pending test results. Depending on the severity of the pain, intravenous opiates, acetaminophen with codeine, meperidine, nonsteroidal antiinflammatory agents (NSAIDs), or morphine may be necessary. **NSAIDs should be used with caution in patients with renal insufficiency, in older patients, and in those with diabetes mellitus.** Evaluation of the patient's volume status will determine how much and what kind of intravenous fluids are necessary. Excessive hydration to dislodge a stone is not therapeutic and should not be attempted. Because definitive therapy is guided by the type of stones that are being formed, recovery of any passed stones and straining all urine is important for long-term management.

Table 20-3
RISK FACTORS FOR NEPHROTOXICITY WITH CONTRAST DYE

Age >60 years

Dehydration

Hypotension

Multiple myeloma

Hyperuricemia

History of intravenous contrast within 72 hours

Debilitated condition

Known cardiovascular disease, especially on a diuretic

Asthma

Renal insufficiency

Diabetes mellitus

Conservative management, including analgesics, hydration, and antibiotics if urinary tract infection is suspected, may be all the patient needs. **Indications for urgent urological consultation** are **inadequate oral pain control, persistent nausea and vomiting, associated pyelonephritis, large stone (>5–8 mm), solitary kidney, or complete obstruction.** If the patient is being managed expectantly, the patient should be instructed to increase fluid intake and strain the urine until the stone is passed. Surgery is indicated on patients with stones larger than 5–8 mm, persistent pain, or failure to pass the stone despite conservative management. Stones located in the lower urinary tract system may be removed using a ureteroscope; upper urinary tract stones can be treated by ESWL.

Comprehension Questions

[20.1] After passing a kidney stone, a 38-year-old female is told by her primary care physician that she had passed a magnesium ammonium phosphate stone. She is most likely to have had a urinary infection caused by which of the following organisms?

A. *Proteus*
B. *Escherichia coli*
C. *Enterococcus* species
D. Group B streptococcus

[20.2] A 55-year-old male presents to the emergency department complaining of right flank pain for the past 2 weeks. He has noted some gross hematuria and has been unable to eat anything secondary to nausea and vomiting. Which of the following is an indication for hospitalization?

A. Gross hematuria
B. Right flank pain
C. Nausea and vomiting despite antiemetics
D. Age greater than 50 years

[20.3] A 39-year-old female complains of the sudden onset of severe left flank pain after running a marathon. She describes the pain as constant with radiation to her left groin area. A urinalysis shows microscopic hematuria and the presence of cystine crystals. Where is the stone most likely to be located?

A. Renal pelvis
B. Proximal ureter
C. Distal ureter
D. Ureterovesicular junction

[20.4] A 33-year-old woman is pregnant at 14 weeks' gestation and presents with right flank pain and gross hematuria. She is afebrile. Which of the following imaging tests is most appropriate for this patient?

A. Ultrasonography
B. KUB
C. IVP
D. Retrograde pyelography
E. Helical CT imaging without contrast

Answers

[20.1] **A.** This woman has a magnesium ammonium phosphate stone, which is common in women and is associated with urease-producing organisms. *Proteus, Pseudomonas*, and *Klebsiella* are all urease-producing organisms.

[20.2] **C.** Hospitalization is required if the patient is unable to tolerate anything by mouth. Gross hematuria and flank pain are expected with nephrolithiasis. Appropriate analgesics should be prescribed for patients if they will not be hospitalized.

[20.3] **A.** Constant pain is most likely to be located in the kidney. Colicky pain is most likely to be located in the ureter and is caused by the stretching caused by the stone and inflammatory processes in the lumen of the ureter.

[20.4] **A.** Because the patient is pregnant, the initial imaging test should be sonography to avoid the radiation risks to the fetus.

CLINICAL PEARLS

❖ The acute presentation of nephrolithiasis resembles other pathologies; the correct studies and appropriate interpretation of laboratory data will help to establish the diagnosis.

❖ Any patient with severe nausea, vomiting, fever, or signs of infection should be hospitalized.

❖ Adequate pain control for patients with suspected nephrolithiasis is a priority even before all test results return.

❖ All urine should be strained to confirm the diagnosis and for the stone composition to be discerned.

❖ The absence of pain does not mean followup is unnecessary. Identifying the etiology of stone formation is important to prevent recurrence.

REFERENCES

Massry, SG, Glassrock RJ. Nephrolithiasis. In: Textbook of nephrology, 4th ed. Baltimore: Lippincott Williams & Wilkins, 2001:1017–38.

Pahira JJ, Schwartz GR. Renal calculi (kidney stones). In: Schwartz GR, Hanke BK, Mayer TA, eds. Principles and practice of emergency medicine, 4th ed. Lippincott Williams & Wilkins, 2001:766–70.

Tanagho EA. Urinary stone disease. In: Smith's general urology, 15th ed. New York: McGraw-Hill, 2000:291–317.

Tintinalli JE, Kelen GD, Stapczynski JS, eds. Emergency medicine, 6th ed. New York: McGraw-Hill, 2004:624–6.

A 64-year-old white male presents to the emergency department complaining of the inability to urinate for the past 24 hours. In addition, he complains of being constipated for the past 4 weeks, weight loss of 20 lb in the past 6 months, a decrease in energy, and occasional night sweats. He has not seen a physician in the past 6 years. On examination, he is thin and in moderate distress. His blood pressure is 168/92 mmHg, heart rate is 95 beats per minute, temperature is 37.7°C (98.8°F), and respiratory rate is 22 breaths per minute. His cardiovascular exam reveals a regular rate and rhythm without murmurs. His lung exam is clear to auscultation. The abdominal examination reveals tenderness to palpation in the suprapubic area with normal bowel sounds. Rectal examination demonstrates guaiac positive stool and a firm somewhat irregular prostate gland. A basic metabolic panel demonstrates an elevated blood urea nitrogen (BUN) level.

◆ **What is the most likely diagnosis?**

◆ **How would you confirm the diagnosis?**

◆ **What is the next step in treatment?**

ANSWERS TO CASE 21: Acute Urinary Retention

Summary: A 64-year-old male presents to the emergency department with a complete inability to void for the past 24 hours and tenderness in the lower abdomen. The patient also has symptoms highly suggestive of prostate cancer, including weight loss, decrease in energy, night sweats, and an enlarged irregular prostate gland.

◆ **Most likely diagnosis:** acute urinary retention likely caused by prostatic carcinoma.

◆ **Confirming the diagnosis:** thorough history and physical examination including a rectal examination, insertion of a urethral catheter, urinalysis, blood count, electrolytes and renal function tests, prostate-specific antigen.

◆ **Next therapeutic step:** relieving pain associated with urinary retention by inserting a urethral catheter and treating the underlying etiology.

Analysis

Objectives

1. Know how to treat and manage acute urinary retention in the emergency department.
2. Recognize typical physical examination signs and symptoms of acute urinary retention.
3. Be able to recognize when it is necessary to admit the patient into the hospital.

Considerations

This patient's history of weight loss, fatigue, and night sweats suggests a prostate carcinoma as the etiology for his acute urinary retention. Although this patient's prostate exam gives typical signs for prostate pathology, a benign exam does not eliminate it as a cause for the obstruction. There are many causes of acute urinary retention (Table 21-1). The patient's inability to void for the past 24 hours was most likely preceded by a history of hesitancy, nocturia, dribbling, prior history of retention, and poor stream. In addition to urinary obstruction, a mass may also cause rectal obstruction causing constipation and abdominal pain. This patient is in moderate distress, his blood pressure and pulse are slightly elevated, and this is most likely related to pain associated with urinary retention. **The patient's BUN level is elevated, suggesting significant reabsorption secondary to the obstruction.** Admission to the hospital may be prudent, because **the elevated BUN increases the likelihood of postobstruction diuresis**. Hematuria may also be present because of stones, tumor, or infection. Passage of a urethral catheter to alleviate the obstruction will bring about pain relief. Lubrication of the catheter with lidocaine jelly is often appreciated.

Table 21-1
COMMON CAUSES OF URINARY RETENTION

Phimosis	Calculus
Meatal stenosis	Hematoma
Foreign body	Benign prostatic hypertrophy
Carcinoma	Bladder neck contracture
Prostatitis	Spinal cord syndromes
Diabetes	Multiple sclerosis
Herpes zoster	Medications

APPROACH TO ACUTE URINARY RETENTION

Definitions

Acute urinary retention: complete inability to void accompanied by abdominal discomfort, with a palpable or percussible bladder containing greater than 150 mL of urine.

Azotemia: presence of nitrogenous bodies, especially urea, in the blood that develops in urinary tract obstruction when overall excretion function is impaired.

Benign prostatic hyperplasia: overgrowth and proliferation of the epithelium and fibromuscular tissue of the prostate.

Hydronephrosis: dilation of the renal pyelocalyceal system because of obstruction of the urinary tract system.

Clinical Approach

Because untreated urinary obstruction may lead to chronic renal failure, relieving the blockage is critical. Loss of urinary concentrating ability, azotemia, renal tubular acidosis, hyperkalemia, and renal salt wasting may occur. Hypertension is common in acute urinary retention because of the increased release of renin by the involved kidneys. The most common presenting symptoms are **urinary hesitancy, decreased force, terminal dribbling, nocturia, and overflow incontinence** (Table 21-2). Pain is the symptom that usually provokes the need for an emergency department evaluation. A detailed history and physical will help to identify the exact cause of the obstruction. History of previous stricture, trauma, neurological disease, prostatectomy, or venereal disease may aid in the proper diagnosis and treatment. Evaluation of medications taken may help in identifying pharmacological agents that may contribute to urinary retention (Table 21-3). On physical exam, a palpable mass above the symphysis that disappears after insertion of a urethral catheter is highly suggestive of acute urinary retention. Digital rectal examination may reveal prostatic nodules, asymmetry, hardened ridges, indurated areas, tenderness, bogginess or the typical stony

Table 21-2

SYMPTOMS OF URINARY RETENTION

Hesitancy	Straining to void
Decrease in force of stream	Sensation of incomplete emptying
Dribble	Urinary frequency
Urinary urgency	Nocturia

Table 21-3

MEDICATIONS THAT MAY CONTRIBUTE TO URINARY RETENTION

Isoproterenol	Atropine
Morphine	Cogentin
Meperidine	Cyclic antidepressants
Dilaudid	Antihistamines
Belladonna	Phenothiazines
Nifedipine	Bentyl
Ditropan	Hyoscyamine
Indomethacin	Diazepam

hard enlargement of prostate cancer. **A urinalysis, electrolytes, and BUN/creatinine levels should be obtained.**

Management   Any individual with acute urinary retention requires relief of the obstruction immediately to prevent progressive renal dysfunction. Initial efforts to relieve painful urinary retention should be attempted with a standard urethral catheter. Lidocaine gel should be placed into the urethra before inserting a 16-French or 18-French catheter. The lidocaine gel will anesthetize, lubricate, and distend the urethra. A 16- or 18-French catheter should pass if a stricture is not present. If the emergency department physician is unable to pass the catheter because of obstruction caused by an enlarged prostate, a finger inserted into the rectum and directing the catheter tip over the median lobe of the prostate while someone inserts the catheter may be helpful. If catheterization attempts fail with a soft rubber catheter, then a coudé catheter may be helpful. Occasionally a catheter may not pass secondary to urethral strictures. **A urethral catheter should never be forced, because urethral trauma and false passages may be created!** In these situations a urologist should be consulted and filiforms followed by sounds may be used. Care should be taken to avoid perforating the urethra or bladder by the rigid instruments. If consultation is not available, a suprapubic catheter may be placed, or percutaneous bladder aspiration may be performed. The bladder should be easily palpable and distended to lessen the risk of complications. After successful bladder drainage, the patient's disposition depends on the risk of postobstructive diuresis that can cause profound fluid loss and electrolyte abnormalities. Prolonged bladder obstruction, older age, or logistic limitations are indications for admission. Many patients, however, can usually be discharged home with an indwelling catheter and be followed up in an outpatient setting. **Patients who have evidence of serious infection, decreased renal function, volume overload, or inability to care for themselves should be admitted.**

Comprehension Questions

[21.1] An 88-year-old female is seen in the ED complaining of significant lower abdominal pain and inability to void. She is noted to have a very full bladder, and urethral catheter is placed with 1400 mL of urine drained. Her blood pressure is 130/64 mmHg, pulse 74 beats per minute, respiratory rate is 20 breaths per minute, temp 37.7°C (99.8°F). Laboratory values include BUN of 65 mg/dL, K 3.4 mEq/L, and urinalysis with moderate leukocyte esterase and many bacteria. What is the next step with this patient?

A. Discharge home with oral hydration and recheck the BUN level in 48 hours
B. Discharge home with home health nurse visits
C. Place the patient on oral antibiotic therapy and followup in 1 week
D. Admit to the hospital for further therapy

[21.2] A 65-year-old male presents to the ED with progressive inability to void, pain, and a lower abdominal mass. He has never experienced this type of pain before and is in moderate discomfort. What is your next step in management?

A. Rectal examination
B. Decompression of bladder with a urethral rubber catheter
C. Computed tomography (CT) scan of the abdomen
D. Percutaneous bladder aspiration

[21.3] A 35-year-old female without any previous medical problems presents to the ED with acute urinary retention. She reports a history of increased fatigue with exertion and paresthesias but denies a history of diabetes, hypertension, or recurrent urinary infections. One year ago, she had some difficulty with double vision, but that completely resolved. What is the most likely diagnosis?

A. Ovarian cancer
B. Multiple sclerosis
C. Drug abuse
D. Spastic bladder

[21.4] A 22-year-old woman complains of acute urinary retention, associated with vulvar burning and tingling. A urethral catheter is placed and the bladder decompressed. Which of the following is the best therapy for this patient?

A. Penicillin
B. Azithromycin
C. Doxycycline
D. Acyclovir
E. Ceftriaxone

Answers

[21.1] **D.** This patient needs to be hospitalized because of inability to care for herself, urinary tract infection, and electrolyte abnormalities.

[21.2] **B.** Decompression of bladder with a rubber urethral catheter should be performed before examination of the prostate. Percutaneous bladder stick is not indicated unless other attempts to decompress the bladder have failed.

[21.3] **B.** Acute urinary retention may be the presenting symptom in a young healthy female with no previous medical problems. Multiple sclerosus is characterized by chronic waxing and waning of symptoms.

[21.4] **D.** This is likely herpes simplex virus, which is associated with acute urinary retention. The treatment would be acyclovir.

CLINICAL PEARLS

❖ Physical examination can provide the information necessary for the accurate diagnosis in most patients with acute urinary retention.

❖ Any patient with evidence of serious infection, decreased renal function, volume overload, or inability to care for themselves should be admitted to the hospital.

❖ Consultation with a urologist may be necessary if catheterization is not accomplished.

❖ Decompression of the bladder should be performed as quickly as possible to prevent further damage to the urinary system.

REFERENCES

Karafin L, Schwartz GR. Renal calculi (kidney stones) In: Principles and practice of emergency medicine, 4th ed. Williams & Wilkins, 2001:762–3.

Harwood-Nuss AL. Selected urologic problems. In: Marx J, Hockberger R, Walls R. Emergency medicine concepts and clinical practice, 5th ed. Mosby, 2002:2245–46.

A 67-year-old man presents with painful blisters over the front of the right chest. The man noticed pain for 2 to 3 days prior to the onset of the blisters. This is the first time he has had these symptoms. He had fever, malaise, congestion, and runny nose for a few days before the onset of the pain and the blisters. He has history of hypertension that is well controlled with hydrochlorothiazide. He is not taking any other medications. He does not have any drug allergies. He does not report contact with poison ivy. On examination, the skin overlying the right fifth rib has a few erythematous maculopapular lesions and a few vesicular lesions.

◆ **What is the most likely diagnosis?**

◆ **What are the complications of this condition?**

◆ **What is the best therapy?**

ANSWERS TO CASE 22: Herpes Zoster

Summary: A 67-year-old man has a 2- to 3-day history of blisters that are painful and that have erupted over his right anterior chest.

 Most likely diagnosis: herpes zoster.

 Associated complications: the complications include pain associated with acute neuritis, postherpetic neuralgia, meningoencephalitis, transverse myelitis, and death, which occurs in 10 percent of patients with bone marrow transplant and varicella-zoster virus (VZV) infection.

 Best therapy: the treatment of herpes zoster includes symptomatic relief and antiviral agents to accelerate resolution of symptoms and to reduce the incidence of postherpetic neuralgia.

Analysis

Objectives

1. Know the clinical features of herpes zoster.
2. Learn about the possible complications of this condition.
3. Understand the treatment of herpes zoster.

Considerations

This 67-year-old man has symptoms of herpes zoster or shingles. His symptoms reflect the reactivation of the latent VZV. The virus infects the dorsal root ganglia during chickenpox where it remains dormant until reactivation, and causes pain in the distribution of the affected dermatome. The pain associated with herpes zoster is often intense, and can persist months, or even years, afterward, particularly in older individuals. Complications that tend to be more common in immunocompromised individuals include meningoencephalitis, disseminated infection, hepatitis, pneumonitis, or ophthalmic involvement. Thus, the patient should be warned about these corresponding symptoms. The diagnosis is largely clinical, and in a straightforward case as above, no further testing is necessary. In unclear cases, a Tzanck smear of the lesion or antigen assays of scrapings may be helpful. This patient may benefit from acyclovir; glucocorticoid therapy is also an option, but has more side effects.

APPROACH TO HERPES ZOSTER

Herpes zoster, or shingles, is a reactivation of the VZV, a deoxyribonucleic acid (DNA) virus that is part of the *Herpesviridae* family. Herpes zoster is **more common in the elderly,** although it can occur in individuals of all ages. It is characterized by **unilateral vesicular eruption of grouped vesicles on an erythematous base within a dermatome.** The eruption is preceded by **pain,**

itching, tingling, or burning sensation within the dermatome, although sometimes bilateral dermatomes or multiple dermatomes can be affected. The initial lesions are erythematous and maculopapular. The lesions are initially few in number and continue to form over 3 to 5 days. The lesions become cloudy after a few days, and become dry, crusted, and scaly after 5 to 10 days. In most cases, pain and dysesthesia last for 1 to 4 weeks; but in others the pain persists for months or years. In immunocompromised individuals, the condition is more severe and protracted.

Virtually any dermatome may be involved in herpes zoster, but the most frequently affected sites are the dermatomes from T3 to L3. Involvement of the ophthalmic branch of the trigeminal nerve causes zoster ophthalmicus. When the sensory branch of the sensory nerve is involved, lesions appear on the ear canal and tongue.

Complications   The most common complications of herpes zoster are pain caused by acute neuritis and postherpetic neuralgia. **Postherpetic neuralgia occurs in 50 percent of patients older than age 50 years, and the symptoms may persist for months after the resolution of the cutaneous lesions.** Central nervous system involvement may occur following localized herpes zoster. Even patients without any signs of meningeal irritation may have changes in the cerebrospinal fluid. Patients with central nervous system involvement show signs of meningeal irritation, such as headache, fever, photophobia, and vomiting.

Cutaneous dissemination of virus, which more often occurs in immunocompromised individuals, is typically associated with pneumonitis, meningoencephalitis, hepatitis and other serious complications. Coxsackievirus infections also cause dermatomal vesicular lesions. Tzanck smear and serological tests can be used to differentiate herpes zoster from coxsackievirus infections.

Treatment   During the acute stage, analgesics and drying, and soothing lotions, such as calamine, help with the pain. After the lesions have dried, repeated application of capsaicin lotion may relieve pain by causing cutaneous anesthesia. **Acyclovir also shortens the duration of acute pain** and speeds the healing of vesicles provided the treatment is begun within 48 hours of the appearance of the rash. **Oral acyclovir (800 mg 5 times daily for 7 to 10 days) seems to be helpful in decreasing the duration of the reactivation**. All patients with **ophthalmic zoster** should receive acyclovir orally; in addition, acyclovir applied topically to the eye is also recommended. **Consultation with an ophthalmologist** may be prudent because visual impairment is a risk. **Immunocompromised patients, or patients with disseminated herpes, should be admitted for intravenous acyclovir. Corticosteroids** such as prednisone (60 mg/d for 7 days, then 30 mg/d for 7 days, then 15 mg/d for 7 days) **may decrease the severity of the postherpetic neuralgia.** It should be used only in healthy individuals because of the side effects, and should not be used concomitantly with acyclovir.

The pain of postherpetic neuralgia is treated with amitriptyline, while carbamazepine is added especially if the pain is of a burning quality. Postherpetic neuralgia eventually subsides even in the most severe and persistent cases. Many of the patients with the most persistent complaints have the symptoms of a depressive state and will often be helped by appropriate antidepressant medications.

Comprehension Questions

[22.1] A 25-year-old healthy man is diagnosed with shingles. Which of the following is the most likely etiology?

    A. Coming in contact with a person with chicken pox
    B. Undiagnosed diabetes mellitus
    C. Stress from work
    D. Undiagnosed immunocompromised state

[22.2] A 58-year-old woman has an outbreak of herpes zoster on her chest wall. One day later, she has photophobia, headache, and nausea. Which of the following is the best next step?

    A. Oral acyclovir
    B. Oral famciclovir
    C. Intravenous acyclovir
    D. Oral prednisone and carbamazepine

[22.3] A 35-year-old man has a macular rash on his chest wall which is possibly caused by herpes zoster. Which of the following would be supportive evidence that this is caused by herpes zoster?

    A. The rash erupted 2 days ago, and now there is a burning sensation
    B. The rash crosses the midline
    C. The rash seems to follow a dermatome distribution
    D. The rash is also on the arms and lower legs

Answers

[22.1] **D.** Young persons under age 40 with herpes zoster should be considered at risk for human immunodeficiency virus (HIV) infection. Although diabetes mellitus can be asymptomatic, it would be less likely than HIV in this circumstance.

[22.2] **C.** This patient likely has meningoencephalitis from the herpes zoster. Admission to the ICU and treatment with intravenous acyclovir is the next step.

[22.3] **C.** The rash of herpes zoster generally comes on after the burning and paresthesias, follows the distribution of a dermatome, and does not often coexist with rashes on the arms and legs.

CLINICAL PEARLS

❖ Herpes zoster in a young, apparently healthy patient should suggest the possibility of HIV infection.

❖ Meningeal symptoms in an individual with herpes zoster may be life-threatening.

❖ Acyclovir therapy likely shortens the length of acute neuralgia and may decrease the likelihood of postherpetic neuralgia.

❖ Herpes zoster in an immunocompromised patient may be life-threatening.

❖ Herpes zoster ophthalmicus should be suspected when lesions appear at the tip of the nose.

REFERENCES

Gilden DH, Mahalingam R, Dueland AN, Cohrs R. Herpes zoster: Pathogenesis and latency. In: Melnick JL, ed. Progress in medical virology, vol. 39. Basel: Karger, 1992:19–75.

Hope-Simpson RE. The nature of herpes zoster: A long-term study and a new hypothesis. Proc R Soc Med 1965;58:9.

Mahalingam R, Wellis M, Wolf W, et al. Latent varicella-zoster viral DNA in human trigeminal and thoracic ganglia. N Engl J Med 1990;323:627.

McKenderick MW, McGill JI, White JE, Wood MJ. Oral Acyclovir in acute herpes zoster. Br Med J 1986;293:1529.

McKenderick MW, McGill JI, Wood MJ. Lack of effect of acyclovir on postherpetic neuralgia. BMJ 1989;298:431.

An 18-year-old female presents to the emergency department complaining of a 1-week history of abdominal pain. She tells you that she and her friends recently returned from spring break vacation in Mexico, and she has noticed a constant ache that is worse on her right side. The patient's mother is worried because her daughter has been unable to eat or drink anything for 2 days and thinks she may have become sick from drinking the water while on vacation. After asking the mother to step out of the room while you examine the girl, she tells you that she has had five sexual partners, occasionally uses condoms for birth control, and has never been pregnant. Her last menstrual period was 2 weeks ago and was heavier than normal. On physical exam, her blood pressure was 100/70 mmHg, pulse 110 beats per minute, respirations 22 breaths per minute, and temperature 38.9°C (102.1°F). Her heart has a regular rate and rhythm without murmurs. Lungs are clear to auscultation bilaterally. The abdominal exam reveals a diffusely tender lower abdomen, greater on the right than left and the patient exhibits voluntary guarding. Examination of the pelvis reveals a greenish, foul-smelling discharge with a friable appearing cervix. Bimanual exam reveals an exquisitely tender cervix with fullness and pain in the right adnexa. Cultures for gonorrhea and chlamydia are collected. The wet prep shows many white blood cells (WBCs), no clue cells, no trichomonas, and no *Candida*. The urine pregnancy test is negative.

◆ **What is the most likely diagnosis?**

◆ **What is your next diagnostic step?**

◆ **What is the next step in your treatment?**

ANSWERS TO CASE 23: Acute Pelvic Inflammatory Disease

Summary: An 18-year-old nulliparous female complains of severe abdominal pain, vaginal discharge, fever, nausea, and vomiting. She displays cervical motion tenderness and her right adnexa is full on examination.

 Most likely diagnosis: pelvic inflammatory disease.

 Next diagnostic step: transvaginal ultrasound to rule out tuboovarian abscess, complete blood count (CBC).

 Next treatment step: admit the patient and start IV antibiotic therapy.

Analysis

Objectives

1. Understand the diagnosis and workup of pelvic inflammatory disease.
2. Know the criteria and treatment for both outpatient and inpatient pelvic inflammatory disease.
3. Know the common differential diagnoses for lower abdominal pain and be able to consult the appropriate specialties based on the physical exam and laboratory studies.

Considerations

This nulliparous woman has lower abdominal pain, fever, abnormal vaginal discharge, adnexal tenderness/fullness, and cervical motion tenderness. Although these symptoms may occur with other diagnoses such as appendicitis, ovarian torsion, ectopic pregnancy, or inflammatory bowel disease, the clinical symptoms are most consistent with pelvic inflammatory disease (PID). **PID is defined as an ascending infection from the vagina or cervix to the upper genital tract,** such as the endometrium, fallopian tubes, or ovaries. Although the etiology may be **polymicrobial**, sexually transmitted organisms such as ***Neisseria gonorrhoeae* or *Chlamydia trachomatis* are implicated in many cases.** Because the disease may mimic other common conditions, a meticulous physical exam, and use of transvaginal ultrasound must be performed to correctly differentiate a gynecological disease from that of a general surgery process.

APPROACH TO PELVIC INFLAMMATORY DISEASE

Definitions

Cervical motion tenderness: also referred to as a "Chandelier sign." Motion of the cervix during bimanual exam elicits extreme tenderness, so as to cause the patient to jump off the bed and "hit the chandelier."

Pelvic inflammatory disease: an ascending infection of microorganisms from the lower genital tract to the upper genital tract that is polymicrobial, but is commonly caused by *N. gonorrhoeae* or *C. trachomatis*. PID may also be termed salpingitis.

Tuboovarian abscess (TOA): a collection of purulent material encompassing the fallopian tube and ovary comprised of predominantly anaerobic organisms. TOAs are a major complication of pelvic inflammatory disease.

Clinical Approach

Pelvic inflammatory disease is an ascending infection from the lower genital tract to the upper genital tract that may be difficult to diagnose due to the variety and severity of presenting symptoms. Risk factors for the development of PID are young age, recent menstruation, multiple sexual partners, no use of barrier contraception, and lower socioeconomic status. Criteria for diagnosis must include **lower abdominal tenderness, adnexal tenderness, and cervical motion tenderness.** Usually, the clinical diagnosis is accurate, but occasionally, the presentation is atypical. Ultrasound imaging or computed tomography (CT) imaging of the abdomen and pelvis may be helpful. The differential diagnosis of acute PID includes appendicitis, ectopic pregnancy, endometriosis, ovarian torsion, hemorrhagic corpus luteum cyst, benign ovarian tumor, and inflammatory bowel disease. Finally, laparoscopy is considered the "gold standard" in establishing the diagnosis, by visualizing purulent discharge from the tube.

The etiology of PID is polymicrobial as many different bacteria are harbored in the vagina. Most commonly, *N. gonorrhoeae* and *C. trachomatis* are isolated from a cervical culture, but other organisms, such as *Bacteroides fragilis, Escherichia coli, Peptostreptococci* sp., *Haemophilus influenzae*, and aerobic streptococci, have been isolated from acute cases of PID. Thus, organisms may be classified as either sexually transmitted organisms or endogenous.

The pathogenesis of PID may include many mechanisms. First, for ascension of infection to develop from the vagina, through the cervical canal, to the endometrium of the uterus, through the fallopian tubes and to the ovaries or peritoneum, there must be a breakdown of the natural host defense system. For instance, hormonal changes unique to a woman's cycle may play a role in the ascending infection. During a normal menstrual cycle, the cervical mucus changes depending on the dominating hormone, either estrogen or progesterone. At mid-cycle, when estrogen predominates and progesterone is low, cervical mucus is thin and may facilitate easy ascension of bacteria. Whereas after ovulation, when progesterone is higher, the cervical mucus is thick and more difficult for bacteria to penetrate. Menses is another time when woman are at greater risk for developing PID because the cervical mucus plug is lost due to outward menstrual flow and organisms may also ascend to the upper genital tract. Retrograde menstrual flow has also been attributed to the risk of bacteria ascending from the uterus into the fallopian tubes, ovaries, or peritoneal cavity.

Table 23-1

CRITERIA FOR HOSPITALIZATION

Surgical emergencies (e.g., appendicitis) cannot be excluded

Pregnancy

Lack of response clinically to oral antimicrobial therapy

Patient is unable to follow or tolerate an outpatient oral regimen

Severe illness, nausea, and vomiting, or high fever

Tuboovarian abscess

Adolescent, nulliparous, or questionable compliance

Presence of an intrauterine device

Table 23-2

THERAPY FOR PELVIC INFLAMMATORY DISEASE

Outpatient therapy
1. Ofloxacin 400 mg PO bid for 14 days or levofloxacin 500 mg PO qd for 14 days (preferably >18 years of age because of concern regarding adverse effects on cartilage) with or without metronidazole 500 mg PO bid for 14 days
2. Ceftriaxone 250 mg IM once or cefoxitin 2g IM once and probenecid 1g PO once and doxycycline 100 mg PO bid for 14 days with or without metronidazole 500 mg PO bid for 14 days

Inpatient therapy
1. Cefotetan 2 IV q12h or cefoxitin 2g IV q6h *and* doxycycline 100 mg PO or IV q12h
2. Clindamycin 900 mg IV q8h *and* gentamicin 2 mg/kg IV loading dose followed by 1.5 mg/kg q8h
3. Ofloxacin 400 mg IV q12h *or* levofloxacin 500 mg IV q24h (preferably >18 years of age because of concern regarding adverse effects on cartilage) *with or without* metronidazole 500 mg IV q8h *or* ampicillin-sulbactam 3g IV q6h and doxycycline 100 mg PO or IV q12h

Source: Centers for Disease Control and Prevention. 2002 Guidelines for treatment of sexually transmitted diseases. MMWR Morb Mortal Wkly Rep 2002; 51(RR-6):1

Treatment of PID varies widely depending on the clinical symptoms of the patient. Treatment should be initiated as soon as a presumptive diagnosis has been made in order to prevent long-term sequelae or complications from acute PID. **Uncomplicated PID in a compliant patient may be treated as an outpatient.** However, **certain criteria for hospitalization** exist for the management of complicated PID (Table 23-1). Although IV antibiotics are used to treat the symptoms of PID, laparoscopy is useful in cases with an uncertain diagnosis, suspicion of a ruptured TOA, or when a patient fails to respond to IV antibiotics.

Treatment options can be divided into **oral treatment and parenteral treatment**. Outpatient management includes **ofloxacin 400 mg twice daily (with or without metronidazole 500 mg twice daily) for 14 days** (see Table 23-2). **Followup and treatment of a known sexual partner** is essential for decreasing the incidence of recurrence of PID. Known **complications are infertility, pelvic adhesions leading to chronic pelvic pain, risk of ectopic pregnancy, Fitz-Hugh–Curtis syndrome, and chronic PID.**

Comprehension Questions

Match the following diseases (A to F) to the clinical situation [23.1] to [23.4]:

A. Ectopic pregnancy
B. Appendicitis
C. Gastroesophageal reflux disease (GERD)
D. Crohn disease
E. Cholelithiasis
F. Pancreatitis
G. Ovarian torsion

[23.1] A 21-year-old woman experiences crampy abdominal pain that begins near the umbilicus and moves to the lower right quadrant. The pain has progressed over days, and is intermittent and crampy. The patient is afebrile and complains of some nausea.

[23.2] A 41-year-old woman complains of pain in the upper abdomen especially after eating. The pain seems to travel to her right shoulder. She has bloating at times.

[23.3] A 35-year-old male complains of epigastric abdominal pain which seems to "bore straight to the back." He has nausea and vomiting.

[23.4] A 22-year-old woman complains of intermittent severe abdominal pain with diarrhea. She also has some joint pain.

[23.5] A 22-year-old woman is noted to have lower abdominal pain associated with some dysuria and abnormal menses. Her appetite has decreased recently. The pregnancy test is negative. Which of the following findings would most likely suggest pelvic inflammatory disease?

A. Endometrial biopsy showing atypical cells
B. Vaginal wet mount demonstrating clue cells
C. Cervical motion tenderness on physical examination
D. Pain on rectal examination

Answers

[23.1] **G.** The intermittent crampy abdominal pain is classic for ovarian torsion. Although this patient's pain moves from the umbilicus to the lower quadrant area, it has lasted longer than 24 hours, without fever.

[23.2]   **E.** The right upper quadrant abdominal pain following meals (especially fatty meals) is very typical of cholelithiasis. The pain often radiates to the right scapula. If she had fever, cholecystitis would be suspected.

[23.3]   **F.** Pancreatitis usually presents with mid-epigastric pain that penetrates straight to the back, is constant in nature, and is associated with nausea and vomiting. Common etiologies include alcohol abuse and gallstones.

[23.4]   **D.** Inflammatory bowel disease often affects individuals in their teens or twenties, with abdominal pain, diarrhea (often bloody), and extraintestinal manifestations such as joint pain or eye findings.

[23.5]   **C.** Although cervical motional tenderness is not specific for acute salpingitis, and can be seen with other acute inflammatory conditions of the lower abdomen such as diverticulitis and appendicitis, it is a classic finding of pelvic inflammatory disease.

CLINICAL PEARLS

❖ The classic triad of symptoms for diagnosing PID include lower abdominal tenderness, adnexal tenderness, and cervical motion tenderness.

❖ Laparoscopy remains the gold standard for diagnosing PID.

❖ Long-term sequelae of PID include infertility, pelvic adhesions, chronic pelvic pain, risk of ectopic pregnancy, and Fitz-Hugh–Curtis syndrome.

❖ Disseminated gonococcal infection, although uncommon, is a serious complication of untreated gonorrhea, which is a very common infection. Persons found to have a positive gonorrhea culture should also be treated for chlamydia because concomitant infection is found in as many as 40 percent of patients. In any person presenting with asymmetric polyarthritis, tenosynovitis, and pustular skin lesions, disseminated gonococcal infection should be considered in the differential diagnosis.

REFERENCES

Centers for Disease Control and Prevention. 2002 Guidelines for treatment of sexually transmitted diseases. MMWR Morb Mortal Wkly Rep 2002;51(RR-6):1.

Stenchever MA, Droegmueller W, Herbst AL, Mishell DR, eds. Comprehensive gynecology. 4th ed. St. Louis: Mosby-Year Book, Inc 2001:707-739.

Sweet RL, Gibbs RS. Infectious diseases of the female genital tract, 4th ed. Baltimore: Lippincott Williams & Wilkins, 2002.

A 27-year-old woman noticed that since 1 day ago, her mouth droops in the right corner, she cannot close her right eye, and that these symptoms have persisted. She also noticed that her right eye is tearing. She denies having headaches, visual disturbances, nausea, vomiting. She does not have a history of trauma. Her past medical history is unremarkable. She is currently not on any medications. She states that she was born in Michigan and has not been traveling. She does not recall being bitten by ticks. Her mother had a stroke when she was age 60 years. On physical examination, the right corner of her mouth droops, the facial creases are absent, and the right lower eyelid is sagging. The patient cannot close her right eye, and on attempts to close the right eye, the eye rolls upwards. The patient also cannot crease her forehead. The other cranial nerves seem to be normal, and the neurological examination reveals no deficits other than as stated.

◆ **What is the most likely diagnosis?**

◆ **How will you manage this condition?**

ANSWERS TO CASE 24: Bell Palsy

Summary: A 27-year-old woman has acute onset of right facial weakness and excess tearing from the right eye. She denies trauma and has no other cranial nerve or neurological problems.

 Most Likely Diagnosis: facial nerve palsy most likely idiopathic (Bell palsy).

 Management of condition: protection of the eye, splint to prevent drooping of the lower face, and consider a course of prednisone and/or acyclovir.

Analysis

Objectives

1. Know the differential diagnosis of facial nerve paralysis, particularly to differentiate an upper motor neuron process from a lower motor neuron process.
2. Understand the clinical presentation of Bell palsy.
3. Learn the management of Bell palsy.

Considerations

This 27-year-old woman is affected by the abrupt onset of right facial weakness. Notably, her **upper facial muscles are affected, which is consistent with a peripheral neuropathy**. She has none of the findings suggestive of a more complicated process (Table 24-1). Her symptoms are likely caused by the paralysis of the seventh cranial nerve, which is mainly a motor nerve supplying all the ipsilateral muscles of facial expression. The drooping of the right corner of the mouth represents paralysis of the orbicularis oris muscle. Tearing of the right eye is because of the paralysis of the orbicularis oculi muscle; this prevents closure of the eyelids and also causes the lacrimal duct opening to sag

Table 24-1
RED FLAGS FOR SUSPECTED FACIAL NERVE PALSY

Cranial nerve involvement other than cranial nerve VII

Bilateral facial weakness

Weakness, numbness of arms or legs

Unaffected upper facial muscles (forehead)

Headache, visual deficits, nausea, or vomiting

History of travel through woods, tick bite

Ulceration or blisters near ear

away from the conjunctiva. The uncreasing of the forehead is a result of paralysis of the frontalis muscle. Affected individuals will often have the Bell phenomenon: upon attempted closure of the eyelids, the eye on the paralyzed side rolls upward. Treatment includes a patch for the eye and placement of eye ointment to prevent corneal abrasions, a splint for the lower face, and consideration of a course of corticosteroids and/or acyclovir.

APPROACH TO BELL PALSY

Clinical Approach

The **seventh cranial nerve** exits the cranium through the stylomastoid foramen and supplies all the **muscles concerned with facial expression.** It also has a small sensory component which conveys taste sensation from the anterior two-thirds of the tongue and cutaneous impulses from the anterior wall of the external auditory meatus. A complete interruption of the facial nerve at the stylomastoid foramen paralyzes all the muscles of the face on the affected side. Taste sensation is intact because the lesion is beyond the site where the chorda tympani has separated from the main trunk of the facial nerve. If the nerve to the stapedius muscle is involved, there is often hyperacusis. If the geniculate ganglion or the motor root proximal to it is involved, lacrimation and salivation may be reduced.

Although the most common form of facial paralysis is called Bell palsy, this is a diagnosis of exclusion. In other words**, the emergency department (ED) physician should guard against too quickly presuming a facial palsy is Bell palsy.** The cause was suspected to be a viral infection, and in the past few years, such a mechanism has been established with a reasonable degree of certainty. The genome of herpes simplex has been isolated in the geniculate ganglion of patients with Bell palsy. Other causes of nuclear or peripheral facial palsy include Lyme disease, tumors of the temporal bone (carotid body, cholesteatoma, dermoid), Ramsey Hunt syndrome (herpes zoster of the geniculate ganglion), acoustic neuromas, and pontine lesions (tumors or infarcts). Stroke, Guillain-Barré syndrome, polio, sarcoid, and human immunodeficiency virus (HIV) infection are other processes that must be considered.

All forms of peripheral facial palsy must be distinguished from the supranuclear type. In the latter, the frontalis and orbicularis oculi muscles are spared, because the corticopontine innervation of the upper facial muscles is bilateral, and that of the lower facial muscles is mainly contralateral. In other words, **if the patient has drooping of the mouth, but is able to wrinkle his or her forehead, an intracranial process should be suspected!** In supranuclear lesions, there may also be a dissociation of emotional and voluntary facial movements. Because Bell palsy is a diagnosis of exclusion, a very careful history and physical examination are critical to assess for other even subtle neurological abnormalities.

The onset of Bell palsy is abrupt, with maximum weakness occurring within 48 hours. The paralysis may be preceded by pain behind the ear. Taste sensation may be lost on the side of the paralysis, and hyperacusis may be present. The patient may complain of heaviness and numbness on the affected side; however, no sensory loss is demonstrable. Eighty percent of the patients recover within weeks to a few months. The presence of incomplete paralysis in the first week is the most favorable prognostic sign.

Treatment   **Protection of the eye** during sleep to prevent corneal drying or abrasions is accomplished with an eye patch and lubricants to the affected eye. Massaging of the weakened muscles may have some role in recovery and muscle tone. A splint to prevent drooping of the lower face has been used by some practitioners. **Corticosteroid use is controversial**. Some advocate its use in older individuals, while others prescribe it widely. **Prednisone** 50 mg daily for the first 5 days and then tapered over the next 5 days is one regimen; if more than 5 days have elapsed since the symptoms began, corticosteroids are unlikely to be effective. **Acyclovir** 200 mg orally 5 times a day for 10 days with/without corticosteroids has also been used by some physicians. **The prognosis is usually very good. Persistent weakness, the appearance of other neurological deficits, or blisters that appear on the ear are indications for referral.**

Comprehension Questions

[24.1] A 32-year-old woman complains of facial weakness for several weeks that has gradually worsened. The upper face and lower face are both affected. She does not have weakness of the arms or legs. Which of the following would suggest a diagnosis other than Bell palsy?

A. Upper facial weakness
B. The onset is insidious, over several weeks
C. Absence of symptoms of arms
D. Absence of symptoms of legs

[24.2] A 55-year-old woman complains of weakness of her facial muscles on the right side of her face along with numbness of her right cheek region. Which of the following is the next step?

A. Recommend eye protection and observation
B. Obtain an rapid plasma reagin (RPR) serology
C. Lumbar puncture
D. Magnetic resonance imaging (MRI) of the brain

Match one of the following mechanisms (A to E) to each of the clinical scenarios presented in questions [24.3] to [24.5]:

A. Pressure on the cerebellopontine nucleus
B. Edema of the nerve at the stylomastoid foramen
C. Immunoglobulins against the acetylcholine receptor
D. Multifocal myelin central nervous system (CNS) destruction
E. Autoimmune attack on myelinated motor nerves particularly of the lower extremities

[24.3] A 22-year-old woman is on the ventilator because of inability to breathe. This condition began 3 weeks ago when she had weakness of the legs. Her deep tendon reflexes are absent.

[24.4] A 32-year-old woman has a 5-year history of progressive weakness during the day. She cannot look upward for a long time because of fatigue.

[24.5] A 35-year-old man had eye weakness 2 years ago with full resolution. Now he has difficulty with his right handgrip. His deep tendon reflexes are normal to increased.

Answers

[24.1]   **B.** The onset of Bell palsy is abrupt with the maximum weakness being attained within 48 hours. Facial nerve palsy as a consequence of tumors of the temporal bone is insidious and the symptoms are progressive.

[24.2]   **D.** The numbness over the cheek is concerning and inconsistent with Bell palsy. The facial nerve supplies all the muscles of the face. Injury of the nerve produces paralysis of the facial muscles, drooping of the corner of the mouth is one of the findings. The tongue is supplied by the hypoglossal nerve. Middle ear lesions producing facial palsy will cause loss of taste over the anterior two-thirds of the tongue, but alteration of taste sensation does not occur. The sensory component of the facial nerve is limited to the anterior wall of the external auditory meatus.

[24.3]   **E.** This presentation of ascending paralysis is very classic for Guillain-Barré syndrome, and typically the deep tendon reflexes are absent.

[24.4]   **C.** Myasthenia gravis is characterized by progressive weakness throughout the day, particularly with the eye muscles. The mechanism is immunoglobulin (Ig) G antibodies against the acetylcholine receptors.

[24.5]   **D.** Multiple sclerosis typically involves young individuals with waxing and waning weakness, with full recovery between exacerbations. The mechanism is multifocal destruction of the myelin.

CLINICAL PEARLS

❖ Bell palsy is an idiopathic seventh cranial nerve peripheral neuropathy, leading to both upper facial and lower facial weakness.

❖ The diagnosis of Bell palsy is one of exclusion.

❖ The most important assessment in a patient who presents with possible Bell palsy is to rule out serious disorders such as intracranial tumors.

❖ Protection of the eye during sleep and to prevent corneal drying or abrasions is accomplished with an eye patch and lubricants to the affected eye.

❖ The prognosis of Bell palsy is usually very good, but persistent weakness, the appearance of other neurological deficits, or blisters that appear on the ear are indications for referral.

REFERENCES

Brodal A. The cranial nerves. In: Neurological anatomy in relation to clinical medicine, 3rd ed. New York: Oxford University Press, 1980:448–577.

Groves J. Bell's (idiopathic) facial palsy. In: Hinchcliff R, Harrison D, eds. Scientific foundations of otolaryngology. London: Heinemann, 1976:446–59

Hauser WA, et al. Incidence and prognosis of Bell's palsy in the population of Rochester, Minnesota. Mayo Clin Proc 1971;46:258.

Karnes WE. Diseases of the seventh cranial nerve. In: Dyck PJ, Thomas PK, eds. Peripheral neuropathy, 2nd ed. Philadelphia: WB Saunders, 1984:1266–99.

Murakami S, Honda N, Mizobuchi M, et al. Rapid diagnosis of varicella zoster virus in acute facial palsy. Neurology 1998;51:1202.

Whitley RJ, Weiss N, Gnann JW, et al. Acyclovir with and without prednisone for the treatment of herpes zoster: a randomized, placebo-controlled trial. Ann Intern Med 1996;125:376.

A 26-year-old female presents to the emergency department with a 6-hour history of worsening abdominal pain. She states the pain initially was near her umbilicus but has since moved to her lower right side. She rates the pain as 8 on a scale of 10 and crampy in nature. The patient states that she noted some vaginal spotting this morning, but denies any passage of clots or tissue. The patient ate breakfast this morning, but states she has not eaten since because she feels nauseous. She denies any fever or chills or any change in her bowel habits. Upon further questioning, the patient states her last menstrual period was 2 months ago, but her periods are irregular. She also states that she was told that she had a vaginal infection a year ago but does not recall having been treated for the illness. On physical exam, her blood pressure is 120/76 mmHg, heart rate is 105 beats per minute, and she is afebrile. In general, she is in mild distress. The abdomen reveals tenderness to palpation in her right lower quadrant that is greater than that in the left lower quadrant. The exam reveals some minimal voluntary guarding, but no rebound tenderness is appreciated. On pelvic examination, the uterus appears mildly enlarged without cervical motion tenderness. There are no masses or tenderness in the adnexal region. Her complete blood count (CBC) reveals a mildly elevated white blood cell count with a left shift. A beta human chorionic gonadotropin (hCG) level was 4658 mIU/mL. A transvaginal sonogram reveals an empty uterus but no adnexal masses or free fluid is noted.

◆ **What is the most likely diagnosis?**

◆ **What is your next step?**

◆ **What is the your initial treatment?**

ANSWERS TO CASE 25: Ectopic Pregnancy

Summary: A 26-year-old female complains of severe abdominal pain, nausea, and vaginal spotting. She has a positive pregnancy test, a quantitative hCG level of 4658 mIU/mL with no intrauterine pregnancy.

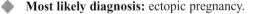 **Most likely diagnosis:** ectopic pregnancy.

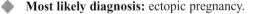 **Next step:** diagnostic versus operative laparoscopy.

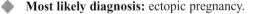 **Initial treatment:** establish an IV line and stabilize the patient in preparation for surgery.

Analysis

Objectives

1. Understand the diagnosis and workup of ectopic pregnancy.
2. Know the different sonographic appearances of ectopic pregnancy.
3. Know the common differential diagnoses for lower abdominal pain and be able to consult the appropriate specialties based on the physical exam.

Considerations

This patient presents to the emergency department with complaints of vaginal bleeding, abdominal pain, and a positive pregnancy examination. Her quantitative **hCG level is above the threshold of 1500 to 2000 mIU/mL**, and **no intrauterine pregnancy** is seen on **transvaginal** sonography; thus, her **risk for an ectopic pregnancy approaches 85 percent.** Other diagnoses should be considered, such as threatened abortion, incomplete abortion, pelvic inflammatory disease, or appendicitis. Ectopic pregnancy is defined as a pregnancy that develops after implantation of the blastocyst anywhere other than in the lining of the uterine cavity.

APPROACH TO ECTOPIC PREGNANCY

Definitions

Ectopic pregnancy: pregnancy that develops after implantation anywhere other than the lining of the uterus.

Ruptured ectopic pregnancy: ectopic pregnancy that has eroded through the tissue in which it has implanted, producing hemorrhage from exposed vessels.

Salpingectomy: surgical excision and removal of the oviduct and ectopic pregnancy.

Clinical Approach

Ectopic pregnancy is defined as a pregnancy outside the lining of the uterus, most commonly occurring in the oviduct, but it may also be found in the abdomen, ovary, or cervix. The incidence of the ectopic pregnancy has increased in the United States for two reasons: (a) the increased incidence of salpingitis caused by more infections with *Chlamydia trachomatis* or other sexually transmitted disease, and (b) improved diagnostic techniques. Other risk factors include prior tubal surgery, previous ectopic pregnancy, use of exogenous progesterone, and a history of infertility agents. The most common presenting symptoms are abdominal pain, absence of menses, and irregular vaginal bleeding. Other symptoms found on physical examination may include a palpable adnexal tenderness, uterine enlargement, tachycardia, hypotension, syncope, peritoneal signs, and fever.

Approximately half of the episodes of ectopic pregnancy are linked to previous salpingitis. Prior infections are likely to lead to anatomic tubal pathology that prevents the normal passage of an embryo into the uterus. In the remaining cases of ectopic pregnancy, an identifying factor cannot be determined and may be linked to a physiological disorder. Increased levels of estrogen and progesterone interfere with tubal motility and increase the chance of ectopic pregnancy.

Approximately 97 percent of ectopic pregnancies occur in the oviduct. The remainder of ectopic pregnancies implant in the abdomen, cervix, or ovary. The ampullary region of the oviduct is the site where most tubal pregnancies are found. Pathogenesis of ectopic pregnancy begins as the embryo invades the lumen of the tube and its peritoneal covering. As the embryo continues to grow, surrounding vessels may bleed into the peritoneal cavity, resulting in a hemoperitoneum. The stretching of the peritoneum results in abdominal pain until necrosis ensues and results in rupture of the ectopic pregnancy.

The differential diagnosis of ectopic pregnancy includes many other gynecological and surgical illnesses. Most common are salpingitis, threatened or incomplete abortion, ruptured corpus luteum, adnexal torsion, and appendicitis. The diagnosis of ectopic pregnancy must be considered in any woman of reproductive age with abnormal vaginal bleeding and abdominal pain.

Diagnosis of ectopic pregnancy may be aided with the use of transvaginal ultrasound (See Figure 25–1). Visualization of the pelvic organs may reveal the absence of an intrauterine pregnancy, a complex adnexal mass, or the presence of an embryo in the adnexa. It is important to note that with **the hCG level >1500 to 2000 mIU/mL, an intrauterine pregnancy is almost always seen on transvaginal sonography.** Lack of an intrauterine gestational sac on transvaginal sonography confers up to an 85 percent risk of an ectopic pregnancy. At times, sonography can visualize an ectopic pregnancy even with hCG levels lower than this threshold; the **level of hCG does not reliably correlate with the size of the ectopic pregnancy.** When hCG levels are lower than the above threshold, the ED physician should rely on the clinical impression to diagnose an ectopic pregnancy. In a reliable and asymptomatic patient whose initial hCG level is below the threshold, a repeat hCG level can be obtained in 48 hours. The **hCG should increase by at least 66 percent over 48 hours**; lack of normal rise strongly implies an abnormal pregnancy, although the test does not indicate the location of the pregnancy (ectopic or miscarriage). A definitive diagnosis of ectopic pregnancy can almost always be made by direct visualization of the pelvic organs using laparoscopy if the diagnosis remains uncertain.

Treatment options include both medical and surgical therapy. Medical treatment consists of using **methotrexate**, a folinic acid antagonist that interferes with deoxyribonucleic acid (DNA) synthesis, repair, and cellular replication. Actively dividing tissue, such as fetal cell growth is susceptible to methotrex-

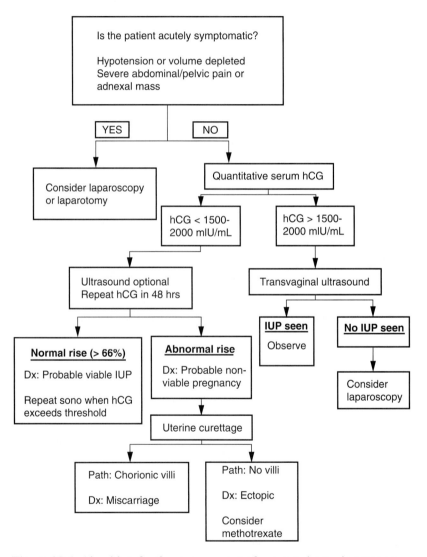

Figure 25-1. Algorithm for the management of suspected ectopic pregnancy.

ate and may be used for treatment of ectopic pregnancy under specific conditions. Potential problems associated with medical management of ectopic pregnancy include drug side effects and treatment failure. If medical therapy fails, surgical intervention is necessary. Surgical management commonly consists of laparoscopy and/or laparotomy. A few common surgical techniques used for treatment of ectopic pregnancy include salpingotomy, salpingostomy, and partial salpingectomy. These techniques can be used to treat the majority of unruptured ectopic pregnancy, whereas exploratory laparotomy may be used in cases of ruptured ectopic pregnancies.

Comprehension Questions

[25.1] A 22-year-old woman complains of lower abdominal pain and vaginal spotting. Which of the following tests is the first priority?

    A. Pelvic ultrasound

    B. KUB (kidneys, ureters, bladder) radiograph

    C. hCG level

    D. *Chlamydia* antigen test of the cervix

[25.2] A 22-year-old woman underwent methotrexate treatment for an ectopic pregnancy 1 week ago and complains of lower abdominal cramping. She denies vaginal bleeding, dizziness, or vomiting. On examination, her blood pressure is 120/80 mmHg and her heart rate is 80 beats per minute. The abdomen reveals mild tenderness. Which of the following is the best management?

    A. Observation

    B. Surgical management of the ectopic pregnancy

    C. Administration of folinic acid

    D. Transfusion of 2 units of red blood cells

[25.3] A 42-year-old woman complains of an acute onset of significant abdominal pain of 6 hours duration. She states that she underwent in vitro fertilization and is currently 8 weeks pregnant. Her blood pressure is 90/60 mmHg and her heart rate is 110 beats per minute. Her quantitative hCG level is 22,800 mIU/mL. Transvaginal sonography reveals a singleton intrauterine gestation with cardiac activity, and a moderate amount of free fluid in the cul de sac. Which of the following is the most likely diagnosis?

    A. Heterotopic pregnancy

    B. Ruptured corpus luteum

    C. Cirrhosis with ascites

    D. Urinary tract infection

[25.4] A 33-year-old woman complains of vaginal bleeding and abdominal cramping. She passed some blood clots. Her last menstrual period was 6 weeks previously. On examination her cervical os is open to 1 cm. Her quantitative hCG level is 2000 mIU/mL. Which of the following is the most likely diagnosis?

A. Ectopic pregnancy
B. Incomplete abortion
C. Completed abortion
D. Incompetent cervix

[25.5] A 28-year-old woman complains of lower abdominal cramping pain for about 3 hours, and passed what was described as "liver-like" tissue, after which her pain resolved. In the ED, her blood pressure is 120/70 mmHg and heart rate is 80 beats per minute. Her uterus is firm and the cervix is closed. The hCG level is 2000 mIU/mL. Transvaginal sonography reveals no intrauterine pregnancy. Which of the following is the next step?

A. Laparoscopy
B. Methotrexate therapy
C. Progesterone level
D. Repeat hCG level in 48 hours

Answers

[25.1] **C.** In general, any woman in the childbearing age group with abdominal pain or abnormal vaginal bleeding should have a pregnancy test. If pregnant, then ectopic pregnancy should be ruled out.

[25.2] **A.** A large number of women who undergo methotrexate treatment of ectopic pregnancy will have some abdominal discomfort. As long as there are no signs of rupture such as hypotension, severe pain, or free fluid on ultrasound, expectant management may be practiced.

[25.3] **A.** In vitro fertilization with embryo transfer produces a rate of coexisting intrauterine pregnancy and ectopic pregnancy of up to 3 percent (markedly higher than the spontaneous rate of 1:10,000). Thus, a woman who has undergone in vitro fertilization who presents with abdominal fluid and hypotension must be suspected as having an ectopic pregnancy, even when an intrauterine pregnancy has been visualized on sonography.

[25.4] **B.** Uterine cramping, vaginal bleeding, passage of tissue, and an open cervical os in a pregnant woman is consistent with an incomplete abortion. Uterine curettage would be the therapy.

[25.5] **D.** This patient likely has a completed abortion with the resolution of symptoms following passage of tissue and now with a small uterus and closed cervical os. Nevertheless, there is still a possibility of ectopic pregnancy and perhaps the "tissue" passed was only a blood clot. The tissue should be sent for pathological analysis. Also, a repeat hCG level should be performed to ensure that all tissue has passed. The hCG level should fall by about 50 percent in 48 hours if all tissue has passed. A plateau in the hCG level may indicate incomplete abortion or ectopic pregnancy. Dilation and curettage would generally be performed, and if chorionic villi were found the diagnosis is miscarriage; absence of chorionic villi establishes the diagnosis of ectopic pregnancy which may be treated by surgery or methotrexate.

CLINICAL PEARLS

❖ In any woman of childbearing age, consider pregnancy. If the pregnancy test is positive, consider an ectopic pregnancy.

❖ Consider pregnancy even when a woman has had a tubal ligation or is using contraception.

❖ When the serum quantitative hCG level is above 1500 to 2000 mIU/mL and transvaginal ultrasound does not reveal an intrauterine pregnancy, the risk of ectopic pregnancy is high.

❖ Surgery, not methotrexate, is the best treatment for the patient who is hemodynamically unstable or with significant abdominal pain.

❖ Laparoscopy remains the gold standard for the diagnosis of ectopic pregnancy.

REFERENCES

American College of Obstetricians and Gynecologists, practice bulletin: medical management of tubal pregnancy. Compendium 2002.

Stenchever MA, Droegmueller W, Herbst AL, Mishell DR, eds. Comprehensive gynecology. 4th ed. St. Louis: Mosby-Year Book, 2001:443–78.

Sweet RL, Gibbs RS. Infectious diseases of the female genital tract, 4th ed. Baltimore: Lippincott Williams & Wilkins, 2002.

A 3-week-old infant presents with a 6-hour history of poor feeding, crankiness, and feeling warm to touch. The mother, a 29-year-old G2 (second pregnancy) woman, reports that he was born vaginally at term after an uneventful pregnancy. His birth weight was 2800 g, and he was discharged on the second hospital day. Mom has bottle fed the infant since birth, reports that he was normal at his 2-week well-child evaluation, and that he had been well until about 6 hours before arrival to the emergency department. The vital signs on the chart include a temperature of 35.8°C (96.5°F) rectally, a heart rate of 180 beats per minute, a respiratory rate of 60 breaths per minute, and a blood pressure of 70/40 mmHg. Your quick glance reveals a lethargic, pale, and ill-appearing infant.

◆ **What is the most likely diagnosis?**

◆ **What is the next step in management?**

◆ **What is the best therapy?**

ANSWERS TO CASE 26: Neonatal Sepsis

Summary: A 3-week-old infant presents with a 6-hour history of poor feeding, crankiness, and feeling warm to touch. He was born vaginally at term weighing 2800 g after an uneventful pregnancy and was discharged on the second hospital day. His temperature is 35.8°C (96.5°F) rectally, heart rate is 180 beats per minute, respiratory rate is 60 breaths per minute, and blood pressure is 70/40 mm Hg. Your quick glance reveals a lethargic, pale, and ill-appearing infant.

◆ **Most likely diagnosis:** neonatal sepsis.

◆ **Next step:** obtain appropriate cultures and initiate antibiotics.

◆ **Best therapy:** depends on local bacterial resistance patterns, but for community-acquired infections, it most commonly includes ampicillin plus either an aminoglycoside or a second-/third-generation cephalosporin.

Analysis

Objectives

1. Understand the common presentations of sepsis in a neonate.
2. Appreciate the variety of organisms responsible for neonatal infections.
3. Learn treatment options for the common infections in the neonate.

Considerations

This 3-week-old neonate has an acute onset of **lethargy, irritability, hypothermia, tachycardia, and tachypnea; these symptoms, in a previously healthy infant, suggest sepsis**. Importantly, the emergency physician must be aware that the neonate will not manifest the same signs of infection as the older infant. A variety of organisms are possible, but initial management would include rapid application of the **ABC**s of resuscitation (maintain **a**irway, control **b**reathing, and ensure adequate **c**irculation). Once these initial resuscitation steps are accomplished, attempts are made to rapidly obtain cultures and to initiate appropriate antibiotic. Admission to the hospital and close observation for cardiovascular stability is warranted (Fig. 26-1).

APPROACH TO NEONATAL SEPSIS

Definitions

Early onset infections: arbitrary definition of a sepsis event in a neonate that occurs in the first 7 days of life. Often these infections are a result of exposure to the pathogen before or during delivery from the mother's genitourinary tract.

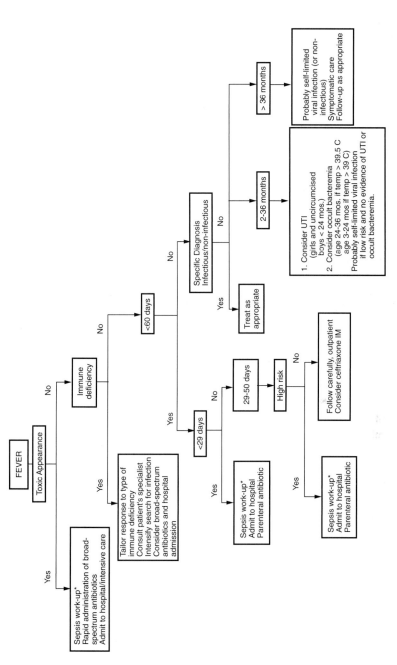

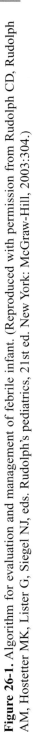

Figure 26-1. Algorithm for evaluation and management of febrile infant. (Reproduced with permission from Rudolph CD, Rudolph AM, Hostetter MK, Lister G, Siegel NJ, eds. Rudolph's pediatrics, 21st ed. New York: McGraw-Hill, 2003:304.)

Late-onset sepsis syndrome: arbitrarily defined as sepsis in a neonate that occurs after about 7 days of life but before about 28 days of life. The source of infection is often from the caregiving environment.

Neonatal sepsis: traditionally includes infections that occur in infants in the first 28 days of life.

Clinical Approach

Signs and Symptoms of Sepsis **The signs and symptoms of sepsis in the neonate can be subtle and nonspecific.** Temperature instability (*hypothermia* is commonly seen), tachypnea, hypotension, and bradycardia are common findings in sepsis and meningitis. Overwhelming shock is manifested by findings of tachycardia, pallor, and poor capillary refill. Neurological findings of impaired level of consciousness, coma, seizures, bulging anterior fontanelle, focal cranial nerve signs, and nuchal rigidity are unusual, but when present hint at meningitis, a condition seen commonly in late-onset disease, as in this case. Tachypnea, grunting, nasal flaring, retractions (costal or substernal), decreased breath sounds, and cyanosis tend to be seen more frequently with pneumonia, a condition more frequently seen in early onset disease.

Evaluation of the Potentially Septic Child Some of the **laboratory findings of neonatal sepsis** can be **nonspecific, including hypoglycemia, metabolic acidosis, and sometimes jaundice.** The complete blood count (CBC) often is used to help guide therapy, although the sensitivity and specificity of these tests are low. Markedly elevated or very low total white blood cell (WBC) count levels, increased neutrophil count, increased immature to total neutrophil (I:T) ratios, and thrombocytopenia with platelet counts less than 100,000/mm^3 have been used as indicators of sepsis. Some physicians use the **C-reactive protein** (an acute-phase protein that is increased with tissue injury) as an adjunct tool to evaluate a potentially septic infant. None of these tests is perfect; a high index of suspicion is the most appropriate screening tool to apply.

Identification of the offending organism requires culture of the body fluids likely infected. All neonates undergoing a sepsis evaluation require a blood culture. Examination of cerebral spinal fluid (CSF) is indicated for infants with signs of late-onset sepsis, but the health care provider must ensure the patient is stable enough to undergo the procedure. Urine is obtained for analysis and culture. Appropriate methods to obtain the urine include bladder catheterization or suprapubic bladder taps; bags attached to the perineum are often contaminated and usually are considered inappropriate specimens. If the patient has diarrhea, culture of the stool may be helpful. Culture of any lesions may also be indicated (i.e., pustules or vesicles) because they may be the source of the symptoms. For the infant with respiratory symptoms, a chest radiograph might identify segmental, lobar, or diffuse reticulogranular patterns of disease.

Pathogens   The organisms commonly causing late-onset sepsis are those that are found in the infant's environment, **such as from the skin, respiratory tract, conjunctivae, gastrointestinal tract, and umbilicus.** Healthy newborns that have been at home (such as the infant in the case) may be infected with group B streptococcus, *Streptococcus pneumoniae,* or *Escherichia coli,* and less commonly with *Staphylococcus aureus, Listeria monocytogenes, Streptococcus* sp., *Citrobacter* sp., and *Haemophilus influenzae.* If the child had been in the neonatal intensive care unit (NICU) for a prolonged time, organisms to which the infant might be exposed include coagulase-negative staphylococci, *S. aureus, E. coli, Klebsiella* sp., *Pseudomonas* sp., *Enterobacter* sp., *Candida* sp., group B streptococcus, *Serratia* sp., *Acinetobacter* sp., and anaerobes. Hospitalized neonates who have catheters (vascular or urinary) are at especially high risk for developing a nosocomial infection.

Treatment   Treatment for the patient in the above case (who may have community-acquired, late-onset disease) includes antibiotics directed at the common pathogens listed above. Choices often include **a combination of intravenous second- or third-generation cephalosporins such as cefuroxime, cefotaxime, or ceftriaxone** (which provide antibiotic coverage for beta-lactamase–producing organisms, some gram-positive organisms, and gram-negative organisms) **and a penicillin (often ampicillin)** for coverage against *Listeria monocytogenes.* Some physicians advocate substitution of gentamicin (or tobramycin) for the cephalosporin, but coverage against beta-lactamase–producing organisms is sacrificed. For hospitalized patients with late-onset disease, therapy often consists of beta-lactamase–resistant antibiotics (such as vancomycin), second- or third-generation cephalosporins, and, sometimes, antifungal agents. In all cases, antibiotic coverage is adjusted depending on the organism identified and the specific antibiotic sensitivities of the organism.

The **duration of antibiotic therapy is at least 48 to 72 hours**. If cultures are negative after that period of time and the patient is otherwise well, antibiotics are often stopped. For infants presenting with convincing signs and symptoms of sepsis (such as in this case) antibiotics may be continued even if the culture results prove to be negative. For infants with positive cultures, therapy continues for 10 to 21 days, depending on the organism and the site of the infection. For all infants, close observation for signs of antibiotic toxicity is important.

Comprehension Questions

[26.1] A 2-week-old, former 35-week-gestation infant presents to the emergency department with maternal concerns of low-grade fever (highest has been 38.2°C [100.8°F]), poor feeding, and lethargy. The mother had prenatal care in Mexico and states that she had no problems during her pregnancy. The mother states that she had low-grade fevers during her labor, that the doctors were concerned that the amniotic fluid had a brown-stained appearance, but that the baby appeared to be normal. The mother and child were discharged after 48 hours in the hospital. You begin a sepsis evaluation and note the child's CBC shows marked monocytosis. This infant most likely had:

A. Disseminated herpes
B. Congenital syphilis
C. Listeriosis
D. Group B streptococcal disease
E. Congenital varicella

[26.2] A 4-week-old infant presents with a 3-day history of increased respiratory rate and cough. The previous 4 weeks have been uneventful with the exception of the infant having mild eye discharge at about 10 days of age; topical antibiotics rapidly resolved the problem. The mother says the child has been eating fairly well, only having to pause occasionally while eating to catch his breath. On examination the child appears to be well, is afebrile, and has a respiratory rate of 60 breaths per minute. He has some rales but no wheezes. The CBC demonstrates an increase in eosinophil count. The chest radiograph shows hyperinflations with minimal interstitial and alveolar infiltrates. The agent most likely to be causing his symptoms is:

A. Group B streptococcus
B. Respiratory syncytial virus (RSV)
C. *Chlamydia*
D. Pneumococcus
E. *Staphylococcus aureus*

[26.3] A 3-week-old infant has had a cough, congestion, and fever for 2 days. She has school-aged siblings who have similar complaints. The child was born via spontaneous vaginal delivery without problems, and was discharged at 2 days of age with her mother. On examination the child is noted to have a temperature of 38.4°C (101.1°F), a respiratory rate of 70 breaths per minute, diffuse wheezes, and subcostal and intercostal retractions. The laboratory test most likely to reveal the etiology of this patient's problem is:

A. Direct fluorescent antibody (DFA) of conjunctiva or nasopharynx specimen for chlamydia
B. Enzyme-linked immunoabsorbent assay (ELISA) of respiratory secretions for RSV
C. Blood culture for *Haemophilus influenzae* B
D. CBC for eosinophils to rule out asthma
E. Tissue culture of rectal secretions for herpes

[26.4] A 3-week-old child presents to the emergency deparment with the complaint of the sudden onset of lethargy, vomiting, poor feeding, and right-sided shaking of the arm. A quick examination reveals an apneic, blue child with an obviously bulging fontanelle; no seizure activity is noted. The child is immediately intubated, and vital signs seem to stabilize. Further history reveals that the child was in the care of the mother's boyfriend when he called to report the child suddenly became lethargic, began to vomit, and would not eat. The child's history is unremarkable with the exception of being treated for colic. The most appropriate next step in the management of this child is to:

A. Perform a lumbar puncture
B. Obtain a stat computed tomography (CT) scan of the head
C. Order serum and urinary organic acids
D. Catheterize the child's bladder for urine culture
E. Initiate intravenous antibiotics

Answers

[26.1] **C.** Listeriosis is a gram-positive rod isolated from soil, streams, sewage, certain foods, silage, dust, and slaughterhouses. The foodborne transmission of disease is related to Mexican (soft ripened) cheese, whole and 2 percent milk, undercooked chicken and hot dogs, raw vegetables, and shellfish. The newborn infant acquires the organism transplacentally or by aspiration or ingestion at the time of delivery. This disease can present as a late-onset disease as described, or as an early onset infection (often with a disseminated erythematous pustular rash, pallor, poor feeding, tachypnea, and cyanosis); mortality rate of early onset disease is approximately 30 percent.

[26.2] **C.** Chlamydial conjunctivitis often presents 5 to 14 days after birth and commonly is treated with topical erythromycin (topical, rather than oral, erythromycin is chosen at this point because oral administration is associated with an increased risk of the infant developing hypertrophic pyloric stenosis). Approximately 25 percent of women whose infants have nasopharyngeal chlamydial infection will progress to have pneumonia, typically presenting between 1 and 3 months of age. An afebrile child with rales but no wheezes suggests chlamydia rather than RSV. The typical radiographic and CBC findings described, along with the history of what appears to have been chlamydial conjunctivitis, supports the diagnosis. The treatment for chlamydial pneumonia is oral erythromycin for about 14 days. Neonates with infections caused by the other organisms presented often have fever, signs and symptoms of sepsis, and often more significant radiographic findings.

[26.3]   **B.** The case is typical of RSV, especially if it occurs between the peak months of October through about March; the exposure to sick, school-aged siblings is typical. The fever, increased respiratory rate, and rales with wheezes suggests RSV. The CBC may be normal or show slightly increased WBCs. The typical radiographic of RSV can be confused with chlamydia (hyperinflations with minimal interstitial and alveolar infiltrates) but the history in this case is more suggestive of RSV. Treatment is supportive and includes oxygen (hypoxia is common), intravenous fluids, and occasionally a trial of bronchodilators. Pneumonia caused by *Haemophilus influenzae* B (and other bacterial agents) more typically lobar consolidations, sometimes with pleural effusion. Herpes presenting as isolated pneumonia without skin or neurological findings would be unusual at this age.

[26.4]   **B.** The history is suspicious for child abuse. A previously healthy child is unlikely to suddenly develop meningitis causing the bulging fontanelle with the other symptoms described. Rather, the history of a demanding (colicky) baby with acute onset of neurological symptoms suggests trauma to the head. A stat CT scan is likely to demonstrate intracranial hemorrhage. After the patient is stabilized, other evaluations might include an ophthalmological examination for retinal hemorrhages, a skeletal survey for evidence of other fractures, and a thorough evaluation of the home situation. Bleeding studies are often obtained to rule out a bleeding disorder; they are rarely found to be the cause of the intracranial problem.

CLINICAL PEARLS

❖ Sepsis in the neonate can present with nonspecific findings of temperature instability (especially hypothermia), tachypnea, poor feeding, bradycardia, hypotension, and hypoglycemia.

❖ Community-acquired, late-onset neonatal infection is often caused by organisms found in the infant's environment, including group B streptococcus, *Streptococcus pneumoniae*, or *Escherichia coli*, and less commonly with *Staphylococcus aureus*, *Listeria monocytogenes*, *Streptococcus* sp., *Citrobacter* sp., and *Haemophilus influenzae*.

❖ Nosocomial, late-onset neonatal infection may be caused by coagulase-negative staphylococci, *S. aureus*, *E. coli*, *Klebsiella* sp., *Pseudomonas* sp., *Enterobacter* sp., *Candida* sp., group B streptococcus, *Serratia* sp., *Acinetobacter* sp., and anaerobes.

❖ Treatment of community-acquired, late-onset disease often includes ampicillin and either a second-/third-generation cephalosporin or gentamicin.

❖ Treatment of hospital-acquired, late-onset disease often includes beta-lactamase–resistant antibiotics (such as vancomycin), second- or third-generation cephalosporins, and sometimes antifungal agents.

REFERENCES

Brady MT. Viral respiratory infections. In: Rudolph CD, Rudolph AM, Hostetter MK, Lister G, Siegel NJ, eds. Rudolph's pediatrics, 21st ed. New York: McGraw-Hill, 2003:1064–75.

Chiriboga CA. Trauma to the nervous system. In: Rudolph CD, Rudolph AM, Hostetter MK, Lister G, Siegel NJ, eds. Rudolph's pediatrics, 21st ed. New York: McGraw-Hill, 2003:2242–52.

Hammerschlag MR. Chlamydial infections. In: McMillan JA, DeAngelis CD, Feigin RD, Warshaw JB, eds. Oski's pediatrics, 3rd ed. Philadelphia: Lippincott Williams & Wilkins, 1999:895–8.

Hammerschlag MR. Chlamydia trachomatis. In: Behrman RE, Kliegman RM, Jenson HB, eds. Nelson textbook of pediatrics, 17th ed. Philadelphia: WB Saunders, 2004:994–9.

Jaffe DM. Assessment of the child with fever. In: Rudolph CD, Rudolph AM, Hostetter MK, Lister G, Siegel NJ, eds. Rudolph's pediatrics, 21st ed. New York: McGraw-Hill, 2003:302–9.

Johnson F. Abuse and neglect of children. In: Behrman RE, Kliegman RM, Jenson HB, eds. Nelson textbook of pediatrics, 17th ed. Philadelphia: WB Saunders, 2004:121–5.

Long SS. Respiratory syncytial virus. In: McMillan JA, DeAngelis CD, Feigin RD, Warshaw JB, eds. Oski's pediatrics, 3rd ed. Philadelphia: Lippincott Williams & Wilkins, 1999:1094–98.

McIntosh K. Respiratory syncytial virus. In: Behrman RE, Kliegman RM, Jenson HB, eds. Nelson textbook of pediatrics, 17th ed. Philadelphia: WB Saunders, 2004:1076–9.

Rosman NP. Acute head trauma. In: McMillan JA, DeAngelis CD, Feigin RD, Warshaw JB, eds. Oski's pediatrics, 3rd ed. Philadelphia: Lippincott Williams & Wilkins, 1999:603–17.

Sanchez Pablo, Siegel JD. Sepsis neonatorum. In: McMillan JA, DeAngelis CD, Feigin RD, Warshaw JB, eds. Oski's pediatrics, 3rd ed. Philadelphia: Lippincott Williams & Wilkins, 1999:404–13.

Staat MA. Chlamydial infections. In: Rudolph CD, Rudolph AM, Hostetter MK, Lister G, Siegel NJ, eds. Rudolph's pediatrics, 21st ed. New York: McGraw-Hill, 2003:929–31.

Stoll BJ. Infections of the neonatal infant. In: Behrman RE, Kliegman RM, Jenson HB, eds. Nelson textbook of pediatrics, 17th ed. Philadelphia: WB Saunders, 2004:623–40.

A 60-year-old woman presents to the emergency department (ED) with left eye pain, redness, and blurred vision for 3 hours after sewing in a dimly lit room. She initially thought she had eyestrain, but then the eye began to hurt suddenly. Her right eye feels fine and vision seems normal. She also reports that her 10-month-old granddaughter accidentally hit her left eye 3 days ago but no change in vision occurred after this very minor trauma. The patient denies any photophobia, ocular discharge, or increased tearing. She wears glasses to sew because she is farsighted. There are no prior similar events. She also reports seeing halos around the light fixtures in the ED, and has a mild headache, but no nausea, vomiting, dizziness, or weakness.

On examination, she is alert and tolerating the ambient light. She has a left infraorbital contusion and a small, medial conjunctival hemorrhage. The left lower lid is not lacerated, and there is no discharge. Visual acuity is 20/30 in the right eye; finger counting is required for the left eye. Visual fields are grossly intact. Gentle palpation of the closed left eye reveals that it is much firmer than the right. Her left pupil is 5 mm, fixed, and unreactive. Her right eye appears normal; the pupil is 3 mm and briskly reactive. Extraocular movements are intact. The left bulbar conjunctiva has a circumcorneal flush, as well as a medial subconjunctival hemorrhage. The left cornea is slightly cloudy, which makes fundoscopy difficult. The right fundus appears normal. Her temporal arteries are pulsatile and nontender. The rest of the physical examination is also within normal.

◆ **What is your next diagnostic step?**

◆ **What is the most likely diagnosis?**

◆ **What is your next therapeutic step?**

ANSWERS TO CASE 27: Red Eye

Summary: This is a 60-year-old woman with acute onset of left eye redness, pain, and markedly decreased visual acuity. She recalls minor trauma 3 days ago. The left eye palpates as firmer than the right eye, the cornea is edematous and the pupil is fixed and dilated.

 Next diagnostic step: slit-lamp examination should be performed and intraocular pressures must be measured in both eyes. The intraocular pressures, measured using a Tono-Pen are 18 and 52 in the right and left eye, respectively. Slit-lamp examination reveals bilateral narrow anterior chambers.

 Most likely diagnosis: acute angle-closure glaucoma.

 Next therapeutic step: lowering the intraocular pressure (IOP) as quickly as possible to preserve vision.

Analysis

Objectives

1. Become familiar with the vision-threatening causes of a painful red eye.
2. Understand the basic treatment modalities and disposition options for vision-threatening causes of a painful red eye.
3. Recognize the clinical settings, signs, and symptoms, as well as complications, of acute angle-closure glaucoma.
4. Understand the key treatment modalities for angle-closure glaucoma.

Considerations

This 60-year-old woman complains of the acute onset of left eye redness, followed by pain and loss of vision. This case is an example of acute angle-closure glaucoma (AACG), a true ophthalmologic emergency characterized by rapidly elevated intraocular pressure. The patient has a preexisting narrow cornea–iris angle, which became blocked, limiting the outflow of aqueous humor causing a precipitous rise in intraocular pressure. It is also possible that the trauma 3 days prior caused some bleeding in the anterior chamber that further limited outflow of aqueous humor.

APPROACH TO THE RED EYE

Acute Angle-Closure Glaucoma

The **mechanism of AACG or primary angle-closure glaucoma is pupillary block**. Another potential mechanism is plateau iris, in which a convex peripheral iris constantly crowds the trabecular network and completely occludes it when the iris dilates. Many other forms of glaucoma have a far more insidious, benign presentation, with an inexorable loss of vision. **Delay in diagnosis and**

treatment of AACG results in permanent loss of vision. The provider must always consider this diagnosis because it is possible to get side-tracked evaluating the associated symptoms of headache, nausea, and vomiting or abdominal pain. Risk factors for a narrow angle-closure include age-related lens thickening and hyperopia (far-sightedness), which results in a shortened eyeball and a relatively shallow anterior chamber. The incidence of narrow angles is 2 percent in white patients, and the rate of AACG is 0.1 percent. African Americans have much higher rates of chronic angle-closure glaucoma (CACG) but lower rates of AACG. Persons between ages 55 and 65 years have the highest incidence of AACG. The incidence in women is three to four times the rate in men, and AACG is likely to occur in 25 to 33 percent of a patient's first-degree relatives, so they should be informed.

Acute angle-closure glaucoma can occur with stress, fatigue, dim lighting, or sustained near work. The patient may present with mild unilateral eye pain with blurring or intense pain, with nausea, vomiting, diaphoresis, and frontal headache. The **hallmarks of the physical examination** include a **fixed, dilated, mid-position pupil, diffuse conjunctival erythema, corneal edema (clouding), and a shallow anterior chamber** (see Figure 27-1). Slit-lamp examination may reveal mild cell and flare. The IOP will be elevated (normal is 9 to 21 mmHg); pressures can reach 80 mmHg in AACG. The other eye must always be examined for anterior chamber depth (the angle is usually narrow), IOP, and for an increased cup:disc ratio in the optic nerve.

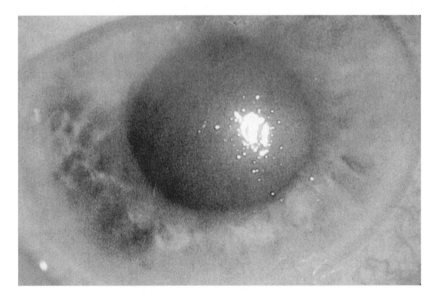

Figure 27-1. Acute angle-closure glaucoma. Pupil is mid-dilated, fixed, and the cornea is cloudy. (Reproduced with permission from Tintinalli JE, Kelen GD, Stapczynski JS, eds. Emergency medicine, 6th ed. New York: McGraw-Hill, 2004:1460.)

IOP depends on the balance between aqueous humor production and outflow. Pressure increases when outflow is blocked or production increases. Conversely IOP decreases when outflow increases and production decreases. The therapeutic goal of the initial management of acute angle-closure glaucoma is decreased IOP. The principal treatment modalities include aqueous suppressants, osmotic agents, and miotic agents. After the corneal edema subsides, **the definitive treatment is a laser peripheral iridectomy.**

Management

Treatment should be initiated in the ED to **lower the intraocular pressure** in **consultation with an ophthalmologist.** Intraocular pressure is lowered by decreasing aqueous humor production with agents such as **carbonic anhydrase inhibitors (acetazolamide) and beta blockers (timolol).** **Alpha$_2$-agonists** will decrease aqueous secretion. **Miotics (pilocarpine)** enhance trabecular outflow, the primary pathway while prostaglandin F$_{2alpha}$ increases uveoscleral outflow, the secondary pathway. Osmotic agents, such as mannitol, glycerol, and isosorbide, are used to dehydrate the vitreous humor, which decreases intraocular fluid volume, thus lowering IOP. Systemic concerns related to topical beta-blocker administration include asthma, severe chronic obstructive pulmonary disease (COPD), bradycardia, heart block, congestive heart failure, and myasthenia gravis. Systemic absorption of topical agents can be reduced up to 70 percent by instructing the patient to close his or her eyes while occluding the lower tear ducts at the root of the nose after applying the drops. Punctal occlusion decreases drug absorption by the nasal mucosa.

Differential Diagnosis of the Red Eye

The diagnosis of AACG is suggested by a painful red eye, with blurry vision, a fixed, mid-dilated pupil, shallow anterior chamber, a cloudy/steamy cornea and elevated intraocular pressure (see Table 27-1 for differential diagnosis). The other vision-threatening causes of red eye include severe conjunctivitis, corneal ulcer, anterior uveitis, orbital cellulitis, and scleritis. The absence of any discharge makes the possibility of conjunctivitis highly unlikely. **Gonococcal conjunctivitis** (the most serious form of bacterial conjunctivitis) produces a copious purulent discharge with an intensely red eye, and may potentially perforate the cornea. A **corneal ulcer** may be visible to the unaided eye as a white defect. Distinguishing an ulcer from a corneal abrasion is clinically significant and can be a challenge. The major distinction is the hazy/cloudy stroma that lies beneath the ulcer in contrast to the clear stroma deep to most abrasions. A slit-lamp examination is a necessary part of the evaluation of all patients with a red eye. Fluorescein staining should be included in every exam and may be the only way to identify the classic dendritic markings found in herpetic keratitis.

Anterior uveitis is associated with photophobia, circumcorneal redness, and cells and flare in the anterior chamber. A hypopyon (layer of white cells) may be

Table 27-1
DIFFERENTIAL DIAGNOSIS OF RED EYE

Processes that usually do not impair vision
    Subconjunctival hemorrhage
    Viral conjunctivitis
    Nongonococcal or nonchlamydial conjunctivitis
    Allergic conjunctivitis
    Blepharitis
    Episcleritis
    Peripheral corneal pterygium

Processes that can impair vision
    Corneal infection (gonococcal infection/chlamydia/herpes simplex virus/herpes-zoster virus)
    Corneal ulcer
    Anterior uveitis
    Scleritis
    Pterygium (encroaching on the paracentral cornea)
    Superficial keratitis

visible. The affected pupil is smaller, irregular, and minimally reactive. IOP can be elevated. Etiologies include idiopathic, infectious (tuberculosis, and syphilis), autoimmune (sarcoid, collagen-vascular diseases), and posttraumatic. Because treatment involves topical corticosteroids with their attendant risk of glaucoma, cataracts, or reactivation of herpes simplex infections, patients should be referred to an ophthalmologist.

Orbital cellulitis, defined as infection deep to the orbital septum is usually associated with blurred vision, diplopia, conjunctival injection, lid swelling, proptosis, fever, toxicity, and limited or painful ocular motility. An orbital computed tomography (CT) (axial and coronal cuts) is diagnostic, and will often reveal sinusitis. Admission and parenteral antibiotics are indicated, because of the potential to invade into the brain. Preseptal or periorbital cellulitis is a superficial and far-less-serious entity that can be difficult to distinguish from orbital cellulitis. In general, these patients are less toxic appearing with less pain. Most of those patients can be discharged on oral antibiotics with close followup to make sure they didn't have an early presentation of the more serious orbital cellulitis.

Subconjunctival hemorrhages should be **painless and not affect vision**. These hemorrhages are often spontaneous or may be associated with minor trauma including coughing and sneezing. In the setting of blunt trauma, continue evaluating for hyphema, or globe rupture or retrobulbar hemorrhage if the patient complains of pain or vision changes. Patients should be informed that the redness might take weeks to resolve.

Blunt trauma to the eye may result in a **hyphema** (blood in the anterior chamber), and painful, blurred vision. The amount of blood may be visible to unaided eye if it layers, or it may only be seen with the slit-lamp (microhyphema) on maximum magnification. Initial treatment includes elevating the head 30 degrees, an eye shield to prevent additional trauma, mydriatics to paralyze the ciliary body allowing the iris to rest, pain medication, and ophthalmologic consultation. Complications include staining of the cornea by the red cells producing a partially opaque cornea, elevated IOP secondary to red blood cells occluding the trabeculae and rebleeding.

Scleritis symptoms include severe eye pain, redness, and decreased vision. An underlying systemic disorder, such as a connective tissue disease, herpes simplex virus (HSV), or syphilis, is frequently the cause. The conjunctival, episcleral, and scleral vessels are inflamed, either diffusely or focally. Unlike episcleral vessels, which blanch with topical vasoconstrictors and move under cotton swabs, scleral vessels do not. Additionally, the entire sclera may have a bluish or violaceous hue. Treatment of the underlying disorder may involve systemic corticosteroids, immunosuppressive therapy, and nonsteroidal antiinflammatory drugs (NSAIDs).

Technically, **temporal arteritis** is associated with **painless vision loss**, but the patient often has associated **scalp tenderness, temporal headache, or jaw claudication**. An ischemic optic neuropathy causes the vision loss. Patients are usually **older than age 50 years**, and will have an **elevated erythrocyte sedimentation rate (ESR)** and an afferent pupillary defect (contracts to indirect light but not to direct light). A temporal artery biopsy showing giant cells is required for definitive diagnosis. Timely treatment with systemic steroids may prevent blindness in the other eye.

Comprehension Questions

[27.1] A 40-year-old man complains of the acute onset of left eye redness with circumcorneal injection (ciliary flush) and pain with bright lights. He states that his eye is painful even when closed. On examination, his pupil is irregular, and minimally reactive. Which of the following is the most likely diagnosis?

A. Acute angle-closure glaucoma
B. Anterior uveitis
C. Herpes simplex virus infection
D. Corneal abrasion

[27.2] A 50-year-old woman is diagnosed with acute angle-closure glaucoma. She has acutely decreased visual acuity. Which of the following is the most likely mechanism for this condition?

A. Increased IOP caused by increased aqueous humor production
B. Nonreactive pupil leading to increased intraocular pressure
C. Decreased outflow of the aqueous humor
D. Separation of the retina leading to decreased visual acuity

[27.3] A 55-year-old man is noted to have acute angle-closure glaucoma. His intraocular pressure is noted to be significantly elevated. His physician prescribes mannitol for treatment of this condition. Which of the following describes the mechanism of action for the mannitol?

A. Decreases production of the aqueous humor
B. Osmotic agent used to decrease intraocular pressure
C. Selective alpha-adrenergic agonists
D. Clears the edema of the cornea

[27.4] A 36-year-old woman has been diagnosed with glaucoma. She also has asthma which has been well controlled. After using the drops prescribed for her glaucoma, she develops an exacerbation of her asthma. Which of the following medications is most likely responsible for her asthmatic exacerbation?

A. Anticholinergic agent
B. Beta-blocker agent
C. Beta-agonist agent
D. Carbonic anhydrase agent

Answers

[27.1]   **B.** Anterior uveitis usually presents as photophobia, red eye with pain, and the affected pupil is smaller, irregular, and minimally reactive.

[27.2]   **C.** In acute angle-closure glaucoma the sudden rise in IOP is a consequence of blocked outflow, and not increased production, of aqueous humor.

[27.3]   **B.** Mannitol is an osmotic agent used to decrease intraocular fluid volume in the vitreous, which helps to lower IOP. All of the other listed agents work by decreasing aqueous humor production.

[27.4]   **B.** Bronchospasm is associated with the use of topical beta blockers.

CLINICAL PEARLS

❖ A useful working differential diagnosis for vision threatening causes of red eye includes acute angle-closure glaucoma, anterior uveitis, corneal ulcer, corneal infection, chlamydial/gonococcal conjunctivitis, orbital cellulitis, hyphema, retrobulbar hemorrhage, and scleritis.

❖ Subconjunctival hemorrhages should be painless and not affect vision. In the setting of blunt trauma, continue evaluating for hyphema, or globe rupture, or retrobulbar hemorrhage if the patient complains of pain or vision changes.

❖   Slit-lamp examination, fluorescein staining, and measurement of
    intraocular pressure are essential elements of a thorough evalua-
    tion of the red eye.
❖   Always assess the depth of the anterior chamber before administering
    a mydriatic to avoid precipitating acute angle-closure glaucoma.

REFERENCES

Barneby HS, Yang-Williams K, Medical considerations in the management of glau-
    coma. In: Gross RL. Clinical glaucoma management. Philadelphia: WB
    Saunders, 2001:255–275.
Leibowitz HM. The red eye. N Engl J Med 2000;343:345–51.
Oram, O. Ciliary Body. In: Gross RL, eds. Clinical glaucoma management: critical
    signs in diagnosis and therapy. Philadelphia: WB Saunders, 2001:19–33.
Rhee DJ. Glaucoma: color atlas and synopsis of clinical ophthalmology. New York:
    McGraw-Hill, 2003.
Shingleton BJ, O'Donoghue MW. Blurred vision. N Engl J Med 2000;343:556–62.
Zimmerman TJ, Kooner KS. Clinical pathways in glaucoma. New York: Thieme,
    2001.

❖ CASE 28

A 26-day-old infant is brought to the emergency department by her concerned mother with a chief complaint of fever. The patient's mother noticed that the baby felt hot to the touch approximately 5 hours ago, at which time she took an oral temperature which measured 38.4°C (101.1°F). Despite a cool bath the infant continued to run a fever, was noted to be more sleepy than usual, and had been feeding poorly for the past 4 hours. Past medical history is unremarkable, including a full-term normal vaginal delivery without complications. In addition, the patient has no sick contacts. Review of systems is negative for cough, rhinorrhea, vomiting, diarrhea, and rash. On physical exam, the infant's vitals are rectal temperature 38.6°C (101.5°F), heart rate 180 beats per minute, blood pressure 95/60 mmHg, respiratory rate 30 breaths per minute, and oxygen saturation 100 percent on room air. The head and neck examination reveals normal tympanic membranes and oropharynx. The lungs are clear bilaterally. The cardiac examination reveals tachycardia, no murmurs, rubs, or gallops. The abdomen is soft, nontender, and nondistended. Capillary refill time is <2 seconds, and there are no petechiae or other rashes. The patient opens eyes spontaneously, cries but is consolable by her mother, and moves all extremities equally. Laboratory studies reveal normal values for the leukocyte count, hemoglobin, hematocrit, platelet count, urinalysis, electrolyte levels, and a chest x-ray. A lumbar puncture is performed and cerebrospinal fluid (CSF) analysis reveals a leukocyte count of 205, with 95 percent neutrophils, red blood cell count of 1 cell/mm^3, protein of 75 mg/dL, and glucose of 37 mg/dL. CSF Gram stain reveals moderate leukocytes and gram-positive cocci in chains. Culture of the CSF is pending.

◆ **What is the most likely diagnosis?**

◆ **What is your next step?**

ANSWERS TO CASE 28: Bacterial Meningitis

Summary: This is a 26-day-old infant with fever and poor feeding for several hours. The patient has a CSF leukocytosis with a positive Gram stain.

◆ **Most likely diagnosis:** bacterial meningitis.

◆ **Next Step:** management of ABCs, including 20 mL/kg IV fluid bolus after the initiation of broad-spectrum antibiotics.

Analysis

Objectives

1. Recognize the clinical setting and the early signs and symptoms of bacterial meningitis.
2. Understand the diagnostic and therapeutic approach to suspected bacterial meningitis.

Considerations

The **classic symptoms of fever, headache, neck stiffness, or nuchal rigidity are often absent in infants, especially in neonates.** Nonspecific signs, such as poor feeding, inconsolability, and/or excessive somnolence may be the physician's only clue that an infectious process is at work. Sometimes the clues can be very subtle and may be nothing more than the parents stating that "my child just isn't acting the right." Given the need for prompt initiation of antibiotics to reduce mortality and to prevent neurological sequelae, a high index of suspicion is essential when dealing with the very young and the possibility of serious bacterial infection.

APPROACH TO SUSPECTED BACTERIAL MENINGITIS

Bacterial meningitis in children and adults is a medical emergency. A delay in diagnosis leads to increased morbidity and mortality; therefore, a high index of suspicion should be maintained. Early administration of intravenous antibiotics can be critical and should be initiated prior to the completion of confirmatory studies including a lumbar puncture. Meningitis (inflammation of the meninges) can be an acute or chronic process. The etiologies of meningitis include chemical, neoplastic, bacterial, viral, mycobacterial, or fungal. Within the pediatric population, the vast majority of cases are acute and infectious (viral or bacterial) in nature. In the preantibiotic era, mortality from bacterial meningitis approached 90 percent. With the advent of antibiotics and pediatric intensive care, the mortality is approximately 5 percent, although the incidence of neurological sequelae (most commonly hearing impairment) remains high at 20 to 30 percent. The infecting organism, and thus the choice of empiric antibiotics, varies greatly with patient age as outlined in Table 28-1. Since the widespread use of vaccination for

Table 28-1

PATIENT AGE, LIKELY ORGANISM, AND EMPIRIC ANTIBIOTIC CHOICE

PATIENT AGE	MOST COMMON ORGANISMS	EMPIRIC ANTIBIOTIC(S)
0–4 weeks	Group B streptococcus, *E. coli*, *Listeria monocytogenes*	Ampicillin + cefotaxime
4–12 weeks	*S. pneumoniae*, group B streptococcus, *E. coli*, *L. monocytogenes*	Ampicillin + third-generation cephalosporin
3 months–18 years	*S. pneumoniae*, *N. meningitidis*, *H. influenzae*	Third-generation cephalosporin
18 years–50 years	*S. pneumoniae*, *N. meningitidis*	Third-generation cephalosporin
>50 years	*S. pneumoniae*, *N. meningitidis*, *L. monocytogenes*, aerobic gram-negative bacilli	Third-generation cephalosporin + ampicillin

Some authors now suggest the addition of vancomycin for patients in whom physicians suspect infection with penicillin-resistant *S. pneumoniae*.

Haemophilus influenzae, bacterial meningitis caused by this organism is rarely seen. *H. influenzae* had been such a common and serious cause of pediatric meningitis. In this postvaccination era, bacterial meningitis is now much more common in adults than in the pediatric population.

Diagnosis

The diagnosis of bacterial meningitis is made by lumbar puncture. Fever, headache, vomiting, neck stiffness, lethargy, irritability, and seizures may or may not be present in the setting of bacterial meningitis. In the neonatal period, poor feeding and lethargy may be the only presenting complaints. Adults, as well as infants, can present with nonspecific signs and symptoms. Physical exam may reveal nuchal rigidity, Kernig sign (inability to completely extend the leg when the hip is flexed to 90 degrees) or Brudzinski sign (severe neck stiffness and pain causes a patient's hips and knees to flex when the neck is flexed), papilledema, or focal neurological deficits. The presence of even a single petechiae may be the only finding in early meningococcemia and should be taken very seriously! Highlighting the difficulty of making this diagnosis, a normal exam is often the case. Hence, these findings are poorly validated and their absence should not deter the physician from initiating antibiotics and performing a lumbar puncture (LP).

Table 28-2

INDICATIONS FOR CT SCAN BEFORE LUMBAR PUNCTURE IN
SUSPECTED BACTERIAL MENINGITIS

Depressed mental status	History or evidence of head trauma*
Evidence of papilledema	Recent seizure
Focal neurological deficit	

*Recent or remote head trauma

Table 28-3

ANALYSIS OF CEREBROSPINAL FLUID

TEST	NORMAL VALUE	SIGNIFICANCE OF ABNORMALITY
Cell count	< 5 WBC/mm^3	Increased WBC in all meningitis
	<1 PMN/mm^3	Increased PMNs suggest bacterial etiology*
	<1 eosinophil/mm^3	Any eosinophil is considered abnormal
Gram stain	no organisms	Identified 80% in bacterial meningitis Identified 60% if patient pretreated
Protein	15–45mg/dL	Elevated in acute bacterial/fungal meningitis
CSF-to-serum glucose	0.6 :1	Depressed in pyogenic meningitis Depressed in hyperglycemia
India ink	Negative	Positive in 33% of cryptococcal meningitis
Cryptococcal antigen	Negative	90% accuracy for cryptococcal disease
Lactic acid	Negative	Elevated in bacterial and tubercular meningitis
Acid-fast stain	Negative	Positive in 80% of tuberculosis meningitis

Abbreviations: CSF, cerebrospinal fluid; PMN, polymorphonuclear leukocyte; WBC, white blood cells
*The typical profile in cases of viral meningitis is a lymphocytic pleocytosis; however, PMNs predominate in the first 48 hours of viral meningitis.

Computed tomography (CT) of the brain is rarely performed prior to LP in the pediatric population unless there are focal neurological signs on examination that could indicate a mass lesion or increased intracranial pressure. While many emergency physicians routinely perform a head CT prior to LP in adults, there is convincing evidence that this may not be necessary in a subset of patients if a careful neurological exam is performed. Table 28-2 presents indications for obtaining a CT scan before lumbar puncture in suspected bacterial meningitis.

A CSF pleocytosis confirms the presence of meningitis, although it does not determine the cause (i.e., bacterial, viral, tubercular, neoplasm, autoimmune). Although the white blood cell differential and the levels of protein and glucose often suggest the etiology of the inflammation, patients with CSF pleocytosis should be admitted and treated with antibiotics while awaiting CSF culture results. Table 28-3 summarizes the analysis of cerebrospinal fluid.

Treatment

If a physician elects to order a CT prior to performing an LP, empiric antibiotics should be given immediately (generally within 30 minutes). If an LP is performed promptly without a CT scan, empiric antibiotics should be administered before the results of the LP are obtained. Do not wait to initiate antibiotics out of fear that they may alter the results of the LP or that the results of the LP will alter the antibiotic selection.

There is much debate in the medical literature over the use of corticosteroids, namely dexamethasone, in the treatment of bacterial meningitis. While dexamethasone has shown benefit in adult and pediatric populations, many of the studies were performed on patients with *H. influenzae* meningitis, which is no longer a primary clinical concern. In addition, the utility of corticosteroids in the treatment of the recently emerging penicillin-resistant *Streptococcus pneumoniae* meningitis has not been demonstrated. Steroid use is indicated in some clinical settings and controversial in others; one should follow institutional guidelines for the use of steroids in one's particular clinical setting.

Comprehension Questions

[28.1] Which organism is the most likely cause of bacterial meningitis in an 18-day-old infant?

  A. *Streptococcus pneumoniae*
  B. *Neisseria meningitidis*
  C. *Listeria monocytogenes*
  D. *Staphylococcus aureus*

[28.2] Which of the following would most likely exclude the presence of bacterial meningitis?

A. Absence of fever and headache
B. Absent Kernig and Brudzinski signs
C. No nuchal rigidity
D. Lumbar puncture

[28.3] Which of the following options represents the best treatment strategy for a 5-year-old child with headache, fever, neck stiffness, and a right hemiplegia on physical exam?

A. Lumbar puncture followed by administration of ceftriaxone
B. Administration of ceftriaxone followed by CT scan and lumbar puncture
C. CT scan followed by administration of ceftriaxone and lumbar puncture
D. Administration of ampicillin and cefotaxime followed by CT scan and lumbar puncture

Answers

[28.1] **C.** *L. Monocytogenes* is a common cause of meningitis in the 0- to 4-week-old infant.

[28.2] **D.** There are no features of the history or physical exam that can reliably exclude bacterial meningitis. Only a lumbar puncture can be used to exclude this diagnosis.

[28.3] **B.** CT scan should be performed prior to LP in patients with focal neurological deficits. Ceftriaxone is an appropriate antibiotic choice in this age group and should not be delayed given the neurological findings.

CLINICAL PEARLS

❖ In the ED setting, when meningitis is suspected, the antibiotics should be generally started within 30 minutes.

❖ The lumbar puncture is the most accurate method to diagnose bacterial meningitis.

❖ Neonates, older patients, and immunocompromised individuals with meningitis may not manifest nuchal rigidity.

❖ In the neonate, Group B streptococcus, *Escherichia coli*, and *Listeria* are the most common etiologies of meningitis. Otherwise, *Streptococcus pneumoniae* is the most common cause.

REFERENCES

de Gans J. Dexamethasone in adults with bacterial meningitis. N Engl J Med 2002;347(20):1549–56.

Hasbun R, Abrahams J, Jekel J, et al. Computed tomography of the head before lumbar puncture in adults with suspected meningitis. N Engl J Med 2001;345:1727–33.

Lavoie FW. Meningitis, encephalitis and central nervous system abscess. In: Rosen P, Barkin R, et al. Emergency medicine concepts and clinical practice 4th ed. Mosby, 1998;2198–209.

Thomas KE. The diagnostic accuracy of Kernig's sign, Brudzinski's sign, and nuchal rigidity in adults with suspected meningitis. Clin Infect Dis 2002;35(1):46–52.

Paramedics are called to the international terminal of the airport for a man seizing. They arrive to find a 30-year-old male in a full tonic-clonic seizure in front of baggage claim. The patient is apparently traveling alone, and medics check for a medical ID bracelet and find none. This patient's past medical history is thus unknown. The medics protect him from injury, manage his airway with assisted bag–value mask, start an IV of normal saline, and administer a total of 10 mg of diazepam per EMS protocol with no resolution of the seizures. The patient continues to seize upon his arrival to the emergency department. The patient's vital signs are blood pressure 200/115 mmHg, heart rate 130 beats per minute, respiratory rate 20 breaths per minute, oxygen saturation of 100 percent on 10 L/min O_2, temperature of 37.8°C (100.1°F). On examination the patient is a well-nourished young male who is having a whole-body seizure. He has blood-tinged sputum about his mouth, and his teeth are clenched. The patient is tachycardic but with normal heart sounds. Lung exam reveals coarse breath sounds throughout. Abdomen is benign. Neurological exam: Patient continues to seize, moving all extremities in a tonic–clonic fashion. The extremities move symmetrically. Cranial nerves are unable to be evaluated. Toes are down-going and deep tendon reflexes are 2+ throughout. Rectal exam reveals a small plastic bag with a white residue on it. Electrocardiogram (EKG) reveals a sinus tachycardia with no acute ST changes. Head computed tomography (CT), chest radiograph, and lumbar puncture are within normal limits. Abnormalities seen on a comprehensive metabolic panel include a bicarbonate level of 10 mEq/L and a creatine phosphokinase (CPK) of 5500 Iu/L. Urine toxicology screen is positive for cocaine.

◆ **What is the most likely diagnosis?**

◆ **What is your next step?**

ANSWERS TO CASE 29: Status Epilepticus Caused by Cocaine

Summary: This is a 30-year-old male with new-onset seizure and status epilepticus secondary to cocaine toxicity. It is likely that this patient was attempting to smuggle cocaine through the country by stuffing a wrapped package of the drug in his rectum.

 Most likely diagnosis: new-onset seizure with status epilepticus secondary to cocaine toxicity.

 Next step: aggressive management of ABCs with rapid sequence intubation to protect the airway, IV hydration, and the use of benzodiazepines and antiepileptic agents for the control of seizures and hypertension.

Analysis

Objectives

1. Develop a methodological approach to the assessment of the patient who presents to the emergency department with first-time seizure and status epilepticus.
2. Understand the diagnostic and therapeutic approach to the patient presenting to the emergency department with first-time seizure and status epilepticus.

Considerations

This 30-year-old man has his first episode of epilepsy, and presents with status epilepticus, likely to be cocaine induced. As always, **the first priority is the ABCs.** The patient should have an **oral airway if possible, prevention from aspiration, be given oxygen, and have his vital signs assessed. Benzodiazepines are the treatment of choice in treating this individual.** His elevated CPK levels indicate rhabdomyolysis. Phenobarbital or neuromuscular blockade may be the only way for successful management. The level of CPK and renal function tests should be followed; alkalization of the urine may be important to keep myoglobin from precipitating in the renal tubules, leading to tubal necrosis.

APPROACH TO SEIZURE DISORDERS

Classification

Any event that disturbs the balance between neuronal excitation and inhibition can produce an excessive discharge of cortical neurons that results in a seizure. Seizures are classified into two broad categories: generalized and partial (focal). Generalized seizures involve both hemispheres of the brain and are accompanied by loss of consciousness. Generalized seizures are further classified according to the presence or absence of various patterns of convulsive movements (tonic, tonic–clonic, atonic, myoclonic). Partial seizures involve the discharge of neurons in a localized area of one cerebral hemisphere. Partial seizures are subclassified according to whether consciousness is maintained (simple partial seizures) or impaired (complex partial seizures). Patients who have recurring seizures without consistent provocation have epilepsy, while patients who have a seizure secondary to a particular toxin, focal central nervous system (CNS) abnormality, or environmental stress have reactive or secondary seizures. Reactive seizures tend to be generalized.

Diagnosis

The medical history of a seizure patient should include a description of the seizure and postictal state, pain or injury resulting from the seizure, including tongue biting, and the presence of a preceding aura or incontinence. The physician should also inquire about sleep deprivation, alcohol and drug ingestion, pregnancy, family history, human immunodeficiency virus (HIV) risk factors, and symptoms consistent with infectious, metabolic, or CNS lesions. Patients with a known seizure disorder should be questioned about the type and etiology of their seizures, as well as medication compliance.

Patients presenting to the emergency department with seizure require a thorough physical exam, noting any findings of trauma, as well as a detailed neurological evaluation. Injuries often associated with seizure include tongue lacerations, shoulder dislocations, and head and facial trauma.

Imaging and Laboratory   Most patients with **new-onset seizure,** or those who have **a known seizure disorder but have new symptoms or physical exam findings**, should undergo either **emergent head computed tomography (CT) or magnetic resonance imaging (MRI)** based upon availability. However, patients who resolve spontaneously from their first-time seizure without neurological sequelae may be safely discharged to home with an outpatient CT scan, MRI, and/or electroencephalogram (EEG) scheduled if the practice environment allows for dependable followup.

Because most life-threatening conditions associated with seizures are related to hemorrhage, brain swelling, or mass effect, a noncontrast CT scan may be all that is necessary on an emergent basis. **Patients older than 40 years of age have an increased likelihood of having an abnormal CT. Tumor** is the most common abnormality in **patients between the ages of 40 and 60 years,** while **cardiovascular accident (CVA) is the most common abnormality** in patients **older than 60 years of age.** Seizures in immunosuppressed patients are frequently associated with mass lesions from infectious causes.

Use of the EEG is uncommon in the emergency department evaluation of first-time seizure except in the assessment of nonconvulsive status epilepticus, or to establish status epilepticus in a patient who has been given long-acting paralytic agents. In the majority of cases, a complete history will reveal the etiology of the seizure and laboratory testing will not be required. Seizures caused by electrolyte abnormalities are quite rare, with hypoglycemia and hyperglycemia accounting for the greatest number, both of which can be evaluated by bedside glucose analysis. Calcium abnormalities are an infrequent cause of seizure, but are more prevalent in patients with a history of malignancy (see Table 29-1 for common causes of reactive seizures).

Status Epilepticus Classically, **status epilepticus has been defined as more than 30 minutes of continuous seizure activity or two or more sequential seizures without full recovery of consciousness between seizures.** The **most common cause of status epilepticus is discontinuation of anticonvulsant medications.** It should also be noted that status epilepticus is the initial presentation of a seizure disorder in approximately one-third of cases. The catecholamine surge that accompanies status epilepticus can cause tachycardia, hypertension, hypotension, cardiac arrhythmias, respiratory failure, hyperglycemia, acidosis, and rhabdomyolysis. Status epilepticus requires prompt recognition and treatment. An aggressive search for the underlying cause is critical as it is the most important factor in determining prognosis. Status epilepticus must be ruled out in any patient who does not regain consciousness within 20 to 30 minutes of cessation of a generalized seizure, and should be considered in any patient with unexplained confusion or coma.

Postictal State A decreased level of arousal and responsiveness, disorientation, amnesia, and headache characterizes the postictal state that follows most generalized seizures. These conditions may persist for only a few minutes or many hours, and may vary from seizure to seizure. Patients who fail to have a steady improvement in their mental status during the postictal period should be carefully evaluated for possible causes of reactive seizures.

Table 29-1
COMMON CAUSES OF REACTIVE SEIZURES

Metabolic encephalopathies: hypomagnesemia, hyponatremia, hypocalcemia, hypoglycemia, hepatic or renal failure

Infectious encephalopathies: central nervous system abscess, meningitis, encephalitis

Central nervous system lesions: neoplasm, arteriovenous malformations, vasculitis, acute hydrocephalus, intracerebral hematomas, cerebrovascular accident, posttraumatic seizures. migraine/vascular headache, degenerative disease (Multiple Sclerosis)

Intoxications: medications (tricyclic antidepressants, isoniazid, theophylline), recreational drugs (cocaine), alcohol and drug withdrawal, lead, strychnine, camphor, eclampsia

---

Differential Diagnosis

Transient alteration in level of consciousness may be mistaken for an epileptic seizure; therefore, obtaining a clear history from witnesses is critical in establishing the diagnosis. Disorders that mimic seizure include syncope, migraines, transient global amnesia, cerebral vascular disease, narcolepsy, psychogenic seizures, hyperventilation, and breath-holding spells in children.

Febrile Seizures **Febrile seizures are the most common type of seizure in childhood** and account for 30 percent of all seizures in children. There appears to be a **family predilection** for febrile seizure and 25 to 30 percent of children who have a single febrile seizure will have another. **Febrile seizures generally occur during the initial 24 hours of fever activity in children between the ages of 6 months and 5 years**. There also appears to be a correlation between the degree of temperature elevation and incidence of seizure, but less evidence supporting the theory that febrile seizures are caused by a precipitous rise in temperature. Either way, patients are often brought to the emergency department for seizure before the family has identified a febrile illness.

The goal of the emergency physician in evaluating a child with febrile seizure is to determine the cause of the fever and to rule out meningitis. Patients with a febrile seizure are not at higher risk for a serious bacterial illness than similarly aged febrile patients, and viral illness is usually the cause of the fever. The need for significant diagnostic testing including lumbar puncture will be determined by the history and physical exam.

While toxic-appearing children require a full septic workup including lumbar puncture, the patient presenting with the classic signs and symptoms of a febrile seizure may be safely discharged to home after identification and treatment of the precipitating illness. Parents must be provided with instructions regarding aggressive fever control and reassurance that this does not represent a lifelong seizure disorder.

Drug-Induced Seizures Because of lack of history and a risk for trauma, most drug-induced seizures will require diagnostic imaging and laboratory testing. In most cases, therapy for drug-induced seizures is guided by general seizure-management principles. However, in some cases, drug-induced seizures necessitate therapy that is specific to the etiological agent. **Cocaine is one of the most frequent causes of drug-induced seizures.** Approximately 15 percent of cocaine users will experience a drug-induced seizure and the development of status epilepticus is a major determinant of mortality in cocaine intoxication. Seizures caused by cocaine are a result of a combination of a lowered seizure threshold and hypersympathetic state, and are often associated with hyperthermia and high lactate levels. These seizures are usually self-limited, but in cases **of status epilepticus, should be treated with high doses of benzodiazepines.** Use of beta blockers or labetalol is inadvisable in the treatment of severe hypertension and tachycardia associated with cocaine toxicity because of the risk of unopposed alpha-adrenergic stimulation. **In other words, benzodiazepines should be used in maximum doses before another agent is contemplated for cocaine-induced seizures.**

Tricyclic antidepressants cause seizures as a consequence of their anti-cholinergic properties. In addition to standard seizure therapy, patients with status epilepticus secondary to tricyclic overdose should be treated with sodium bicarbonate in an effort to obtain a blood pH of approximately 7.5. This will decrease the free form of the drug in the patient's CNS as well as mitigate the drug's sodium channel blocking effect at the heart.

Isoniazid-induced seizures are associated with a high mortality rate and typically occur within 120 minutes of an acute overdose. Isoniazid toxicity overwhelms the body's ability to bind the drug with **vitamin B$_6$ (pyridoxine)** and often results in status epilepticus by depleting the CNS inhibitory transmitter gamma-aminobutyric acid (GABA). Treatment of seizures secondary to isoniazid toxicity is often refractory to standard measures and **should be treated with IV pyridoxine.** The dose of pyridoxine is based upon the amount of drug ingested.

Theophylline-induced seizures frequently result in status epilepticus and are associated with a mortality of up to 50 percent. Theophylline antagonizes adenosine and causes an increased sympathetic state. Serum theophylline levels do not correlate well with the risk of seizures, and chronic intoxication carries a greater risk of seizure than does acute ingestion. Charcoal hemoperfusion should be considered in patients with high serum theophylline levels in whom standard therapy has not abated their seizures.

Alcohol Withdrawal Seizures   **Alcohol withdrawal seizures are a leading cause of seizures in adults**. Alcohol withdrawal seizures **typically occur 6 to 48 hours after the last drink**, but may occur up to 7 days status post alcohol cessation. The use of CT scan in the evaluation of an alcoholic with first-time seizure is prudent because of the high risk of head trauma and intracerebral bleeding in these patients. Alcoholism is a common cause of hypoglycemia and hypomagnesemia, thus electrolytes in these patients should be checked. Most alcohol withdrawal seizures can be effectively managed with the use of **benzodiazepines**, as they are notoriously unresponsive to anticonvulsants. IV hydration with a glucose-containing solution in addition to thiamine, magnesium, potassium, and multivitamins is also indicated. Alcohol withdrawal is relatively unlikely to cause status epilepticus, and in the case of status, should prompt the physician to rule out other causes of seizure in the alcoholic patient.

Pseudoseizures   Pseudoseizures are defined as episodes of altered movement, sensation, or experience similar to epilepsy, but caused by a psychological process and not associated with abnormal electrical discharges in the brain. The incidence of psychogenic seizures appears to decrease after age 35 years and is rare after age 50 years. Unlike patients with true neurogenic seizures, patients with **psychogenic seizures tend to have multiple seizure patterns**, which are usually **not followed by a postictal period**. Distinguishing between neurogenic seizures and pseudoseizures can be a challenge. Urinary incontinence and injury such as tongue biting has been reported in up to 20 percent of patients with psychogenic seizure. Nonnoxious and noxious stimuli such as ammonia capsules may elicit responses from patients having psychogenic seizures, which is not the case for those experiencing true neurogenic seizures. The observation of purposeful movement during the seizure also is atypical of neurogenic seizure. Blood gas analysis is useful in identifying patients with true neurogenic seizures, because many of these patients will demonstrate some degree of metabolic acidosis that rapidly resolves following the event.

The gold standard for the diagnosis of pseudoseizures is the use of synchronized video EEG, although the diagnosis is ultimately based upon the combination of history and seizure observation, and the lack of an organic explanation for the seizures.

Treatment of Seizures

Initial stabilization of a patient with seizure requires (a) **ABCs**, (b) bedside **glucose** analysis, (c) **pulse oximetry and electrocardiogram (EKG) monitoring**, (d) initial treatment with **benzodiazepines**, and (e) **laboratory testing and diagnostic imaging** as indicated by the history and physical exam.

A seizing patient has a decreased gag reflex and is at **risk for aspiration**. **Aggressive airway protection** is indicated and should include appropriate positioning of the patient and frequent **suctioning**. Patients who continue to seize or whose airway is unable to be protected with conservative measures should be intubated using a benzodiazepine as the induction agent in hopes of abating the seizure. If the patient requires **paralysis** for management purposes, it cannot be assumed that the patient's seizure has been terminated. In this situation, anticonvulsant therapy should be continued and **EEG monitoring** of the patient should be arranged (see Table 29-2).

Pharmacological Therapy

The **first-line therapy of any active seizure is a parenteral benzodiazepine**. Benzodiazepines suppress seizure activity by **directly enhancing GABA-related neuronal inhibition**. They are effective in terminating seizures in 75 to 90 percent of patients. Drugs commonly used by the emergency physician in the treatment of seizure include **diazepam, lorazepam, and midazolam.** No one drug is clearly superior in the treatment of seizures, although many physicians favor lorazepam because of its relatively longer duration of seizure-suppression activity. All of the benzodiazepines have the potential to cause sedation, hypotension, and respiratory depression.

Table 29-2
ACUTE SEIZURE MANAGEMENT: DRUG THERAPY

First-line therapy

DRUG	ADULT DOSE	PEDIATRIC DOSE	DURATION OF ACTION	COMMENTS
Lorazepam	0.1 mg/kg IV at 1–2 mg/min up to 10 mg	0.05–0.1 mg/kg IV	2–8 hours	Rapid acting; longer duration of action than diazepam; prolonged CNS depression possible
Diazepam	0.2 mg/kg IV at 2 mg/min up to 20 mg	0.2–0.5 mg/kg IV up to 20 mg	5–15 minutes	Rapid acting; short effective half-life
Midazolam	2.5–15 mg IV 0.2 mg/kg IM	0.15 mg/kg IV then 2–10 μg/kg/min	1–15 minutes	Significant amnestic effect

Second-line therapy

DRUG	ADULT DOSE	PEDIATRIC DOSE	DURATION OF ACTION	COMMENTS
Phenytoin	20 mg/kg IV at <50 mg/min	20 mg/kg IV at 1 mg/kg/min	24 hours	Hypotension and arrhythmias at high infusion rates; cardiac monitoring required
Phenobarbital	20 mg/kg IV at 60–100 mg/min		1–3 days	Long lasting; may be given as IM loading dose

Third-line therapy

DRUG	ADULT DOSE	PEDIATRIC DOSE	DURATION OF ACTION	COMMENTS
Pentobarbital	5 mg/kg IV at 25 mg/min, then titrate to EEG		Minutes	Intubation, ventilation, and pressor support required; respiratory arrest, hypotension, and myocardial depression common
Isoflurane	Via general endotracheal anesthesia		Minutes	Monitor with EEG

The anticonvulsant drugs **phenytoin and phenobarbital** are considered second-line agents in the abortive treatment of seizures. Phenytoin does not directly suppress electrical activity at the seizure focus, but rather suppresses neuronal recruitment, thus concurrent benzodiazepine administration is necessary when treating active seizures. Phenytoin's onset of action is 10 to 30 minutes and its duration of action is 24 hours. Slow IV administration is necessary to avoid **hypotension** and **cardiac dysrhythmias** associated with its propylene glycol diluent. **The phenytoin prodrug fosphenytoin is water-soluble and can be administered quickly without significant toxicity.** Cerebellar symptoms, such as nystagmus and ataxia, are the most common neurological side effects associated with phenytoin. Oral loading is appropriate in patients who present to the emergency department for medication refills and report medical noncompliance. **Oral doses of 18 mg/kg of phenytoin will achieve therapeutic blood levels in approximately 10 to 24 hours**, which is why most physicians reserve this approach for patients who present to the ED without a history of recent seizure.

Phenobarbital is a CNS depressant that **directly suppresses cortical electrical activity** and is often used after benzodiazepines and phenytoin have failed. The **onset of action of phenobarbital is 15 to 30 minutes and its duration of action is 48 hours.** Phenobarbital is **extremely sedating** and often accompanied by **respiratory depression and hypotension**, which is why many physicians will attempt seizure control with phenytoin prior to using this drug.

The patient in status epilepticus who continues to seize despite aggressive therapy with parenteral benzodiazepines and anticonvulsants requires third-line agents such as **barbiturate coma and/or inhalational anesthesia.** Barbiturates, such as pentobarbital, directly enhance GABA-mediated neuronal inhibition while also suppressing all brainstem function. This is useful in decreasing intracranial pressure and increasing cerebral brain flow, but may also induce respiratory arrest, myocardial depression, and hypotension. **Patients undergoing barbiturate coma require intubation and ventilatory management, as well as careful hemodynamic monitoring and support.**

Isoflurane anesthesia suppresses electrical seizure foci and is **the treatment of last resort** for the patient in status epilepticus.

Patient Disposition and Long-Term Management

The **underlying condition responsible** for the **reactive seizure should be aggressively addressed**. The patient may be discharged from the emergency department following consultation with the patient's primary care provider and/or neurologist. First-time seizure patients will likely receive **an MRI and EEG** as part of their outpatient neurological evaluation. The institution of an antiepileptic drug from the emergency department may affect the usefulness of subsequent EEG analysis. Patients need to be provided detailed **seizure precautions**, and locally mandated reporting requirements must be meticulously noted in the patient's chart. The risk of seizure recurrence after a first, unprovoked generalized seizure is approximately 42 percent at 2 years. Neurological abnormalities or epileptiform activity on the EEG double the risk of recurrence. The decision regarding the long-term management of seizure must take into account factors such as side effects, costs, quality of life, patient's occupation, aversion to the risk of recurrent seizures, and requirement of a driver's license.

Patients with Established Seizure Disorder

The majority of patients evaluated in the emergency department for seizure have an established history of epilepsy. Patients should be questioned carefully about their **medical compliance** and their seizure history and pattern. Common seizure triggers should be elicited from the patient, and a careful evaluation for signs of trauma from the event should be undertaken. Patients with previously diagnosed epilepsy who are awake and alert following a typical convulsion require little diagnostic workup other than a thorough history and consideration of measurement of antiepileptic drug levels. Subtherapeutic levels of antiseizure medication can be a result of medical noncompliance or increased metabolism, often caused by concurrent medication intake, and increased drug metabolism. Patients who are found to have **subtherapeutic blood levels** of their antiseizure medication can usually be **loaded with the medication and discharged safely to home**. Any history or physical exam findings consistent with a **new seizure pattern should be addressed, as would the first-time seizure.**

Comprehension Questions

[29.1] A 34-year-old man is brought into the ED with a seizure of new onset. It is determined that it was likely to be metabolic in etiology. Which of the following is the most likely diagnosis?

A. Hyperthyroidism
B. Hypocalcemia
C. Hypoglycemia
D. Hypomagnesemia

[29.2] A 28-year-old woman is brought into the ED by paramedics because of seizure activity that has persisted for 40 minutes despite intravenous Valium at the house and en route. What is the most likely reason for this patient's condition?

A. Meningitis
B. Noncompliance with seizure medications
C. Cocaine
D. Benzodiazepine allergy

[29.3] A 21-year-old man is brought into the ED for a seizure which was witnessed. It was described as tonic–clonic and lasting for 3 minutes. Currently, the patient appears alert, oriented, and with normal vital signs. He has no nuchal rigidity. He admits to being diagnosed with HIV disease, but otherwise has no medical problems. He denies head trauma, or alcohol or illicit drug use. He denies headache. Which of the following is the best next step?

A. Emergent CT or MRI imaging of the brain
B. Begin fosphenytoin for seizure disorder
C. Observation because this is his first seizure
D. Stat EEG

Answers

[29.1] **C.** New-onset seizure in the ED caused by metabolic abnormalities is rare. Hypoglycemia is considered the most common metabolic cause of seizure. Symptomatic hypoglycemia occurs most commonly as a complication of insulin or oral hypoglycemic therapy in diabetics. Hyperglycemia, hypocalcemia, and hypomagnesemia are other, less-common metabolic causes of seizure.

[29.2] **B.** A patient who experiences 30 minutes of continuous seizure activity or a series of seizures without return to full consciousness between seizures is considered to be in status epilepticus. The most common cause of status epilepticus is discontinuation of anticonvulsant medications.

[29.3] **A.** Diagnostic imaging with head CT or MRI is recommended for seizure patients with suspicion of head trauma, elevated intracranial pressure, intracranial mass, persistently abnormal mental status, focal neurological abnormality, or HIV disease.

CLINICAL PEARLS

❖ Identifying the patient within one of the following subgroups facilitates the evaluation and management of the seizure patient in the emergency department: (a) new-onset (first-time) seizure, (b) recurrent seizures in patients with epilepsy, (c) febrile seizures, (d) posttraumatic seizures, and (e) alcohol- and drug-related seizures.

❖ The possibility of reactive seizures should be considered in all seizure patients who present to the ED, including patients with a history of epilepsy. Failure to treat the underlying cause of reactive seizure is a major pitfall.

❖ Seizures may be confused with other nonictal states such as syncope, hyperventilation, and breath-holding spells in children, migraines, transient global amnesia, cerebral vascular disease, narcolepsy, and psychogenic seizures.

❖ Prolonged altered mental status following a seizure should not be attributed to an uncomplicated postictal state.

REFERENCES

Armon K, Stephenson T, MacFaul R, et al. An evidence and consensus based guideline for the management of a child after a seizure. Emerg Med J 2003;20(1):13–20.

Pollack CV, Pollack ES. Seizures. In: Marx J, Hockberger R, Walls R, eds. Emergency medicine: concepts and clinical Practice, 5th ed. St Louis: Mosby-Year Book, 2002.

Scheuer ML, Pedley TA. The evaluation and treatment of seizures. N Engl J Med 1990;323(21):1468–74.

Seamans CM, Slovis CM. Seizures: classification and diagnosis, patient stabilization and pharmacologic interventions. In: EMR textbook, 2002 (http://www.emronline.com/articles/textbook/44).

Turnbull TL, Vanden Hoek TL, Howes DS. Utility of laboratory studies in the emergency department patient with a new-onset seizure. Ann Emerg Med 1990;19(4):373–7.

A 40-year-old woman wandered into a convenience store. She was disheveled in appearance, seemed to be confused, and had been incontinent of urine. Paramedics were called. The patient's vital signs upon arrival in the emergency department are temperature 37.4°C (99.3°F), heart rate 104 beats per minute, blood pressure 138/68 mmHg, respiratory rate 32 breaths per minute, and oxygen saturation 97 percent on room air. Her finger glucose test was 98 mg/dL in the field. On your exam, she appears sleepy and smells of alcohol; however, she is unable to participate with the breathalyzer test. She complains of a headache, but cannot elaborate further or provide any other history. On physical exam, her skin is warm and dry with no apparent rashes. She has no signs of head trauma and no hemotympanum. Her pupils are normal-sized and symmetrical, but minimally reactive. Her oropharynx is unremarkable. Her neck is supple, without thyromegaly. She is tachypneic, but her lung sounds are clear and she has no accessory muscle use. She is mildly tachycardic, but her cardiac exam is otherwise normal. Her abdomen is benign. Neurologically, her speech is slurred and she appears drowsy, however her exam is nonfocal. A complete blood count (CBC) shows a white blood cell count of 8000 cells/mm³. Her electrolyte panel reveals Na 145 mEq/L, K 4.2 mEq/L, Cl 105mEq/L, bicarbonate 15 mEq/L, blood urea nitrogen (BUN) 10 mg/dL, creatinine 1.1 mg/dL, and glucose 100 mg/dL. Urine toxicology screen is negative for cocaine, opiates, and amphetamines. Serum alcohol level is 0.02.

◆ **What is the most likely diagnosis?**

◆ **What is the next lab test that should be ordered?**

◆ **What important component of the physical exam was omitted and what would you have been looking for?**

ANSWERS TO CASE 30: Altered Mental Status (Alcohol Ingestion)

Summary: This is a 40-year-old woman with a toxic alcohol ingestion (methanol vs. ethylene glycol). She presented confused and tachypneic with a significant anion gap in her electrolytes.

 Most likely diagnosis: toxic alcohol ingestion, likely methanol and less likely ethylene glycol.

 Next lab test: serum osmolality, serum methanol, and ethylene glycol levels.

 Omitted step: fundoscopic exam to assess optic disk hyperemia.

Analysis

Objectives

1. To establish a practical approach to the evaluation of patients with altered mental status, incorporating a focused physical exam with bedside lab tests.
2. To recognize which altered patients warrant a more extensive workup beyond this practical approach.
3. To develop a comprehensive yet clinically relevant differential diagnosis for patients with altered level of consciousness.

Considerations

This 40-year-old woman is disoriented, smells of alcohol, and has an anion gap acidosis. The serum alcohol level is low, and does not account for her altered mental status. Two concerns include ethylene glycol or methanol ingestion. **Ethylene glycol, which is in antifreeze, is odorless, colorless, and sweet tasting.** It turns into toxic metabolites, leading to metabolic acidosis and kidney and liver injury. Typically, ethylene glycol induces the **slurred speech and ataxia, but without the smell of alcohol**. Also, the optic fundus is usually normal. This patient's alcohol breath makes ethylene glycol poisoning less likely. Serum levels would yield a definitive diagnosis. Methanol or wood alcohol is the likely culprit in this patient's case. **Methanol** is metabolized to formaldehyde and formic acid. It is **colorless but has a distinct odor**, and can be absorbed orally and through the lungs. Toxic levels can lead to **optic papillitis** and **blindness**. Thus, a fundoscopic examination should be performed in this patient to assess the optic disc. Although definitive diagnosis is made by assaying serum levels, treatment should not be delayed. The treatment rests on administration of ethanol or fomepizole to decrease the conversion to toxic metabolites (by inhibiting alcohol dehydrogenase), and consideration of dialysis for severe disease.

APPROACH TO ALTERED MENTAL STATUS

Altered level of consciousness presents a serious diagnostic dilemma for emergency physicians. Many of the potential etiologies are serious and life-threatening. Between 5 and 10 percent of emergency department (ED) patients present with altered mental status and 80 percent of these have an underlying systemic or metabolic disorder. As with all patients presenting to the ED, the initial evaluation of affected patients relies on history, physical examination, and auxiliary testing or imaging when appropriate. Clearly, these patients are more challenging because they cannot provide a reliable history and are often unable to fully participate with the physical exam.

History

The differential diagnosis for altered mental status is so broad that any historical information that can be learned may be very helpful. Providers need to search for information related to the rate of onset of recent behavioral changes, recent illnesses or trauma, past medical history, current medications, substance abuse, and a history of depression or suicidality. It can be helpful to interview any friends or family members who arrived with the patient. If no one familiar with the patient can be contacted, one should not hesitate to look through the patient's belongings for clues such as phone numbers, medication bottles, and medic alert bracelets. If the patient arrived by ambulance, the EMS run sheet will provide details about the conditions under which the patient was found. Were there empty alcohol bottles? Did witnesses see the patient convulsing? Was the patient found in a closed room next to a furnace? Finally, check with the medical records department at your hospital and the local psychiatric facility to explore the availability of any old charts.

Physical Exam

The importance of the physical exam for patients with altered levels of consciousness cannot be overemphasized. The patient's **vital signs** may offer key clues to the underlying diagnosis. In conjunction with oxygen saturation, the respiratory rate and pattern may suggest conditions ranging from opiate intoxication to pulmonary emboli to metabolic acidosis. The heart rate and rhythm may indicate sepsis, electrolyte abnormalities (changes in potassium or calcium), ingestions (sympathomimetics, digoxin, tricyclics), or closed head injuries. Bradycardia, along with an elevated blood pressure, suggests a Cushing reflex indicative of increased intracranial pressure. Abnormal temperature values may point towards infection, heat stroke, or hypothermia.

In addition to the standard cardiac, respiratory, and abdominal surveys, a directed physical exam for this patient population includes the head, pupils, breath, neck, and skin, as well as a focused neurological exam. Assess the

head for signs of **trauma** (laceration, cephalohematoma, hemotympanum, Battle sign, and raccoon eyes). The **size, symmetry, and reactivity** of the **pupils** provide information about both metabolic and structural processes such as opiate use and space-occupying lesions with herniation, respectively. Often overlooked, the **fundoscopic exam** can reveal signs of **increased intracranial pressure, hypertensive crisis, and methanol ingestion**. **Breath odor** may suggest diabetic ketoacidosis, liver failure, and toxins such as cyanide (almond odor), alcohol, and insecticides (onion odor). Look inside the oropharynx and at the tongue for lacerations if you suspect seizure activity. Check the **neck** for meningismus and thyroid abnormalities such as a goiter or an operative scar. The patient's **skin** is an underused source of important information; rashes may suggest meningococcemia, endocarditis or vasculitis; color may indicate hypoxia, anemia, or uremia; hydration status may range from the cool clamminess of shock to the hot, dry, flushed changes associated with anticholinergic toxicity; needle marks indicate recent substance use. A pregnancy test should be performed if appropriate.

As altered patients are typically unable to participate in formal neurological exam, the directed exam assesses **gross focality** of the cranial nerves, **movement of all extremities**, **reflexes** (especially plantar or Babinski), **rectal tone**, **muscular tone**, and **mental status**. The evaluation of mental status includes orientation to person/place/time/situation, short-term recall, and level of alertness, as denoted by the mnemonic AVPU—awake and alert, responsive to verbal stimuli, responsive to painful stimuli, or unresponsive. The Confusion Assessment Method (CAM) is a formalized tool used to help differentiate delirium from dementia. It assess five parameters: acuity of onset, fluctuating course, inattention, disorganized thinking, and altered level of consciousness. It may be helpful to assign a Glasgow Coma Scale (GCS) score in order to allow for comparison on reexamination.

Diagnostic Testing

The vast majority of patients with altered sensorium will have a presumptive diagnosis after the history and physical exam are supplemented with rapid bedside tests, including **finger blood glucose; pulse oximetry; breathalyzer or serum ethanol level; cardiac monitor and electrocardiogram; urinalysis.** If these studies do not reveal the underlying etiology, other useful tests include a complete blood count to look for leukocytosis or anemia, basic urine toxicology, a chemistry panel to assess electrolytes, blood urea nitrogen (BUN), creatinine, calcium, magnesium, and serum osmolality to look for the presence of alcohols such as methanol and ethylene glycol.

More extensive and directed testing may be appropriate in specific clinical scenarios. Suspected hepatic failure warrants liver function tests, an ammonia level, and paracentesis if infected ascites is a consideration. Hypoxic patients may benefit from a chest x-ray and an arterial blood gas. Other focused studies based on clinical judgment include thyroid function tests, carboxyhemoglobin levels, directed drug or toxin screening, lumbar puncture when subarachnoid hemorrhage or meningitis is a consideration, and computed tomography (CT) scan of the head.

Differential Diagnosis

With such an extensive range of disorders manifesting as altered mental status, clinicians need to identify their own organized, systematic approach to best generate a comprehensive list of potential diagnoses. The two most common systems are the mnemonic AEIOU TIPS, and the "head-to-toe" technique, in which one starts at the head and progresses down the body, generating diagnostic possibilities in association with each anatomic location or body system encountered (Tables 30-1 and 30-2).

TABLE 30-1
DIFFERENTIAL DIAGNOSIS OF ALTERED MENTAL STATUS

AEIOU TIPS

A—alcohol, drugs, toxins
E—endocrine, electrolytes
I—infection
O—oxygen, opiates
U—uremia (renal, including hypertension)

T—trauma, temperature
I—insulin (diabetes)
P—psychiatric, porphyria
S—subarachnoid, space-occupying lesion

Table 30-2
HEAD-TO-TOE APPROACH

HEAD: space-occupying lesions, encephalitis/abscess, head trauma, seizure, cerebrovascular accident, psychiatric, subarachnoid hemorrhage

MOUTH: (ingestions/medications): alcohols, heavy metals, anticholinergics, opiates, anticonvulsants, phenothiazines, barbiturates, salicylates, carbon monoxide, sedative–hypnotics, cyanide, sympathomimetics, hallucinogens, tricyclics

NECK: meningitis, thyroid

CHEST: hypoxia, hypercarbia, pulmonary embolus, congestive heart failure, anemia

ABDOMEN: liver (encephalopathy, Wernicke), pancreas (diabetes), kidneys (uremia, electrolytes), adrenals (endocrine), peritonitis

SKIN: rash (endocarditis, toxic shock, vasculitis, thrombotic thrombocytopenic purpura), color (uremic frost, hypoxia, hepatic failure), temperature (hypothermia, heat stroke)

Management

As with all ED patients, **management begins with the ABCs.** The treatment for patients with altered mental status is generally supportive, focusing on stabilization and symptom relief. When indicated, specific interventions can be added to treat the underlying etiology. Common interventions include **oxygen for hypoxia, thiamine for ethanol-related disorders, dextrose for hypoglycemia, naloxone (Narcan)** for hypoventilating patients with **suspected opiate ingestions, IV fluids for dehydration, and antibiotics for suspected infections.** The Poison Control Center may be consulted for any suspected toxic exposure or ingestion; the patient in our case, for example, would have warranted treatment with **ethanol or fomepizole (antidote for ethylene glycol and methanol).** All patients with altered mental status warrant high-visibility beds within the ED as well as repeated neurological checks. A broad differential diagnosis must be kept in mind. CT or magnetic resonance imaging (MRI) imaging of the brain may be indicated.

Comprehension Questions

[30.1] A 63-year-old male presents with 2 days of bizarre behavior and agitation. The history and physical examination demonstrates a low-grade fever, tachycardia, periods of somnolence followed by agitation, disorganized thinking and auditory hallucinations. Which aspect of this presentation is *least* consistent with the diagnosis of delirium?

   A. Abnormal vital signs
   B. Fluctuating mental status
   C. Disorganized thinking
   D. Auditory hallucinations

[30.2] An 18-year-old male is brought into the ED by police for being combative and agitated in a department store. He is disoriented and verbally abusive. The ED physician requests the police to help restrain the patient so that the physician can perform an eye examination because this assessment often gives important information in cases of altered mental status. Which of the following statements regarding the ophthalmic examination is most accurate?

   A. The earliest sign of papilledema is the loss of arterial pulsations
   B. Slowly roving eye movements are a finding consistent with hysteria
   C. A unilateral dilated pupil in an alert patient usually indicates a serious disease
   D. A mass causing herniation is usually on the same side as the dilated pupil

[30.3] Reversal agents or antidotes can be used to diagnose or treat a number of conditions that can affect an individual's mental status. With respect to these agents, which of the following statements is accurate?

A. For patients with hypoglycemia, 1 dose of intravenous D50 (50% dextrose injection) is always adequate because it will usually raise the blood sugar by at least 130 mg/dL.

B. Naloxone is to be used with caution because its half-life may be shorter than the ingested drug.

C. Flumazenil is dangerous because of the risk of causing bone marrow suppression.

D. Korsakoff psychosis can be successfully reversed with thiamine.

[30.4] An 80-year-old male is brought into the ED for confusion. The ED physician is attempting to evaluate for possible delirium and uses the Confusion Assessment Method (CAM). Which of the following statements is most likely to indicate delirium rather than dementia with this examination?

A. Subacute onset with gradual but progressive deficits
B. Easily distracted, inattentive
C. Normotensive and normal heart rate
D. Normal level of consciousness

Answers

[30.1]   **D.** Auditory hallucinations are uncommon in patients with delirium. If hallucinations occur, they are usually visual. The other signs and symptoms are consistent with delirium but can also be present in patients that present with acute psychosis.

[30.2]   **D.** The abnormal pupil is usually on the same side as the uncal herniation. Eye movements tend to be slowly roving in the comatose patient. Hysterical patients usually fix their eyes in one direction or they move them about in a "herky-jerky" manner. Eyelid tone follows a similar pattern. When the lids are pried open, the comatose patient will slowly close the lids or leave them partially open. The hysterical patient will usually close the lids quickly and completely. Early sign of papilledema is absence of venous pulses.

[30.3]   **B.** One of the advantages of naloxone (Narcan) in the emergency department is that its half-life is shorter (about 1 hour) than most of the opioids that the patient could have ingested. Therefore, if patients are watched in the ED for more than a couple of hours with a stable respiratory system, it is safe to send them home without fear of subsequent respiratory depression. Naloxone has a shorter half-life and thus is preferable to naltrexone in the ED setting.

[30.4]   **B.** Abnormal vital signs are common in patients with delirium, but are not part of the CAM. An acute onset, fluctuation of mental status, inattention, and altered mental status suggest delirium.

CLINICAL PEARLS

❖ Remember to assess the basics: glucose and alcohol level, and vital signs including oxygen saturation.

❖ With altered mental status, be a detective: call family members, consult past medical records, call the local psychiatric hospital, search the patient's belongings for phone numbers and diagnostic clues.

❖ Make sure your physical exam includes assessment of the patient's pupils, skin signs, and breath odor.

❖ Because altered mental status has such a broad differential, the clinician should not narrow the possibilities too early.

REFERENCES

Berk WA, Henderson WV. Alcohols. In: Tintinalli JE, Kelen GD, Stapczynski JS, eds. Emergency medicine, 6th ed. New York: McGraw-Hill, 2004:1069–70.

Starkman S, Wright S. Altered mental status. In: Hamilton GC, Sanders AB, Strange G, Trott A, eds. Emergency Medicine: an approach to clinical problem solving. Philadelphia: WB Saunders, 1991:517–533.

A 4-year-old boy is brought to the emergency department (ED) after having a limp for 5 days and fever for 2 days. The limp began after he tripped while playing and has worsened progressively to the point where he can no longer bear weight on his left leg. Low-grade fever began 2 days prior to presentation. He was treated for otitis media with Augmentin (amoxicillin and clavulanate potassium) 2 weeks ago. There has been no nausea, vomiting, rhinorrhea, cough, congestion, abdominal pain, recent traveling, or insect bites. His blood pressure is 115/68 mmHg, pulse is 108 beats per minute, respiration is 22 breaths per minute, and temperature is 38.8°C (101.8°F). On physical exam, he appears ill. His left hip is flexed with slight abduction and external rotation and is warm to touch. There is limited range of motion of the left hip with passive motion. The left knee is normal. There are no other findings on physical exam.

◆ **What is your next step?**

◆ **What is the most likely diagnosis?**

◆ **What is the best treatment for this problem?**

ANSWERS TO CASE 31: Septic Arthritis (Child)

Summary: A 4-year-old boy has left hip pain and fever.

◆ **Next step:** radiograph of the left lower extremity including the hip and knee joints, ultrasound of the hip joint and consider arthrocentesis.

◆ **Most likely diagnosis:** septic arthritis.

◆ **Best treatment for this problem:** if this proves to be septic arthritis, immediate surgical consultation for surgical drainage and intravenous antibiotics are the best treatments.

Analysis

Objectives

1. Be familiar with the clinical presentation of septic arthritis.
2. Learn about the diagnosis and treatment of suspected septic arthritis.
3. Be familiar with other causes of limp in children.

Considerations

This 4-year-old child has a 5-day history of progressive hip pain, to the point where he cannot put any weight on it, and fever. This is clearly abnormal and demands investigation. On physical exam, he appears ill. His left hip is flexed with slight abduction and external rotation, and appears to be inflamed (warm to touch). There is limited range of motion of the left hip with passive motion. Septic arthritis is very likely given all these findings. Other considerations are hip fracture, which would not present with fever, but would cause pain, swelling, and decreased range of motion, and slipped capital epiphysis (SCFE), which usually affects adolescents but can present with subacute or chronic hip pain. These latter two diagnoses would be established by radiography.

APPROACH TO THE CHILD WITH A LIMP

Limp is an uneven, jerky, or laborious gait, usually caused by pain, weakness, or deformity. It is not an **uncommon complaint in childhood**, accounting for about 1 visit of every 200 pediatric patients presenting to the emergency department. The differential diagnosis of a child with a limp is broad but only a few conditions require emergent treatment. The emergency physician must have a systematic approach to quickly identify such conditions. History taking is difficult because very young children are unable to communicate verbally and children who can talk may not be able to localize the site of pain. The following information may help to identify the causes of limping that require emergent treatment (Table 31-1).

There is a lot of overlap among age groups, but knowing which diseases are common in each group can help in generating the list of possible diagnoses

Table 31-1
KEY QUESTIONS FOR THE CHILD WITH A LIMP

Age (age-specific diagnoses)

Onset of pain (acute vs. chronic)

Duration of pain (intermittent vs. constant)

Location of pain (referred pain is common)

History of trauma (may be misleading)

Constitutional symptoms (fever, malaise, weight loss)

(Table 31-2). For example, **the obese teenager with a limp is likely to have slipped capital femoral epiphysis,** whereas the **7-year-old with gradual onset hip pain** is more likely to have **Legg-Calvé-Perthes disease.** Constitutional signs and symptoms are common in patients with a septic joint or transient synovitis, and uncommon in most other causes of joint pain. Table 31-3 lists the causes of hip pain.

A child with a limp rarely requires laboratory testing; however, a complete blood count (CBC) and erythrocyte sedimentation rate (ESR) may be helpful with entities such as osteomyelitis, neoplasm, septic joint, and transient synovitis. A urinalysis may also assist the practitioner. Hematuria may suggest acute glomerulonephritis or lupus. Pyuria is associated with appendicitis or salpingitis, both of which may result in a shuffling gait, and the presence of uric acid crystals may support the diagnosis of gout.

In the emergency department, **plain films should be taken of the entire limb in question,** bearing weight when possible, with **the joint above and below the affected joint included.** An ultrasound is particularly useful for diagnosing joint pathology and confirming the presence of an effusion. Other imaging studies that will be considered as an outpatient or after admission include bone scan with IV technetium 99m-labeled methylene diphosphonate tracer, which accumulates in areas of increased cellular activity and blood flow; scintigraphy, which is useful in detecting early Legg-Calvé-Perthes disease, osteomyelitis, stress fractures, and osteoid osteomas (scintigraphy is 84 to 100 percent sensitive and 70 to 96 percent specific for osteomyelitis); and magnetic resonance imaging, which can detect bone infarction and is helpful in conditions such as Legg-Calvé-Perthes disease or avascular necrosis.

Septic Arthritis

The **most serious acute cause of joint pain is a septic joint**. Bacteria and the inflammatory response can rapidly destroy the articular cartilage resulting in long-term morbidity if diagnosis and treatment are delayed. Approximately 3 percent of children who are evaluated in the emergency department for a limp will have septic arthritis. Joints of the lower extremity are affected in more

Table 31-2

DIFFERENTIAL DIAGNOSIS OF HIP PAIN BASED ON AGE

AGE (YR)	INFECTIOUS	TRAUMA	INFLAMMATORY	DEVELOPMENTAL	NEOPLASIA
Toddler (1–3)	Septic arthritis Osteomyelitis	Toddler fracture Child abuse	Transient synovitis Juvenile rheumatoid arthritis	Developmental dysplasia of the hip Clubfoot	Leukemia
Juvenile (4–10)	Septic arthritis Osteomyelitis	Fracture Legg-Calvé-Perthes disease	Transient synovitis Juvenile rheumatoid arthritis	Developmental dysplasia of the hip	Ewing sarcoma Osteoid osteoma
Adolescent (11–17)	Septic or gonococcal arthritis Osteomyelitis	Fracture Slipped capital femoral epiphysis	Juvenile rheumatoid arthritis Osgood-Schlatter disease	Osteochondritis desiccans Osteoid osteoma	Osteosarcoma Ewing sarcoma

Table 31-3
CAUSES OF HIP PAIN

Sickle cell disease

Juvenile rheumatoid arthritis

Osteosarcoma

Osteoid osteoma

Muscular dystrophy

Rickets

Discitis

Charcot-Marie-Tooth disease

Cerebral palsy

Leg-length discrepancy

Lyme disease

than 90 percent of the cases, with the **knee and hip most commonly involved**. Causative bacterial organisms vary with age group, but *Staphylococcus aureus* **is the most common organism,** followed by *group A streptococci* and *Streptococcus pneumoniae.*

Children with septic arthritis typically are ill-appearing and febrile with limited movement of the affected joint, joint pain and swelling, and refusal to bear weight. Only 8 percent of septic arthritis in children will involve more than one joint. Occasionally the presentation is more subtle, especially in neonates and young infants who may present with misleading irritability and poor feeding. These infants may offer no clue of joint involvement or they may refuse to move the entire limb and present with pseudoparalysis, with or without fever. The presentation of septic arthritis can also be altered by recent use of antibiotics.

On physical examination, the involved joint is typically flexed to limit motion. Local erythema, warmth, swelling, and palpable effusion may be present. In septic arthritis of the hip these findings will be more subtle, the joint is usually flexed with slight abduction and external rotation, and limitation of internal rotation with passive motion. There may be referred pain to the knee.

When septic arthritis is suspected, diagnostic studies should include a CBC, blood cultures, ESR, and plain radiographs. The white blood cell count (WBC) is elevated in 30 to 60 percent of cases, but lacks both sensitivity and specificity. ESR, the most sensitive test, is elevated in 90 percent of cases, but lacks specificity. A combination of ESR >20 mm/h and/or temperature >37.5°C (99.5°F) detected 97 percent of those with septic arthritis, but 50 percent had unnecessary arthrocentesis. Findings on plain radiograph may include joint space widening, increased opacity of the joint space, local soft-tissue swelling, distortion of periarticular fat or muscle, and osteomyelitis. The **definitive diagnosis of septic arthritis** is made **by examination of synovial fluid obtained by arthrocentesis.**

Treatment of septic arthritis includes immediate surgical drainage and intravenous antibiotics. Choice of antibiotic therapy should be based partly on the age of the patient to ensure coverage of the most likely causative organism. Empiric coverage should include an antistaphylococcal agent in neonates and gram-negative coverage in adolescents.

Transient Synovitis

Transient (or toxic) synovitis (TS) is the most common cause of acute hip pain in children ages 3 to 10 years. The disease causes arthralgia and arthritis secondary to a transient inflammation of the synovium of the hip. Unilateral hip or groin pain is the most common complaint; however, some patients with TS may complain of medial thigh or knee pain. TS is difficult to clinically differentiate from septic arthritis and often presents a diagnostic dilemma for emergency physicians. Both entities can have an effusion identified with an ultrasound study and an elevated WBC along with a low-grade fever. At the two ends of the clinical spectrum it is relatively safe and easy to distinguish the two entities. Toxic-looking children with a high fever and significant WBC elevation are likely to have a septic arthritis, whereas those that appear well with a **low-grade fever and minimal changes in the WBC** likely have TS. The group in the middle may need to have arthrocentesis with joint fluid analysis to distinguish between the two. Once other causes of hip pain have been excluded, the child can be treated for transient synovitis with bed rest for 7 to 10 days and antiinflammatory agents.

Developmental Dysplasia of the Hip

Developmental dysplasia of the hip (DDH) is a malformation of the hip joint found in babies or young children. There are several maneuvers that can detect a dislocatable hip. The *Ortolani maneuver* is done with the hip flexed to 90 degrees and abducted. The femoral head is lifted forward and a clunk is heard as the head slides into the acetabulum (sign of entry). The *Barlow maneuver* is performed with the hip adducted and pressing posteriory feeling for a clunk which is the femoral head sliding out of the joint (sign of exit). Ultrasound of the hip will demonstrate the hip deformity. Plain films of the hip can be done in infants older than 6 months. Infants are often placed in a brace like the Pavlik Harness, which keeps the legs abducted and maintains the femoral head in the acetabulum. If the infant is too large or strong for the harness, a cast can be applied and changed every few weeks as the child grows. If early measures fail or the dislocation is detected at a later age, surgery can be performed.

Legg-Calvé-Perthes Disease

Legg-Calvé-Perthes (LCP) disease develops when insufficient blood supply to the femoral head leads to necrosis. It is commonly found in **boys ages 4 to**

10 years. The child usually presents with a limp and may complain of hip or knee pain. During a physical exam, **decreased range of motion** will be noted at the affected hip. Plain films will reveal the abnormality in most cases (Fig. 31-1).

The aim of treatment is to protect the bone and joint from further stress and injury while the healing process takes place. Bed rest or crutches may be needed during the initial phase. A brace, cast, or splint to immobilize the hip's position may be used while bone regrowth takes place. Surgery may be performed to keep the hip in its socket.

Slipped Capital Femoral Epiphysis

Slipped capital femoral epiphysis (SCFE) remains one of the most common disorders affecting the hip in adolescence. SCFE results in displacement of the femoral head through the physeal plate. It is most common in **obese boys ages 11 to 15 years.** Children who grow rapidly and who have hormonal imbalances from other conditions are also at risk. In addition to a limp, patients will complain of hip and/or knee pain. On exam, patients will have pain when practitioners attempt to range the hip. **Plain films of the hip** or pelvis will usually reveal the displacement (Fig. 31-2). The femoral head is described as **the "fallen ice cream from the cone"** (the shaft of the femur). Rarely, a magnetic resonance imaging (MRI) may be needed to show the abnormality. **Most patients require surgery where a screw is placed to secure the femoral head.**

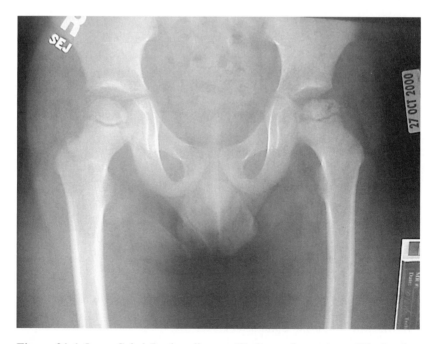

Figure 31-1. Legg-Calvé-Perthes disease. (Radiograph courtesy of Dr. Jocelyn Freeman Garrick)

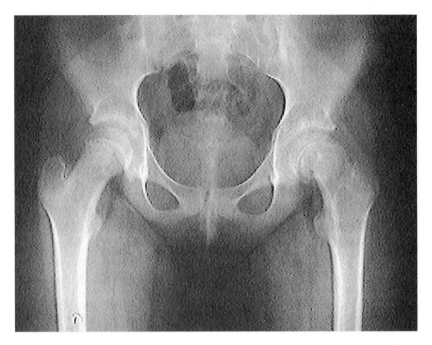

Figure 31-2. Slipped femoral capital epiphysis. (Radiograph courtesy of Dr. Barry Simon)

Toddler's Fractures

Toddler's fractures occur most commonly in children younger than age 2 years who are learning to walk. Frequently, there is no definite history of a traumatic event, and the child is brought to the emergency department because of a limp or reluctance to bear weight on the leg. Examine the hip, thigh, and knee first to rule out other causes of limping as well as possible child abuse. A thorough physical examination may be limited by the child's cooperation, but maximal tenderness can usually be elicited over the fracture site. If you suspect a toddler's fracture, obtain anteroposterior (AP) and lateral views of the entire tibia and fibula. The typical findings are a nondisplaced spiral fracture of the tibia and no fibular fracture. It is not uncommon for initial radiographs to be normal and the diagnosis of this fracture made several days after the injury when followup radiographs show a lucent line or periosteal reaction.

Osgood-Schlatter Disease

This disease is caused by a **reaction of the bone and cartilage of the tibial tubercle** to **repetitive stress (e.g., jumping)** and is believed to represent tiny stress fractures in the apophysis. The condition is also associated with **rapid growth spurts.** Physical examination reveals tenderness and swelling over the tibial tubercle. Running, jumping, and kneeling worsen the symptoms. The condition is managed with **ice, antiinflammatory medication, and a decrease**

in activity. Daily stretching of the quadriceps and hamstrings is also beneficial. Patients with severe pain may require immobilization using crutches or a knee immobilizer. Individual regulation of activity is usually effective; pain may recur until the tubercle matures (i.e., ossifies completely).

There are a host of other diseases that can cause a limp in the pediatric population.

Comprehension Questions

[31.1] A mother states that her 2-year-old child won't bear weight on her left leg and has had a fever up to 38.7°C (101.6°F). The child seems to have significant pain when you attempt to assess the range of motion of the left hip. An ultrasound is performed revealing fluid in the left hip joint. A left hip radiograph is normal. An aspiration of the hip joint shows a low level of protein concentration. Which of the following is the most likely diagnosis?

    A. Osteomyelitis
    B. Septic joint
    C. Transient synovitis
    D. Legg-Calvé-Perthes disease

[31.2] A 9-year-old boy complains of mild right hip pain over 12 months that has progressed to a limp. He denies trauma to the leg. Which of the following describes the probable etiology of his condition?

    A. Femoral dislocation
    B. Femoral subluxation
    C. Femoral avascular necrosis
    D. Femoral head dysplasia

[31.3] An 8-year-old boy is brought into the ED by his mother for left hip pain of 2 days duration. She states that no trauma was involved. Which of the following is the most likely cause?

    A. Subacute osteomyelitis
    B. Transient synovitis
    C. Developmental dysplasia of the hip
    D. Slipped capital femoral epiphysis

[31.4] A 12-year-old active boy complains of bilateral knee pain. He denies trauma to the legs. On examination, he is noted to have tenderness at the patellar region, but full range of motion of the knees. There does not seem to be an effusion. Which of the following is the most likely diagnosis?

    A. Legg-Calvé-Perthes disease
    B. Slipped capital femoral epiphysis
    C. Osgood-Schlatter disease
    D. Transient synovitis

Answers

[31.1]   **C.** Fluid in the hip joint demonstrated by ultrasound can either be a result of septic arthritis or transient synovitis. Joint aspiration showing transudative fluid (low protein, low leukocyte count) is consistent with synovitis, which will resolve.

[31.2]   **C.** Legg-Calvé-Perthes is a insidious disease found commonly in boys ages 4 to 10 years. It results in avascular necrosis of the femoral head.

[31.3]   **B.** Transient synovitis is the most common cause of hip pain in children ages 3 to 10 years. Although a benign process, it must be distinguished from the other more serious entities, such as slipped femoral capital epiphysis, Legg-Calvé-Perthes disease, or septic arthritis.

[31.4]   **C.** Osgood-Schlatter disease is associated with pain of the knees bilaterally with some tenderness at the patellar region.

CLINICAL PEARLS

❖ In general, an ultrasound and/or arthrocentesis should be performed in a child with fever who refuses to move a joint.

❖ A septic joint is the most serious condition associated with a child with a limp.

❖ Consider Legg-Calvé-Perthes disease in boys ages 4 to 10 years who present with a limp.

❖ The frog-leg radiograph in a teenager who presents with a limp will assess for slipped capital femoral epiphysis (SCFE).

❖ Perform a thorough history (with and without the parent) and physical on children who present with fractures to evaluate for possible child abuse.

REFERENCES

Allen BL Jr, Ferguson RL. Topics of interest in pediatric orthopedics. Pediatr Clin North Am 1985;32:1333.

Del Becarro MA, Champoux AN, Bockers T, et al. Septic arthritis versus transient synovitis of the hip: the value of screening laboratory tests. Ann Emerg Med 1992;21:1418.

Kunnamo I, Kallio P, Pelkonen P, Hovi T. Clinical signs and laboratory tests in the differential diagnosis of arthritis in children. Am J Dis Child 1987;141:34.

Nade S. Choice of antibiotics in management of acute osteomyelitis and acute septic arthritis in children. Arch Dis Child 1977;52:672–82.

Nelson JD. Skeletal infections in children. Adv Pediatr Infect Dis 1991;6:59.

Shetty AK, Gedalia A. Septic arthritis in children. Rheum Dis Clin North Am 1998;24:287.

Singer JI. The cause of gait disturbance in 425 pediatric patients. Pediatr Emerg Care 1985;1:7.

Sonnen GM, Henry NK. Pediatric bone and joint infections: diagnosis and antimicrobial management. Pediatr Clin North Am 1996;43:933–47.

Welkon, CJ, Long SS, Fisher MC, Alburger, PD. Pyogenic arthritis in infants and children: a review of 95 cases. Pediatr Infect Dis 1986;5:669.

A 57-year-old man complains of lower back pain of 1-month duration that has been steadily worsening. He states that he worked in a warehouse for 30 years, but has been on light duty for the past month. He denies trauma to his back or prior surgery. The patient states that he has had pain radiating down the back of both legs, but the pain suddenly became worse yesterday. Intermittently, he has numbness to his perianal area and notes that the skin doesn't feel normal when he wipes with toilet tissue. He denies a history of herpes simplex virus. For the past 2 days, he has been having difficulty voiding, and has had some urinary incontinence.

◆ **What is the most likely diagnosis?**

◆ **What is the next diagnostic step?**

ANSWERS TO CASE 32: Low Back Pain

Summary: A 57-year-old warehouse worker has a 1-month history of suddenly worsening lower back pain with radiation bilaterally to his legs. He denies trauma to his back or prior surgery. Intermittently, he has perianal numbness, difficulty voiding, and urinary incontinence.

◆ **Most likely diagnosis:** cauda equina syndrome (CES)

◆ **Next diagnostic step:** magnetic resonance imaging (MRI) of the lumbar and sacral spine

Analysis

Objectives
1. Be familiar with the different causes and a clinical approach to lower back pain.
2. Know the danger signs of lower back pain.
3. Be aware of the clinical presentation of cauda equina syndrome.

Considerations

This 57-year-old man complains of low back pain, which is a common complaint. His occupation as a warehouse worker makes herniated lumbar/sacral disc a likely etiology. Although low back pain is common, and usually a result of a benign condition, this patient has several **"red flag" conditions** that are worrisome. First, the **age of onset being older than 50 years** is more likely to be associated with serious etiologies. Second, he also has **bilateral leg pain.** Finally, he has **perianal numbness and bladder dysfunction**, which is consistent with compression of the sacral nerves, cauda equina syndrome. **The cauda equina is the terminal nerves from the spinal cord and injury or compression typically causes "saddle anesthesia" and bladder or bowel dysfunction.** Sacral nerve dysfunction can be confirmed with a **rectal examination revealing loss of sphincter tone.** CES is a surgical emergency and confirmed with MRI. Rapid decompression is vital to prevent permanent dysfunction.

APPROACH TO LOW BACK PAIN

Definitions
Cauda equina syndrome: compression of sacral nerve bundle that forms the end of the spinal cord with symptoms of bladder or bowel dysfunction and/or pain or weakness of the legs. This disorder should be diagnosed at an early stage to avoid permanent injury.

Entrapment neuropathies: involves compression of a nerve leading to symptoms such as sciatica, when a prolapsed intervertebral disc applies pressure to an adjacent nerve in the lumbosacral plexus.

Mechanical backache: usually chronic and may result in a long-term debilitating illness without any definite or demonstrable cause. Back sprains are usually associated with minor trauma, producing ligamentous or muscular injury.

Clinical Approach

Because low back pain is so common, it is of fundamental importance to differentiate significant from insignificant pain to prevent the onset of chronicity. Pain in spinal disorders may be local or referred, or may occur along the distribution of nerves. Osteoarthritis and rheumatoid arthritis are associated with conditions such as spinal stenosis, spondylolisthesis, and ankylosing spondylitis, which may cause chronic back pain (Table 32-1).

Herniation of the nucleus pulposus, the softer inner part of an intervertebral disc, through the outer tough annulus fibrosus causes **compression of adjacent nerves,** which emanate from the spinal canal. On occasion, fragmentation of the disc may occur without protrusion of the nucleus pulposus, in which case, the annulus itself protrudes. This may cause severe pain, weakness, and sensory loss. The problem may also be caused by the protrusion of osteophytes, bony spurs that occur in osteoarthrosis of the spine. Ultimately, **spinal stenosis** may develop.

With disc prolapse, the severity of symptoms may vary from mild localized back pain to **urgent cauda equina compression resulting in loss of motor and sensory function. The L4-L5 and L5-S1 intervertebral discs are the most commonly involved, thus, pain down the posterior or lateral leg is characteristic (sciatica).** Back pain frequently radiates into the buttock, posterior thigh, or calf. Coughing, sneezing, or straining tends to increase the pain. Other exacerbating factors are bending, sitting, and getting in and out of a vehicle, whereas **lying flat characteristically relieves pain.** Caudal equina compression may effect **bladder and bowel function**, spinal stenosis may produce pain which radiates down both legs.

The paravertebral muscles are often in spasm and there is loss of the normal lumbar lordosis. Straight-leg raising is limited on the side of the lesion and dorsiflexion of the foot, at the limit of straight-leg raising, often exacerbates the discomfort. There may be tenderness to palpation of the central back or buttock. Rectal or perineal examination reveals loss of sphincter tone. Sensory loss and muscular weakness may be present along the appropriate dermatomes; ankle or knee reflexes may be absent. The differential diagnosis includes: fracture, joint subluxation, tumors of bone, joint or the meninges, abscess, arachnoiditis, ankylosing spondylitis, rheumatoid arthritis, aortic occlusion, and peripheral neuropathies. Magnetic resonance imaging may demonstrate the disc protrusion and plain x-rays of the lumbosacral spine may show narrowing of the intervertebral space, but this is not diagnostic.

Bedrest, the application of either heated pads or ice packs, nonsteroidal antiinflammatory drugs and muscle relaxants, and/or physical therapy represent the first line of conservative management. A back brace or corset

TABLE 32-1
ETIOLOGIES OF LOW BACK PAIN

CAUSES OF LOW BACK PAIN	INCIDENCE
Musculoskeletal low back or leg pain	97%
Lumbar sprain or strain	70%
Degenerative disk disease	10%
Herniated disk	4%
Spinal stenosis	3%
Trauma	1%
Congenital disease, e.g., kyphoscoliosis	<1%
Referred or visceral pain	2%
Pelvic disease	
Renal disease	
Aortic aneurysm	
Gastrointestinal disease	
Nonmechanical low back pain	1%
Neoplasia	
Infection	
Inflammatory arthritis	
Paget disease	

Source: Adapted, with permission, from Deyo RA. Low back pain. N Engl J Med 2001; 344(5):365.

may help the patient through the early stages of mobilization. **The indications for surgical decompression are the development of an acute disabling neurological deficit (bladder dysfunction) or intractable severe pain.**

In evaluating patients with low back pain, the clinician needs to exclude potentially serious conditions such as **malignancy, infection**, or dangerous neurological processes such as **spinal cord compression or cauda equina syndrome.** Individuals without these conditions are initially managed with conservative therapy. Nearly all patients recover spontaneously within 4 to 6 weeks; only 3 to 5 percent remain disabled longer than 3 months. If patients do not improve within 4 weeks with conservative management, they should receive further evaluation to rule out systemic or rheumatic disease and to clarify the anatomical cause, especially patients with localized pain, nocturnal pain, or sciatica.

When pain radiates below the knee, it is more likely to indicate a true radiculopathy than radiation only to the posterior thigh; a history of persistent leg numbness or weakness further increases the likelihood of neurologic involvement.

Most cases are idiopathic, and this group in general is referred to as musculoskeletal low back pain. **Imaging studies and other diagnostic tests are generally not helpful in managing these cases**. Studies show that the history and physical exam can help separate the majority of patients with simple and self-limited musculoskeletal back pain from the minority with more serious underlying causes. Finding "red-flag" symptoms can help the physician use diagnostic tests in a more judicious manner (Table 32-2). When the patient has worrisome symptoms or signs, the most effective initial evaluation would still be plain AP and lateral radiographs of the involved area of the spine, a sedimentation rate, and a complete blood count in most cases. More expensive tests, such as MRI, should be reserved for those cases in which surgery is being considered, as it is not required to make most diagnoses.

During the physical exam, palpable point tenderness over the spinous processes may indicate a destructive lesion of the spine itself; however, those with musculoskeletal back pain most often have tenderness in the muscular paraspinal area. Strength, sensation, and reflexes should be assessed,

TABLE 32-2
RED-FLAG SIGNS AND SYMPTOMS OF LOW BACK PAIN

New-onset of pain in a patient older than 50 or younger than 20 years

Fever

Unintentional weight loss

Severe nighttime pain or pain worse in supine position

Bowel or bladder incontinence

History of cancer

Immunosuppression (chemotherapy or human immunodeficiency virus)

Saddle anesthesia

Major motor weakness

IV drug use

Significant trauma

especially in those with complaints of radicular, or radiating pain. **Straight-leg testing**, in which the examiner, holding the patient's ankle, passively elevates the patient's leg to 45 degrees, is helpful if it elicits pain in the lower back radiating down the leg. However, it is **not a very sensitive or specific test.** Patrick maneuver, in which the patient externally rotates the hip, flexes the knee, and crosses the knee of the other leg with the ankle (like a number 4) while the examiner simultaneously presses down on the flexed knee and the opposite side of the pelvis, can help distinguish pain emanating from the sacroiliac joint.

Treatment

In treating idiopathic low back pain, various modalities are equally effective in the long run. Randomized, controlled trials have shown that encouraging patients to **continue their usual activity is superior to recommendations of bed rest.** Patients without disability and without evidence of nerve root compression probably can maintain judicious activity rather than be sent for bed rest. Bed rest is probably only appropriate for individuals with severe pain or with neurological deficits. The patient should be instructed to be positioned as to minimize pain; this usually consists of lying supine with the upper body slightly elevated and with a pillow under the knees. Nonsteroidal antiinflammatory medications (on a scheduled rather than as-needed basis), nonaspirin analgesics, and muscle relaxants may help in the acute phase. Because most cases of disk herniation with radiculopathy will resolve spontaneously within 4 to 6 weeks without surgery, this is the initial regimen recommended for these patients as well. Narcotic analgesics are also an option in cases of severe pain; however, because idiopathic low back pain is often a chronic problem, their prolonged use beyond the initial phase is discouraged. Chiropractors, physical therapists, massage therapists, and acupuncture have been studied (in trials of varying quality) with results comparable to traditional approaches. Referral to a surgeon may be considered in those patients with radicular pain with or without neuropathy that doesn't resolve with 4 to 6 weeks of conservative management.

Comprehension Questions

[32.1] Which of the following describes the most common location of herniated disks of the lumbar spine region?

A. L1-L2
B. L2-L3
C. L3-L4
D. L4-L5

[32.2] A 47-year-old woman complains of lower back pain with radiation to the right leg. She was placed on ibuprofen and bed rest. Over the next 3 weeks, the patient's pain worsens and she complains of difficulty with voiding and bowel movements. Which of the following is the most likely diagnosis?

A. Spinal stenosis
B. Lumbar neoplasm
C. Cauda equina syndrome
D. Tuberculosis of the spine (Pott disease)

[32.3] Each of the following maneuvers would exacerbate the pain from lumbar prolapsed nucleus pulposus *except*:

A. Standing position
B. Straight-leg raising
C. Valsalva
D. Sitting position

Answers

[32.1] **D.** The L4-L5 interspace is the most commonly affected.

[32.2] **C.** The bowel and bladder complaints are typical for cauda equina syndrome.

[32.3] **A.** Standing exacerbates spinal stenosis, but bending over or sitting exacerbates lumbar disc disease.

CLINICAL PEARLS

❖ The most common location of herniated lumbar disc disease is at the L4-L5 and L5-S1 levels.

❖ Bowel and bladder complaints with lower back pain are suspicious for cauda equina syndrome, which must be diagnosed early to avoid permanent damage.

❖ The initial treatment for herniated lumbar pulposus is bed rest and nonsteroidal antiinflammatory agents.

❖ In 90 percent of patients, acute low back pain, even with sciatic nerve involvement, resolves within 4 to 6 weeks.

❖ Analgesics such as nonsteroidal antiinflammatory drugs or narcotics, as well as muscle relaxants, and trying to maintain some level of activity, are helpful in managing acute low back pain; bed rest does not help.

❖ Pain that interferes with sleep, significant unintentional weight loss, or fever suggest an infectious or neoplastic cause of back pain.

❖   Imaging studies such as MRI are only of use if surgery is being
    considered (persistent pain and neurological symptoms after 4
    to 6 weeks of conservative care in patients with herniated
    disks), or if a neoplastic or inflammatory cause of back pain is
    being considered.

REFERENCES

Deyo RA, Weinstein JN. Low back pain. N Engl J Med 2001;344(5):363–70.
Hoff JT, Boland MF. Neurosurgery. In: Schwarz SI, Shires GT, Spencer FC, et al.,
    eds. Principles of surgery, 7th ed. New York: McGraw-Hill, 1999:1896–9.
Jarvik JG, Deyo RA. Diagnostic evaluation of low back pain with emphasis on
    imaging. Ann Intern Med 2002;137:586–97.

A 26-year-old woman is brought by EMS to the emergency department (ED) complaining of difficulty breathing. She is noticeably short of breath, even on a nonrebreather mask on 100 percent oxygen, and only able to answer questions with three to four words at a time. She also complains of subjective fever and chills and nonproductive cough. She denies any chest pain.

She admits to being human immunodeficiency virus (HIV)-positive but has not had followup in the last year or so. She does not know her last CD4 count or viral load and is not taking any medications. To her knowledge, she has not had any opportunistic infections.

On exam, her vital signs are temperature 38.3°C (100.9°F), blood pressure 105/66 mmHg, heart rate 107 beats per minute, respiratory rate 28 breaths per minute, and O_2 saturation 93 percent on nonrebreather. She is in moderate respiratory distress. Her examination is notable for crackles in both lung fields with supraclavicular retractions. Although she does have thrush in her oropharynx, she does not have any pretibial edema nor any skin lesions. She is placed on monitors and has an IV established. Her portable chest x-ray has prominent interstitial markings although there are no lobar consolidations.

◆ **What is the most appropriate next step?**

◆ **What are the potential complications of this disease process?**

◆ **What is the best therapy?**

ANSWERS TO CASE 33: *Pneumocystis carinii* Pneumonia

Summary: This is a 26-year-old who is HIV-positive complaining of fever and cough. She is hypoxic and in respiratory distress with interstitial disease shown on her chest x-ray.

◆ **Next step:** stabilization of ABCs

◆ **Potential complications:** pneumothorax, respiratory failure, pleural effusion, hematogenous spread, death

◆ **Best therapy:** trimethoprim-sulfamethoxazole, steroids

Analysis

Objectives

1. Learn the differential diagnosis of pneumonia in the HIV-positive patient.
2. Understand the clinical presentation, x-ray findings, and management of *Pneumocystis carinii* pneumonia (PCP).

Considerations

This young woman who is HIV-positive complains of fever and cough. Her respiratory distress is striking, and is alarming even in an immunocompetent individual. In a patient who is HIV infected, these symptoms indicate a critical emergency. Typically, *Pneumocystis carinii* pneumonia presents as mild dyspnea and cough with a paucity of pulmonary findings. The clinician is usually surprised by the dramatic findings on the chest radiograph or arterial blood gas. This individual, however, has dramatic clinical findings. Aggressive therapy is important because PCP has up to a 20 percent mortality rate. This patient should be transferred to the intensive care setting. Therapy should include trimethoprim-sulfamethoxazole, or pentamidine, or clindamycin plus primaquine. Steroids are sometimes helpful to decrease the inflammation. This patient is in severe respiratory distress and may benefit from steroid therapy. Depending on her response in the ensuing 2 to 3 hours, she may require intubation and mechanical ventilation.

APPROACH TO PNEUMOCYSTIS PNEUMONIA

Respiratory complaints in the HIV-positive patient can be attributed to a host of causes including PCP, bacterial pneumonia (*Streptococcus pneumoniae, Haemophilus influenzae*), tuberculosis, fungal infections (*Cryptococcus neoformans, Histoplasma capsulatum, Coccidioides immitis*), and malignancies (Kaposi sarcoma, lymphoma) (Table 33-1).

Table 33-1
ETIOLOGIES OF RESPIRATORY COMPLAINTS IN HIV-POSITIVE PATIENTS

ETIOLOGY	CD4 COUNT (CELLS/MM³)	CHEST X-RAY FINDINGS
Community-acquired organisms	800	Lobar or diffuse interstitial infiltrates
Pneumocystis carinii	<200	Diffuse interstitial infiltrates, nodular densities, cavitations, pneumothorax, normal x-ray
Mycobacterium tuberculosis	250–500	Hilar or mediastinal adenopathy, lobar or diffuse interstitial infiltrates
Cryptococus neoformans	250–500	Local, diffuse, or miliary infiltrates; cavitations; nodules; effusions
Histoplasma capsulatum	250–500	Local, diffuse, or miliary infiltrates
Cancer	Variable	Mass lesions, adenopathy, nodules

As with immunocompetent patients, **community-acquired pathogens are the most common cause of pneumonia in HIV-infected individuals, with *Streptococcus pneumoniae* the leading cause. *Pneumocystis carinii* is a common pathogen, particularly in patients with a CD4 count <200 cells/mm³.** The presentation of PCP is highly variable, ranging from mild shortness of breath to respiratory failure. Classically patients complain of a gradual onset of fever, dyspnea, and a nonproductive cough. Other symptoms include chest pain, weight loss, lethargy, and decreased exercise tolerance.

Clinical Findings

On exam, patients are often febrile and tachypneic. They may show signs of respiratory distress such as cyanosis and hypoxia. Lung examination varies from normal to rhonchi and rales. The physician should also check for other stigmata of HIV/acquired immunodeficiency syndrome (AIDS) (e.g., thrush).

Testing should include pulse oximetry, arterial blood gases (ABGs), **lactic dehydrogenase (LDH) levels**, and chest x-rays. Although resting pulse oximetry may be normal in early or mild disease, exercise-induced desaturation is suspicious for PCP. The ABG often reveals hypoxemia and hypocarbia as well as an increased A-a gradient. LDH levels are commonly elevated in patients with PCP (>220 IU/L) and reflect disease progression (high at onset and decreased with successful treatment). Classically, **the chest x-ray shows diffuse interstitial or alveolar infiltrates, spreading from the perihilar area to the periphery in a "bat wing" distribution.** However, the x-ray may be normal in up to 20 percent of patients. **The gold standard for diagnosis is bronchoscopy with biopsy or bronchoalveolar lavage.** An alternative is fluorescent antibody staining of induced sputum.

Treatment

As always, treatment begins with management of the ABCs. In more mild cases, supplemental oxygen via nasal cannula or face mask can be used to correct hypoxia. Intubation should be considered for any patient with a compromised airway, inadequate ventilation, or respiratory failure. The next step is antibiotic administration. **The initial drug of choice is trimethoprim-sulfamethoxazole.** Alternative regimens **include pentamidine, clindamycin plus primaquine, trimethoprim plus dapsone, trimetrexate plus leucovorin, and atovaquone. Steroids** should be used as adjunctive therapy in more-severe cases of PCP (pO_2 <70 mmHg, A-a gradient >35 mmHg). Either oral prednisone or IV methylprednisolone can be given 15 to 30 minutes prior to the initiation of antibiotics.

Comprehension Questions

[33.1] A 24-year-old male is known to be HIV-positive. He arrives at the ED complaining of fever, cough, and dyspnea. Pneumonia is diagnosed. What is the most common cause of pneumonia in this patient?

 A. *Streptococcus pneumoniae*
 B. *Pneumocystis carinii*
 C. Lymphoma
 D. *Cryptococcus neoformans*

[33.2] A 30-year-old woman complains of progressive dyspnea especially with activity. She admits to intravenous drug use and her partner is HIV infected. Her oxygen saturation is 98 percent on room air. Which of the following findings is suspicious for PCP?

 A. Oxygen saturation that continues to be 98 percent with exertion
 B. Exercise-induced desaturation with oxygen saturation in the range of 88 percent on room air
 C. Gram stain of sputum showing gram-positive diplococci
 D. Gold stain positive on the pulmonary biopsy

[33.3] First-line therapy for PCP is:

 A. Pentamidine
 B. Steroids
 C. Trimethoprim plus dapsone
 D. Trimethoprim-sulfamethoxazole

[33.4] A 28-year-old male with HIV is seen in the ED for dyspnea and cough. His chest x-ray is normal. Which of the following statements is most accurate regarding Pneumocystis pneumonia?

    A. PCP is very unlikely in the face of a normal chest radiograph
    B. PCP would be very unlikely unless the CD4 count was <50 cells/mm³
    C. PCP is often seen with a normal chest radiograph
    D. The diagnosis is PCP is usually established with elevated alkaline phosphatase levels

Answers

[33.1] **A.** *Streptococcus pneumoniae* is the most common cause of pneumonia in the HIV-positive patient.

[33.2] **B.** Exercise-induced desaturation is suspicious for PCP.

[33.3] **D.** Trimethoprim-sulfamethoxazole is first-line therapy for PCP. Steroids may be used as an adjunct in more severe cases. The other choices are alternative regimens.

[33.4] **C.** The chest x-ray may be normal in up to 20 percent of patients with PCP.

CLINICAL PEARLS

❖ Because PCP can have an insidious onset and has a 10 to 20 percent mortality rate, the clinician must have a high level of suspicion in HIV-positive patients with CD4 counts <200 cells/mm³.

❖ Classic chest x-ray findings include diffuse interstitial or alveolar infiltrates in a "bat wing" distribution. However, the x-ray may be normal in up to 20 percent of patients. In these cases, exercise-induced desaturation or elevated LDH levels may make the diagnosis of PCP more likely.

❖ First-line treatment is trimethoprim-sulfamethoxazole. Steroids are adjunctive therapy in more severe cases.

REFERENCES

Moran GJ, House HR. HIV-related illnesses: the challenge of ED management. Emerg Med Prac 2002;4(1):1–28.

Rothman RE, Marco CA, Kelen GD. HIV infection and AIDS. In: Tintinalli JE, Kelen GD, Stapczynski JD, eds. Emergency medicine: a comprehensive study guide, 6th ed. New York: McGraw-Hill, 2004:925–37.

Wolff AJ, O'Donnell AE. HIV-related pulmonary infections: a review of the recent literature. Curr Opin Pulm Med 2003;9(3):210–4.

A 43-year-old man is brought in on an EMS stretcher after a syncopal episode. After obtaining a palpated pressure of 80 mmHg systolic and heart rate of 120 beats per minute, EMS started an 18-gauge IV and began infusing normal saline. The patient relates a 3 to 4 day history of dark, tarry stools (about three to four times per day). Today he passed out while having a bowel movement. He does complain of some epigastric pain and light-headedness. He denies any hematemesis, hematochezia, chest pain, shortness of breath, and any similar past episodes. He does admit to drinking a 6-pack to a 12-pack of beer each day and hasn't seen a doctor in years.

On exam, his vital signs are temperature 36.6°C (97.9°F), blood pressure 92/45 mmHg (after 900 mL IV fluid prior to arrival), heart rate 113 beats per minute, and respiratory rate 24 breaths per minute. The patient is noticeably jaundiced and pale with dried, dark stool covering his legs. He has mild tenderness to palpation in the epigastrium but no rebound or guarding. He does not have any obvious spider angioma, gynecomastia, palmar erythema, or ascites. On rectal exam, he has grossly melanic stool.

 What is the most likely diagnosis?

 What is the best therapy?

ANSWERS TO CASE 34: Gastrointestinal Bleeding

Summary: This 43-year-old man presents with tachycardia and hypotension after several episodes of melena.

◆ **Most likely diagnosis:** upper gastrointestinal (GI) bleed with hypovolemic shock.

◆ **Best therapy:** stabilization of the ABCs, including IV access and volume resuscitation. Consider the use of blood products, proton pump inhibitors, and somatostatin or octreotide. Endoscopy is another treatment option.

Analysis

Objectives

1. Learn the differences between upper and lower GI bleeding.
2. Understand the evaluation and management of patients with a GI bleed.

Considerations

This 43-year-old man is in class III shock (see Case 6), because he is hypotensive and has tachycardia. This correlates to a 1500 to 2000 mL blood loss. The most important priorities are stabilization by addressing the ABCs, including placing two large-bore intravenous lines, giving boluses of normal saline, such as 2 L as fast as can be run, and monitoring the blood pressure, heart rate, pulse oximetry, and urine output. Blood work should be sent off, including complete blood count (CBC), electrolytes, renal and liver function tests, coagulation studies, and type and cross for at least 2 units of blood. The main priorities are to determine whether there has been significant blood loss and to maintain hemodynamic stability. After stabilization, a focused history should be taken to determine the probable etiology of the gastrointestinal bleeding. Chronic nonsteroidal antiinflammatory drug (NSAID) or aspirin use may indicate gastritis. This patient is icteric, which likely indicates cirrhosis and possibly coagulopathy or esophageal varices. Room-temperature water lavage via a nasogastric (NG) tube will establish the diagnosis of upper GI bleeding and often slow the bleeding. **Upper endoscopy is likely to be the treatment of choice for these patients.**

APPROACH TO GI BLEEDING

GI bleeding is classified as upper or lower based on whether it arises proximal or distal to the ligament of Treitz. Common causes of upper GI bleeding include peptic ulcer disease, esophageal or gastric varices, Mallory-Weiss tear, esophagitis, and gastritis (Fig. 34-1). The most common etiologies of lower GI bleeding are upper GI bleeding, hemorrhoids, diverticulosis, angiodysplasia, malignancy, inflammatory bowel disease, and infectious conditions (Fig. 34-2).

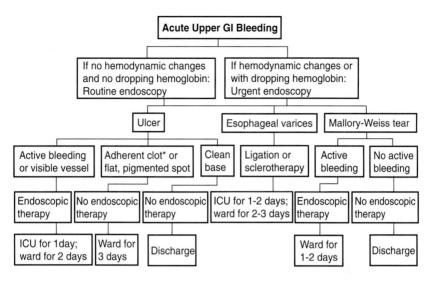

Figure 34-1. Algorithm for upper GI bleeding.

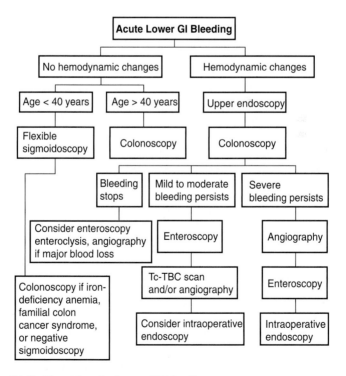

Figure 34-2. Algorithm for lower GI bleeding.

In children, Meckel diverticulum, volvulus, and intussusception are other possible causes.

When taking a history, the clinician should focus on the nature, duration, and amount of bleeding. Classically, patients with an upper GI bleed present with hematemesis and melena, while hematochezia suggests a lower GI source. However, this is not always the case, depending on the speed and amount of bleeding. It is important to ask about syncope, weakness, chest pain, dyspnea, and confusion because these symptoms suggest significant blood loss. In addition, risk factor assessment may help determine the cause of the bleeding (Table 34-1).

During the physical exam, careful attention must be paid to the vital signs, searching for evidence of hypovolemic shock (tachypnea, tachycardia, hypotension). Cool, pale, or diaphoretic skin and pale conjunctiva, nail beds, or mucous membranes suggest anemia. If stigmata of chronic liver disease (jaundice, caput medusae, spider angiomata, palmar erythema, and gynecomastia) are present, variceal bleeding is a strong possibility. The abdominal exam should focus on searching for peritoneal signs, such as guarding and rebound.

Bedside testing includes a rectal exam to check for hemorrhoids, anal fissures, and occult blood in the stool. All patients should have a nasogastric tube with room temperature normal saline (NS) or water lavage. If blood is present (bright red or "coffee ground"), an upper GI source is more likely.

After IV access is obtained, blood should be sent for complete blood count, electrolytes, blood urea nitrogen (BUN)/creatinine, coagulation studies, and type

Table 34-1
ETIOLOGIES OF GI BLEEDING AND RISK FACTORS

ETIOLOGY	RISK FACTORS
Varices	Alcoholism, cirrhosis
Peptic ulcer disease	*Helicobacter pylori* infection, NSAID use, alcohol use, heredity, tobacco use
Gastritis	NSAID use, alcohol use, steroids, burns, major trauma, head injury
Mallory-Weiss syndrome	Recent vomiting or retching, hiatal hernia, alcohol use, esophagitis
Aortoenteric fistula	History of abdominal aortic graft
Diverticulosis	High-fat diet, older age
Colon cancer	Weight loss, change in bowel habits

and screen or crossmatch. In patients with chest pain, dysrhythmia, or risk factors for coronary artery disease; an electrocardiogram (EKG) should be obtained.

Treatment

Treatment begins with stabilizing the ABCs. Intubation may be necessary to protect the patient's airway. **IV access (large-bore peripherals or central) is a high priority.** Volume resuscitation should begin with 2 L of NS or lactated Ringer solution. For patients who are hemodynamically unstable after crystalloid infusion, have ongoing blood loss, or whose hemoglobin is <7 mg/dL, packed red blood cells (PRBCs) should be transfused. **Fresh-frozen plasma and vitamin K** may be indicated in patients with coagulopathies caused by **liver disease** or anticoagulation therapy. As a general rule, **a proton pump inhibitor should be given to patients with upper GI bleeding to decrease rebleeding rates.** Surgery is indicated for massive or refractory bleeding.

With variceal bleeding, somatostatin, octreotide, or vasopressin can be helpful. However, vasopressin has fallen out of favor because of the side effects and the risk of end-organ ischemia. In massive bleeding, balloon tamponade with a **Sengstaken-Blakemore tube may be useful.**

Various modalities exist to identify the source of bleeding. In upper GI bleeds, endoscopy is the study of choice because it can also be used to treat through use of lasers, electrocoagulation, sclerotherapy, or band ligation. For lower GI bleeds, anoscopy, sigmoidoscopy, or colonoscopy are preferred. Tagged red blood cell (RBC) scans are an alternative in stable patients. If there is massive or continuous bleeding, angiography is a better option.

Comprehension Questions

[34.1] Risk factors for peptic ulcer disease include which one of the following?

    A. *Helicobacter pylori* infection
    B. Estrogen replacement therapy
    C. Acetaminophen use
    D. *Chlamydia trachomatis*

[34.2] A 43-year-old male complains of acute onset of vomiting bright red blood. He denies alcohol use and history of peptic ulcer disease. He is anxious, and his blood pressure is 120/70 mmHg and heart rate is 90 beats per minute. Which of the following is the best next step in managing his condition?

    A. Morphine sulfate
    B. Endoscopic examination
    C. Chest radiograph
    D. Intravenous fluid resuscitation

[34.3] In the patient described in question [34.2], which of the following modalities is best to identify the source of bleeding?

A. Tagged RBC scan
B. Endoscopy
C. Angiography
D. Laparotomy

[34.4] A 58-year-old woman is brought into the ED complaining of bright red bleeding per rectum that was of acute onset. She denies abdominal pain. Which of the following is the most likely etiology of her condition?

A. Varices
B. Gastritis
C. Diverticulosis
D. Mallory-Weiss tear

Answers

[35.2] **A.** Risk factors for peptic ulcer disease include *Helicobacter pylori* infection, NSAID use, alcohol use, heredity, and tobacco use.

[35.2] **D.** Stabilization of the patient is always the first priority. The ABCs come first; assuming that his airway and breathing are stable, then circulation is next.

[35.3] **B.** Endoscopy is the preferred modality to identify the source of bleeding in upper GI bleeding.

[35.4] **C.** Common causes of lower GI bleeding are diverticulosis, upper GI bleeding, hemorrhoids, angiodysplasia, malignancy, inflammatory bowel disease, and infectious conditions. Bleeding with diverticulosis is described as painless and abrupt, "as though a water faucet was suddenly turned on." The other choices are common causes of upper GI bleeding.

CLINICAL PEARLS

❖ Although most GI bleeds resolve spontaneously, each case is potentially life-threatening. The main priorities are to determine whether there has been significant blood loss and to maintain hemodynamic stability.

❖ In upper GI bleeds, endoscopy is the study of choice because it can also be used to treat. Anoscopy, sigmoidoscopy, or colonoscopy are preferred in lower GI bleeds.

❖ In general, all patients with GI bleeding are admitted. If hemodynamically unstable or actively bleeding, they should be admitted to an ICU setting.

REFERENCES

Conrad S. Acute upper gastrointestinal bleeding in critically ill patients: causes and treatment modalities. Crit Care Med 2002;30(6):S365–8.

Girmann RA, Emerick ML. Acute gastrointestinal bleeding. In: Hamilton GC, Sanders AB, Strange GR, Trott AT. Emergency medicine: an approach to clinical problem-solving. Philadelphia: WB Saunders, 2003:97–112.

Gosh S, Watts D, Kinnear M. Management of gastrointestinal haemorrhage. Postgrad Med J 2002;78:4–14.

Mick NW, Peters JR, Silvers SM. Blueprints in emergency medicine. Malden, MA: Blackwell Publishing, 2002:95–7.

Overton DT. Gastrointestinal bleeding. In: Tintinalli JE, Kelen GD, Stapczynski JS, eds. Emergency medicine: a comprehensive study guide, 5th ed. New York: McGraw-Hill, 2004:505–8.

A 63-year-old woman arrives in the ED in respiratory distress. The ambulance crew who transported her wasn't able to obtain any information about her past medical history but did bring her bag of medications, which includes furosemide (Lasix).

On exam, her temperature is 37.5°C (99.5°F), blood pressure 220/112 mmHg, heart rate 130 beats per minute, respiratory rate 36 breaths per minute, and oxygen saturation 93 percent on high-flow oxygen. The patient's skin is cool, clammy, and diaphoretic and she can only answer yes-or-no questions because of dyspnea. She has jugular venous distension to the angle of the jaw, rales in both lung fields, and +2 pretibial edema bilaterally. Her heart sounds are regular although tachycardic with an S_4 gallop.

◆ **What is the most likely diagnosis?**

◆ **What is the most appropriate next step?**

ANSWERS TO CASE 35: Congestive Heart Failure/ Pulmonary Edema

Summary: This is a 63-year-old female in respiratory distress with signs of pump failure and fluid overload.

 Most likely diagnosis: congestive heart failure (CHF) and pulmonary edema

 Most appropriate next step: management of the ABCs, preload reduction, and diuresis

Analysis

Objectives

1. Recognize the clinical presentation and complications of CHF.
2. Understand the diagnostic and therapeutic approach to suspected CHF.

Considerations

This 63-year-old woman is brought into the ED with significant congestive heart failure, dyspnea, respiratory distress, hypertension, and tachycardia. Her medication including furosemide (Lasix) strongly suggests congestive heart failure. This clinical presentation is classic for a CHF exacerbation. Rapid assessment of the ABCs, IV access, and prompt initiation of preload reduction and diuresis are the mainstays of therapy. Oxygen should be administered. Endotracheal intubation may be necessary for severe cases and those refractory to treatment. Once the patient is stabilized, it is important to try to determine the precipitant of the exacerbation. Diagnostic tests should be directed at possible myocardial infarction, a common cause of worsening CHF.

APPROACH TO CONGESTIVE HEART FAILURE/PULMONARY EDEMA

The right side of the heart receives blood from the peripheral circulation and sends it to the lungs for oxygenation. The left side subsequently receives oxygenated blood from the lungs and pumps it back into the circulation. Disruption of these functions leads to loss of normal contractile ability and heart failure. The term "congestive" refers to abnormal fluid retention resulting from this loss of contractility. There are many causes of heart failure, the most common of which are coronary artery disease and hypertension.

Failure of the right side of the heart results in increased systemic venous pressures while left-sided failure causes increased pulmonary venous pressures. Thus each has different symptoms and physical findings (Table 35-1).

Table 35-1
COMMON PRESENTATIONS OF HEART FAILURE

TYPE OF FAILURE	SYMPTOMS	EXAM FINDINGS
Right-sided	Peripheral edema, right upper quadrant pain	Dependent edema, right upper quadrant tenderness, hepatomegaly, hepatojugular reflux, jugular venous distension
Left-sided	Dyspnea, orthopnea, paroxysmal nocturnal dyspnea	Tachypnea, pulmonary crackles or wheezes, S_3 or S_4 gallop

Clinical Evaluation

During the evaluation, the clinician must also seek to determine what caused the patient's condition to decompensate. **The most common precipitants are myocardial ischemia or infarction and noncompliance with medications or dietary restrictions.** Other causes are uncontrolled hypertension, valvular dysfunction, arrhythmia, infection, anemia, and thyrotoxicosis.

Although history and physical exam are the most important aspects to diagnosing CHF, chest radiography still provides valuable information for the clinician. In early CHF, the chest x-ray shows upper zone vascular redistribution (cephalization). As the pulmonary congestion increases, interstitial edema and Kerley B lines become prominent, followed by opacification of the air spaces with alveolar edema. Other findings include cardiomegaly and pleural effusions.

Laboratory studies include complete blood count, electrolytes, and blood urea nitrogen (BUN)/creatinine. If there is a suspicion of acute coronary syndrome, cardiac markers should be sent. A newer diagnostic tool is B-type natriuretic peptide (BNP), a hormone released from the ventricles in response to stretch. It is a promising marker of heart failure with higher levels being predictive of CHF. Electrocardiograms (EKGs) are helpful in detecting evidence of cardiac ischemia or infarction and arrhythmias.

Treatment

Treatment of cardiogenic pulmonary edema consists of oxygenation, vasodilation, diuresis, and augmenting cardiac contractility if needed. High-flow oxygen should be the first intervention. Positive pressure ventilation via continuous positive airway pressure (CPAP) may be necessary if hypoxia continues. Ultimately, the patient may require intubation if refractory to the aforementioned interventions. **Vasodilation is obtained by reducing preload.** This is most effectively and rapidly achieved with **nitroglycerin**, which can be given via sublingual, oral, topical, or IV routes. **Diuresis with furosemide or bumetanide effectively reduces intravascular volume and**

preload, thus reducing pulmonary congestion. **Morphine** is useful as an analgesic, anxiolytic, and vasodilator. In addition, **angiotensin-converting enzyme (ACE) inhibitors may play a role in preload reduction** and in the treatment of CHF. If patients do not improve with this therapy, **inotropes,** such as **dobutamine or milrinone,** may be given to increase myocardial contractility. If the patient is **hypotensive, dopamine is the preferred inotrope.**

Comprehension Questions

[35.1] A 62-year-old woman is sent to the ED from her primary physician's office with worsening heart failure. The patient has had congestive heart failure, previously controlled with oral digoxin and Lasix. Which of the following is the most likely reason for the exacerbation of her CHF?

    A. Valvular dysfunction
    B. Arrhythmia
    C. Myocardial ischemia and infarction
    D. Thyrotoxicosis

[35.2] A 55-year-old male has symptoms of worsening orthopnea, tachypnea, and rales on pulmonary examination. The liver is percussed at 6 cm at the midclavicular line. His jugular vein is at +2 cm at 45 degrees. Which of the following is the best description of this patient's disease process?

    A. Right-sided heart failure
    B. Left-sided heart failure
    C. Biventricular heart failure
    D. Acute respiratory distress syndrome

[35.3] A 58-year-old man is brought into the ED by paramedics because of worsening dyspnea. He has congestive heart failure due to cardiovascular disease. On examination, his blood pressure is 150/100 mmHg and heart rate 104 beats per minute. He has jugular venous distension and rales in both lung fields. What is the most effective and most rapid method of reducing preload in this patient?

    A. Diuretics
    B. Nitroglycerin
    C. Dobutamine
    D. Morphine

[35.4] A 54-year-old man complains of acute onset of worsening fatigue and dyspnea. He has alcohol-induced cardiomyopathy and congestive heart failure. Which of the following is the best workup for his CHF exacerbation?

    A. Chest x-ray, cardiac enzymes, EKG
    B. Computed tomography (CT) scan of the chest, EKG, D-dimer test
    C. Echocardiogram of the heart, EKG, thallium stress treadmill of the heart
    D. Arterial blood gas, cardiac enzymes, pulmonary angiography

Answers

[35.1] **C.** Myocardial ischemia and infarction are among the most common precipitants of a CHF exacerbation (as well as noncompliance with medications).

[35.2] **B.** Left-sided heart failure can present with dyspnea, orthopnea, paroxysmal nocturnal dyspnea, tachypnea, crackles or wheezes, and an S_3 or S_4 gallop. The lack of jugular venous distension and/or hepatomegaly suggests absence of right-heart failure.

[35.3] **B.** Nitroglycerin is the most effective and most rapid means of reducing preload in the patient with CHF.

[35.4] **A.** The workup of a CHF exacerbation includes chest x-ray, EKG, electrolytes, BUN/creatinine, and cardiac enzymes. A BNP level may also be sent.

CLINICAL PEARLS

❖ The most common causes of CHF include coronary artery disease and hypertension while the most common causes of an acute exacerbation are myocardial ischemia or infarct and noncompliance.

❖ BNP is a hormone released by the ventricles in response to stretch. It is useful as a marker for heart failure.

❖ Treatment of CHF includes oxygenation, correction of the underlying cause, and relief of symptoms by vasodilation, diuresis, and possibly inotropic support.

REFERENCES

Cairns CB. Heart failure and pulmonary edema. In: Tintinalli JE, Kelen GD, Stapczynski JS, eds. Emergency medicine, 5th ed. New York: McGraw-Hill, 2000:374–8.

Collins SP, Ronan-Bantles S, Storrow AB. Diagnostic and prognostic usefulness of natriuretic peptides in emergency department patients with dyspnea. Ann Emerg Med 2003;41:532–44.

Kosowsky JM, Kobayashi L. Acutely decompensated heart failure: diagnostic and therapeutic strategies for the new millennium. Emerg Med Pract 2002;4(2):1–28.

Maisel AS, Krishnaswamy P, Nowak RM, et al. Rapid measurement of B-type natriuretic peptide in the emergency diagnosis of heart failure. N Engl J Med 2002;347:161–7.

A 25-year-old woman is brought to the emergency room by the police after they picked her up attempting to break into a grocery store. When they apprehended her, they noted her pupils were widely dilated, and that she seemed "high." The patient states that she has been "smoking" for the majority of the past year. She notes that without her "smokes" she craves the drug, becomes very sleepy, depressed, and has a huge appetite. In the emergency department, she complains of chest pain. The patient has a temperature of 38°C (100.4°F), heart rate of 120 beats per minute, and blood pressure of 160/90 mmHg. Her pupils are both dilated and reactive. Her thyroid is normal to palpation. The heart and lung examinations reveal tachycardia. Neurological examination does not elicit any defects.

◆ **What is the most likely diagnosis?**

ANSWER TO CASE 36: Cocaine Intoxication

Summary: This 25-year-old woman was arrested while attempting to burglarize a grocery store. She lost her job because she was late and stealing, secondary to her desire to "smoke." The patient has needed increased amounts of her drug of choice to get high, and she suffers cravings, sleepiness, depression, and hyperphagia when she is unable to take it. While high, the patient notes a feeling of euphoria and heightened energy. The patient has tried to quit "smoking" but has been unsuccessful. Her pupils are widely dilated, she has a low-grade fever, tachycardia, and hypertension. She has lost 30 pounds in 6 months.

◆ **Most Likely Diagnosis:** cocaine intoxication.

Analysis

Objectives

1. Recognize the clinical manifestations of cocaine intoxication.
2. Know the treatment for acute cocaine intoxication.

Considerations

This patient has many of the clinical effects of cocaine intoxication. Cocaine is a stimulant with local anesthetic characteristics, and has potent vasoconstriction properties. **Hyperpyrexia or severely elevated blood pressure** may result. **Myocardial infarction** from coronary artery spasm and **stroke** from cerebral artery effects have also been reported. **Acute cocaine intoxication is a medical emergency and is life-threatening, and is best managed in an intensive care setting. Seizures, ventricular arrhythmias, and myocardial infarction** are all complications. Treatment includes, first and foremost, **benzodiazepines** (many times at high dosages) and supportive measures. Beta blockers are not advisable because of the risk of unopposed alpha-adrenergic stimulation. Other illicit agents should also be suspected.

APPROACH TO COCAINE INTOXICATION

Definitions

Cocaine: A crystalline alkaloid, obtained from the leaves of *Erythroxylum coca* used as a local anesthetic applied topically to mucous membranes. Abuse of cocaine or its salts by snorting the powder form, inhaling the fumes of the crystalloid form ("crack"), or injecting a dissolved crystalline form leads to intoxication, dependence, and withdrawal.

Formication: A tactile hallucination in which there is a sensation of tiny insects crawling over the skin; most commonly seen in cocaine or amphetamine intoxication.

Intoxication: An organic mental syndrome characterized by the presence in the body of an exogenous psychoactive substance that produces a substance-specific syndrome of effects on the central nervous system.

Clinical Approach

Recent studies indicate that 11.3 percent of the U.S. population have used cocaine sometime in their lives. With such widespread use, emergency department visits related to cocaine intoxication and its complications have risen substantially. Before the mid 1980s the main routes of administration were intranasal and intravenous injection of cocaine hydrochloride. When taken in this form, the effects are felt within 1 to 5 minutes, with a peak effect between 20 and 60 minutes. During the 1980s, crack cocaine emerged as the form of choice. Crack is the hydrochloride salt converted to a more volatile form, usually by adding sodium bicarbonate, water, and heat. The onset of the high is quicker (less than 1 minute) and more intense. Frequently on the streets cocaine is combined with other drugs for various effects. Examples include "speedball," which is cocaine mixed with heroin, and "liquid lady," which is cocaine mixed with alcohol.

Approximately two-thirds of the emergency department visits related to cocaine intoxication are for trauma, resulting from risky or violent behaviors associated with cocaine use. The other one-third of visits are for medical complications of intoxication. Symptoms of **cocaine** use include **euphoria, feelings of power or aggression, agitation, anxiety, hallucinations (classically formication), and delusions.** Signs **include mydriasis, tachycardia, hypertension, diaphoresis, irritability, tremors or seizures.** Table 36-1 lists the acute complications of cocaine intoxication. The effects on the cardiovascular and neurological systems are of major concern. **Severe arrhythmias, myocardial infarction, seizures, and subarachnoid hemorrhage** may result and potentially kill the patient. Pulmonary effects include pulmonary hemorrhage, pneumonitis, asthma, and pulmonary edema. Gastrointestinal effects include mesenteric vasospasm and intestinal ischemia, bowel necrosis, and splenic infarction. **Body packers, who swallow relatively pure cocaine to avoid arrest, may die from intoxication if the bag ruptures. Rhabdomyolysis** may result in renal failure, strongly associated with mortality. Serum creatine phosphokinase (CPK) and creatinine levels are reasonable to obtain in suspected cocaine intoxication. **Pregnant** women may experience **abruptio placentae or hepatic rupture.**

Individuals intoxicated with cocaine often present with chest pain. The ED physician must have a high index of suspicion for myocardial infarction. **The young male**, particularly if a **smoker** and **a chronic user of cocaine**, is at risk. The history is many times atypical and the electrocardiogram (EKG) may be normal. Beta blockers should **not** be used when cocaine is involved. Nitroglycerin and calcium channel blockers may be helpful. Treatment for acute coronary syndrome using morphine, nitrates, and aspirin is advisable. Additionally, benzodiazepines, many times in large dosages, are often required. **Thrombolytic therapy is relatively contraindicated** in the presence of cocaine use. The possibility of aortic or coronary dissection should be entertained. Often, emergent coronary artery catheterization may provide the best diagnostic information.

Table 36-1

ACUTE COMPLICATIONS OF COCAINE INTOXICATION

AUTONOMIC	Hyperthermia, rhabdomyolysis, hypertension, hypotension
CARDIAC	Dysrhythmias, myocarditis, cardiomyopathy, myocardial infarction or ischemia
CENTRAL NERVOUS SYSTEM	Seizures, intracranial hemorrhage and infarction, intracranial abscess, altered mental status
PULMONARY	Pulmonary hemorrhages, barotrauma, pneumonitis, asthma, pulmonary edema
GASTROINTESTINAL	Mesenteric vasospasm, intestinal ischemia, bowel necrosis, splenic infarction
RENAL	Renal insufficiency, renal infarction

Treatment for acute cocaine intoxication is generally unnecessary, because the drug is so short-acting. Should progressive, severe toxicity ensue, however, interventions are necessary and critical. Cardiac arrhythmias need to be controlled with the appropriate medication, usually lidocaine. Ventricular fibrillation requires cardioversion. Severe hypertension should be treated with direct vasodilators or alpha antagonists such as **sodium nitroprusside or phentolamine,** respectively. The first-line agent for nearly all cocaine toxicity is **benzodiazepines**, usually with very large doses required; the benzodiazepines should be pushed to maximum doses before another agent is used. In general, **beta-blocking agents should not be used, because unopposed alpha-adrenergic stimulation may lead to myocardial ischemia or seizures.** Even labetalol (mixed alpha- and beta-blocker) administered in the face of cocaine use has been associated with excess mortality in animal studies. Seizures are treated with a short-acting benzodiazepine such as lorazepam. Rhabdomyolysis, metabolic acidosis, and electrolyte imbalances are difficult complications. These patients require close attention for adequate fluid replacement and in cases of severe acidosis, may require mannitol-alkaline diuresis.

The suspected body packer who is asymptomatic may be observed, or given activated charcoal and judicious amounts of polyethylene glycol lavage (GoLYTELY) to gently hasten the passage of the potentially toxic bags of cocaine. If an individual shows signs of severe cocaine intoxication such as severe hypertension, hyperthermia, seizures, or agitation, benzodiazepine administration and surgical consultation should be obtained to possibly remove the cocaine packages operatively. Endoscopy should not be performed, because perforation of the bags is a hazard.

Comprehension Questions

[36.1] A 25-year-old male is brought into the emergency room by police because of suspected cocaine intoxication. He is noted to be very agitated, fighting against five burly policeman, and wild-eyed. On examination, his blood pressure is 180/100 mmHg and heart rate 110 beats per minute. He is noted to have rotational nystagmus. The neurological examination reveals no focal abnormalities. Which of the following is the most likely diagnosis?

A. Cocaine intoxication
B. Cocaine withdrawal
C. Amphetamine intoxication
D. Amphetamine withdrawal
E. Opiate intoxication
F. Opiate withdrawal
G. Phencyclidine intoxication
H. Phencyclidine withdrawal

[36.2] A 28-year-old male is noted to have extremely elevated blood pressures in the 210/130 mmHg range associated with chest pain and dyspnea. His urine drug screen is positive for cocaine metabolites. Which of the following is the best next step?

A. Labetalol intravenously
B. Ephedrine intravenously
C. Lorazepam (Ativan) intravenously
D. Albuterol intravenously

[36.3] A 35-year-old man is brought into the ED with altered level of consciousness, drowsiness, and pinpoint pupils. Which of the following is the most likely therapy for this patient?

A. Benzodiazepines
B. Naloxone
C. Activated charcoal
D. Alkalinization of the urine

Answers

[36.1]   **G.** Phencyclidine intoxication often presents with agitation, superhuman strength, and rotational or vertical nystagmus.

[36.2]   **C.** Benzodiazepines should be used as the first-line agent for nearly all cocaine toxicities. The hypertension is caused by sympathetic stimulation. Beta blockers are contraindicated because it would allow unopposed alpha-adrenergic stimulation and exacerbation of the chest pain and hypertension. Occasionally, hypertension not responsive to sedation requires phentolamine 2.5 mg IV, an alpha-adrenergic antagonist.

[36.3]   **B.** This patient likely has an opiate intoxication with drowsiness and pinpoint pupils. Cocaine intoxication would lead to dilated pupils and agitation. Benzodiazepines are generally given for alcohol withdrawal, usually presenting as agitation, tremulousness, and hallucinations.

CLINICAL PEARLS

❖ Cocaine intoxication has its manifestations by sympathetic overactivity and vasospastic effect.

❖ Cocaine intoxication can cause life-threatening complications, including stroke, myocardial infarction, rhabdomyolysis, and death.

❖ Cocaine can cause a quinidine-like effect prolonging the QT interval, leading to wide-complex dysrhythmia, bradycardia, and hypotension.

❖ Beta blockers are not advisable for cocaine intoxication because of the risk of unopposed alpha-adrenergic stimulation.

REFERENCES

Perrone J, Hoffman RS. Cocaine, amphetamines, caffeine, and nicotine. In: Tintinalli JE, Kelen GD, Stapczynski JS, eds. Emergency medicine, 6th ed. New York: McGraw-Hill, 2004:1075–9.

Zafar H, Vaz A, Carlson R. Acute complications of cocaine intoxication. Hosp Pract 1997:32(2)167–81.

An 18-year-old female is brought by her roommate to the emergency department (ED) about 30 minutes after she took "a bunch" of Tylenol. The patient
states that after an argument with her boyfriend, she "wanted to make him
sorry" and swallowed half a bottle of Extra-Strength Tylenol. She is tearful,
says she was "stupid," and denies any true desire to hurt herself or anyone else.
She has no other complaints and denies any past attempts to hurt herself. On
examination, her blood pressure is 105/60 mmHg, heart rate is 100 beats per
minute, and respiratory rate is 24 breaths per minute (crying). Her pupils are
equal and reactive bilaterally. Her sclera are clear, and her mucous membranes
are moist. The lungs are clear and the heart sounds are regular. The abdominal
exam is benign with normal bowel sounds. She is awake and alert without any
focal neurological deficits.

◆ **What is the most appropriate next step?**

◆ **What are the potential complications of this ingestion?**

◆ **What is the mechanism of acetaminophen toxicity?**

ANSWERS TO CASE 37: Acetaminophen Toxicity

Summary: This is an 18-year-old female with an acute acetaminophen overdose 30 minutes prior to arrival in the ED. She is alert and oriented with stable vital signs.

 Most appropriate next step: obtain IV access, send appropriate laboratory studies; gastric lavage and administer activated charcoal; evaluate need for *N*-acetylcysteine (NAC).

Potential complications: hypoglycemia, metabolic acidosis, **hepatic failure**, and renal failure.

Mechanism: production of toxic metabolite, *N*-acetyl-*p*-benzoquinone-imine (NAPQI).

Analysis

Objectives

1. Learn the general approach to the poisoned patient.
2. Recognize the clinical signs and symptoms of acetaminophen toxicity.
3. Understand the evaluation and treatment of patients with acetaminophen toxicity.

Considerations

Acetaminophen (APAP) is one of the most commonly used analgesics and antipyretics. It is available in a variety of prescription and over-the-counter medications. As a result, it is a very common agent reported in accidental and intentional overdoses, as in the patient described. A toxic exposure to APAP is suspected when 140 mg/kg or more is ingested in a single dose, or 7.5 g over the course of 24 hours. Hepatotoxicity is the most life-threatening complication, but may be indolent; thus, serum acetaminophen level and a precise time of ingestion are important to plot on a nomogram to assess likelihood of toxicity. This patient was forthcoming about the medication used in the overdose; however, many patients will underreport or deny the use of APAP. Consequently, as a general rule, an acetaminophen level should be drawn on all overdose patients. Although clinical evidence of hepatotoxicity may be delayed for 24 to 72 hours, NAC therapy is most effective if started within 8 hours of ingestion. Because this patient reports the ingestion within 30 minutes, there is time for a serum level, activated charcoal decontamination, and then NAC therapy. If time is an issue, NAC treatment should be initiated without delay. Emesis should not be induced because of the possible delay in therapy. After medical stabilization, assessment of suicide potential is important.

APPROACH TO ACETAMINOPHEN TOXICITY

Although APAP is safe at therapeutic dosages, **ingestions >140 mg/kg can lead to liver failure and death.** Under normal circumstances, most APAP is metabolized in the liver and excreted by the kidneys. Of the remainder, approximately 5 percent is excreted unchanged in urine. Another 5 percent is metabolized by the hepatic cytochrome P450 system to form NAPQI. This toxic intermediate is then detoxified by conjugation with glutathione. In **acute APAP overdose, glutathione depletion leads to accumulation of NAPQI and subsequent hepatocellular necrosis.** Individuals with **glutathione deficiency**, such as **alcoholics or those with HIV** infection, are **especially at risk for acetaminophen hepatotoxicity.** APAP toxicity can be divided into four clinical phases (Table 37-1).

Clinical Evaluation

When approaching the poisoned or overdose patient, the clinician's priorities are to perform a **rapid assessment, stabilize the ABCs, decontaminate, minimize absorption**, and administer any **antidotes**. Important historical information includes type, amount, and timing of ingestion, current symptoms, circumstances of the ingestion (accidental or intentional), and possible coingestants. A careful exam is important to determine the extent of the poisoning and to search for any concomitant toxic syndromes (toxidromes) (Table 37-2). Table 37-3 lists common antidotes.

Diagnostic studies include serum electrolytes, blood urea nitrogen (BUN)/creatinine, glucose, and liver enzyme levels, coagulation studies, urinalysis (and pregnancy test if appropriate). Strong suspicion of coingestion is generally the

Table 37-1
CLINICAL PHASES OF APAP TOXICITY

PHASE 1 (30 MINUTES TO 24 HOURS AFTER INGESTION)	PHASE 2 (24 TO 72 HOURS AFTER INGESTION)	PHASE 3 (72 TO 96 HOURS AFTER INGESTION)	PHASE 4 (4 TO 10 DAYS AFTER INGESTION)
Anorexia, nausea, vomiting, malaise, diaphoresis	Decreased gastrointestinal symptoms, right upper quadrant pain and tenderness, elevated liver enzymes, oliguria	Anorexia, nausea, vomiting, peak liver function abnormalities (jaundice, coagulopathy, encephalopathy), renal failure, death	Resolution of hepatic dysfunction or progression to fulminant hepatic failure

Table 37-2

COMMON TOXIDROMES

TOXIDROME	CLINICAL FINDINGS	COMMON AGENTS
Opioid	Coma, respiratory depression, pinpoint pupils	Codeine, heroin, morphine, meperidine, hydrocodone
Anticholinergic	Tachycardia, hyperthermia, dry skin and mucous membranes, delirium, urinary retention, mydriasis, flushed skin, absent bowel sounds	Antihistamines, phenothiazines, tricyclic antidepressants, scopolamine, Jimson weed, belladonna
Cholinergic	Salivation, lacrimation, urination, diarrhea, miosis, bradycardia, emesis	Organophosphate insecticide, pilocarpine, betel nuts
Sympathomimetic	Hypertension, tachycardia, mydriasis, hyperpyrexia, arrhythmias	Cocaine, methamphetamine, ephedrine, ecstasy
Sedative–hypnotic	Decreased level of consciousness, respiratory depression, hypotension, variable pupillary changes, hypothermia, seizures	Barbiturates, benzodiazepines

rule; a toxicology screen and salicylate level should be obtained. If the patient's mental status is altered, a computed tomography (CT) scan of the head is also recommended. However, the single best predictor of the risk of hepatotoxicity is a serum APAP level. This should be drawn 4 hours postingestion, or immediately if the time of ingestion is unknown. Using the APAP level and the Rumack-Matthew nomogram, the clinician can then predict the severity of toxicity and determine the need for NAC therapy (see Figure 37-1). This nomogram is not applicable for chronic ingestions, extended release APAP, or coingestions.

Treatment

Initial treatment of the patient with an APAP overdose consists of stabilizing the ABCs, obtaining IV access, and placing the patient on cardiac and oxygen saturation monitors. If the patient presents within 1 hour of the overdose, gastric lavage is indicated. In addition, administering activated charcoal can reduce gastric absorption of the drug. Then the priority is to decide whether NAC is necessary. **NAC, the antidote for APAP toxicity, acts by replenishing glutathione stores and combining with NAPQI as a glutathione substitute**. It is most effective when given within 8 hours of ingestion. The indications for NAC include a toxic level as determined using the Rumack-Matthew

Table 37-3

COMMON ANTIDOTES: DOSES AND INDICATIONS

ANTIDOTE	PEDIATRICS	ADULT	POISON
N-acetylcysteine	140 mg/kg PO load, followed by 70 mg/kg PO q4h for 18 total doses		Acetaminophen
Activated charcoal		1 g/kg PO	Most ingested poisons
Antivenin Fab	4–6 vials IV initially over 1 h may be repeated. 2 vials every 6 h for 18 h	10–30 mL IV	Envenomation by *Crotalidae*
Calcium gluconate 10% (9 mg/mL elemental calcium) Calcium chloride 10% (27.2 mg/mL elemental calcium)	0.6–0.8 mL/kg IV		Hypermagnesemia, hypocalcemia (ethylene glycol, hydrofluoric acid), calcium channel antagonists, black widow spider venom)
Cyanide antidote kit Amyl nitrate	Not typically used	1 ampule in oxygen chamber of ambu-bag 30 s on/30 s off	Cyanide poisoning
Sodium nitrate	0.33 mL/kg IV (3% solution)	10 mL (3% solution)	Hydrogen sulfide (use only sodium nitrate)
Thiosulfate	Thiosulfate: 1.65 mL/kg IV	Thiosulfate: 12.5 g IV	
Deferoxamine	90 mg/kg IM (1 g max) or 15 mg/kg per h (IV 1 g max)	2 g IM or 15 mg/kg per h (6–8 g/d max)	Iron

Table 37-3 (Continued)
COMMON ANTIDOTES: DOSES AND INDICATIONS

ANTIDOTE	PEDIATRICS	ADULT	POISON
Dextrose		1 g/kg IV	Hypoglycemia
Digoxin immune Fab			Digoxin and cardiac glycosides
Acute	1–2 vials IV	10–20 vials IV	
Chronic		3–6 vials IV	
Ethanol 10% for IV administration	10 mL/kg over 30 min, then 1.5 mL/h*		Ethylene glycol, methanol
Folic acid/leucovorin		1–2 mg/kg q 4–6h IV	Methanol, methotrexate (only leucovorin)
Fomepizole		15 mg/kg IV, then 10 mg/kg q 12h	Methanol, ethylene glycol, disulfiram
Glucagon	50 µg/kg	1–10 mg IV	Calcium channel blocker, β-blocker
Methylene blue	1–2 mg/kg Neonates: 0.3–1 mg/kg	1–2 mg/kg	Oxidizing chemicals (e.g., nitrates, benzocaine, sulfonamides)
Octreotide	1 µg/kg q6h SC	5–100 µg SC q6h	Refractory hypoglycemia after oral hypo-glycemic agent ingestion
Naloxone	As much as is needed. Typical starting dose 0.4 mg–10 mg IV		Opioid, clonidine

Physostigmine	0.2 mg/kg IV	Anticholinergic substances (not tricyclic antidepressants)
Pralidoxime (2-PAM)	20–40 mg/kg IV	Cholinergic substances
Protamine	1 mg neutralizes 100 U of administered heparin; administered over 15 min; 0.6 mg/kg 25–50 mg IV: empiric	Heparin
Pyridoxine	Gram for gram ingestion if amount of isoniazid is known 70 mg/kg IV 5 g IV	Isoniazid, Gyromitra esculenta, rocket fuel
Sodium bicarbonate	1–2 mEq/kg IV bolus followed by 2 mEq/kg per h	Sodium channel blockers, alkalinization of urine or serum
Thiamine	100 mg IV	Ethylene glycol, Wernicke syndrome, "wet" beri-beri
Vitamin K_1	2–5 mg/d PO 25–50 mg TID	Anticoagulants
Whole-bowel irrigation	0.5 L/h PO 1.5–2 L/h PO	Multiple indications

* This is an approximation. Doses should be titrated to level.
Reprinted, with permission, from Tintinalli JE, Kelen GD, Stapczynski JS, eds. Emergency medicine, 6th ed. New York: McGraw-Hill, 2004:1017.

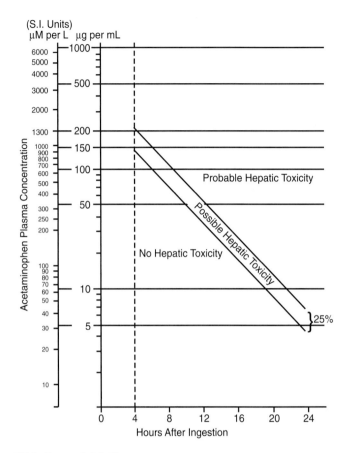

Figure 37-1. Rumack-Matthew nomogram

nomogram or an ingestion of >140 mg/kg more than 8 hours prior to arrival in the ED. In the latter instance, NAC can be discontinued if the level is non-toxic and the patient is asymptomatic. Any patient who requires NAC treatment should be admitted to the hospital. Importantly, although the nomogram may not be applicable for ingestions greater than 24 hours postingestion, NAC therapy may still be helpful.

The standard 72-hour NAC regimen is an oral loading dose of 140 mg/kg followed by maintenance doses of 70 mg/kg every 4 hours for 17 additional doses. Because of its acrid smell and taste, NAC often induces nausea and vomiting. Dilution in fruit juice or a chilled drink is helpful. A small fraction of patients will develop fulminant hepatic failure, associated with a 60 to 80 percent mortality rate. **Most deaths associated with liver failure occur 3 to 5 days postingestion, attributed to shock, cerebral edema, hemorrhage, or acute respiratory distress syndrome (ARDS).**

Comprehension Questions

[37.1] A 16-year-old female is brought into the ED after taking a number of pills from her parents' medicine cabinet. The parents have brought in all the medication bottles. Which of the following is most concerning for toxicity?

A. Diphenhydramine
B. Theophylline
C. Ampicillin
D. Prozac

[37.2] A 34-year-old man admits taking "the whole bottle" of acetaminophen over the course of 36 hours because of a severe headache. Which of the following is the best guide as to whether to initiate NAC therapy?

A. Plotting the serum APAP level on the nomogram
B. Serum APAP and liver function tests
C. If fairly certain that 24 hours have elapsed, NAC therapy is not efficacious
D. Clinical assessment of icterus
E. At 24 hours postingestion, NAC therapy may be helpful especially in the presence of alcoholism or human immunodeficiency virus (HIV) infection

[37.3] A 25-year-old male is brought into the ED 1 hour after a witnessed overdose of 20 to 25 pills of acetaminophen tablets. At what time would be the best time to draw the APAP level?

A. As soon as the patient arrives in the ED
B. At 2 hours postingestion
C. At 4 hours postingestion
D. At 8 hours postingestion

[37.4] A 38-year-old school teacher took a "large number of Tylenol tablets" and is found to have a APAP level of 200 mcg/mL. The estimated time postingestion is 8 hours. The first dose of NAC is given. Which of the following is the next step to guide therapy?

A. Check APAP level 4 hours after the first NAC dose and if below the toxicity line, no further NAC needed
B. Check the APAP level 12 hours after the first NAC dose and if below the toxicity line, no further NAC needed
C. Check the APAP level and liver function tests 8 hours after the first NAC dose and if in the normal/nontoxic range, then no further NAC needed.
D. Give the entire course of NAC and no further APAP levels are necessary

Match the following antidotes (A to H) to the clinical situation (questions [37.5] to [37.8]):

    A. *N*-acetylcysteine
    B. Calcium gluconate
    C. Deferoxamine
    D. Digoxin Fab
    E. Glucagon
    F. Naloxone
    G. Physostigmine
    H. Vitamin K

[37.5] A 45-year-old man takes too many of his antihypertensive pills and is noted to have a heart rate of 40 beats per minute.

[37.6] A 22-year-old pregnant woman with preeclampsia receiving intravenous medication to prevent seizures develops weakness and difficulty breathing.

[37.7] A 24-year-old man is brought into the ED with somnolence, pinpoint pupils, and track marks on his arm.

[37.8] A 56-year-old woman taking tablets to "thin her blood" is noted to be bleeding from her gums and has multiple bruises on her arms and legs.

Answers

[37.1] **B.** Theophylline has a very narrow therapeutic index, with toxic effects of tachycardia, nausea, vomiting, and seizures.

[37.2] **E.** At 24 hours postingestion, NAC therapy has not been proven to be helpful but still may be useful; thus, many ED clinicians will administer it in this situation. It definitely has a role in patients at increased risk for hepatotoxicity such as alcoholics or acquired immunodeficiency syndrome (AIDS) patients who have relative glutathione deficiency.

[37.3] **C.** A serum APAP should be drawn 4 hours postingestion; the nomogram has relevance between 4 hours and 24 hours postingestion.

[37.4] **D.** Once it is determined by the nomogram that the APAP dose is potentially toxic, the entire NAC regimen is given. No further APAP levels need to be drawn.

[37.5] **E.** Glucagon is effective in treating calcium channel blocker or beta-blocker overdose.

[37.6] **B.** This patient is likely receiving magnesium sulfate for seizure prophylaxis, and the antidote for hypermagnesemia is calcium gluconate.

[37.7] **F.** Naloxone is the treatment of choice for opiate overdose. This individual likely is a heroin abuser.

[37.8] **H.** This patient likely has warfarin overdose, which is treated by vitamin K.

> ## CLINICAL PEARLS
>
> ❖ Because the devastating effects of APAP toxicity may be delayed for 24 to 72 hours and antidotal therapy is most effective if started within 8 hours of ingestion, the clinician must have a high level of suspicion for APAP toxicity in any poisoned patient.
>
> ❖ APAP toxicity is caused by the formation of a toxic metabolite, *N*-acetyl-*p*-benzoquinone-imine (NAPQI).
>
> ❖ *N*-acetylcysteine (NAC) is the antidote for APAP toxicity and should be given if a toxic ingestion is suspected (based on ingested dose or APAP level and Rumack-Matthew nomogram).
>
> ❖ The priorities when dealing with a patient with an APAP overdose are to perform a rapid assessment, stabilize the ABCs, decontaminate, minimize absorption, and administer NAC if appropriate.
>
> ❖ In general, an APAP level should be drawn on any patient with an overdose history even when APAP ingestion is denied.

REFERENCES

Ford MD, ed. Clinical toxicology, 1st ed. Philadelphia: WB Saunders, 2000:265–73.

Mick NW, Peters JR, Silvers SM. Blueprints in emergency medicine. Malden, MA: Blackwell Publishing, 2002:273–6.

Rosen P, Barkin RM, Hayden SR, Schaider JJ, Wolfe R. The 5-minute emergency medicine consult. Philadelphia: Lippincott Williams & Wilkins, 1999:24–5.

Tintinalli JE, Kelen GD, Stapczynski JS, eds. Emergency medicine, 5th ed. New York: McGraw-Hill, 2000:1125–31.

Wilson R, Wolf L. The poisoned patient. In: Hamilton GC, Sanders AB, Strange GR, Trott AT, eds. Emergency medicine: an approach to clinical problem-solving. Philadelphia: WB Saunders, 2003:259–71.

A 30-year-old woman with a history of sickle cell disease presents complaining of chest pain. She states this pain is right-sided, worsens on inspiration, and is more severe than her usual "crisis pain." She has been having subjective fevers, mild shortness of breath, and a cough productive of yellow phlegm. She denies any vomiting, hemoptysis, leg swelling, and pain elsewhere. She has no other past medical history besides her sickle cell disease, with her last pain crisis about 3 months ago. She usually takes Vicodin at home for pain but has not had sufficient relief with this episode. On examination, her temperature is 38.3°C (101°F), blood pressure 126/65 mmHg, heart rate 98 beats per minute, respiratory rate 22 breaths per minute, and oxygen saturation 94 percent on room air. Her examination is unremarkable except for crackles in her lower right lung field. She does not have any jugular venous distension, calf tenderness, or lower extremity edema.

 What is the most likely diagnosis?

What is the best treatment?

ANSWERS TO CASE 38: Sickle Cell Crisis

Summary: This is a 30-year-old woman with a history of sickle cell disease who presents with chest pain, shortness of breath, and cough. She is febrile, tachypneic, and hypoxic.

◆　**Most likely diagnosis:** acute chest syndrome.

◆　**Best treatment:** supplemental oxygen, IV hydration, analgesia, and antibiotics.

Analysis

Objectives

1. Recognize the clinical signs and symptoms of sickle cell crisis.
2. Understand the diagnosis and treatment of acute chest syndrome.

Considerations

Sickle cell disease is very common, affecting approximately 1 of every 600 African Americans. It can affect almost any organ system and has a wide variety of clinical presentations. The clinician's priorities are to differentiate the mild from the life-threatening crises and to treat them.

The patient in this case, a 30-year-old woman with known sickle cell disease, **has acute onset of chest pain, cough, fever, and subtle findings on the pulmonary examination.** Her **oxygen saturation is 94 percent on room air**, which is concerning, and should be followed up with an arterial blood gas. Pulmonary embolism, pneumonia, and **acute chest syndrome (ACS)** should be entertained as possible diagnoses. The chest radiograph can be helpful. ACS can result from infectious and noninfectious (pulmonary infarct) causes. It usually presents with some combination of chest pain, fever, hypoxia, and a new pulmonary infiltrate on x-ray. Individualized diagnostic workup and therapy are critical. The arterial blood gas reading and judicious observation of the patient over 20 to 30 minutes should give the clinician sufficient time to consider the likelihood of pulmonary embolism. A V/Q scan or spiral computed tomography (CT) scan should be performed if appropriate. Many times, ACS and pneumonia cannot be sorted out initially, and the patient may require sputum Gram stain and culture, initiation of antibiotic therapy, and admission. The treatment for ACS is supportive: oxygenation, intravenous fluid hydration, and analgesia.

APPROACH TO SICKLE CELL CRISIS

Sickle cell disease is caused by abnormal hemoglobin production. In normal adults, hemoglobin is composed of two alpha and two beta chains. However, in hemoglobin S (HbS), valine is substituted for glutamine in the sixth position of the beta chain. Under hypoxic or acidotic conditions, this abnormal hemoglobin polymerizes and sickles, resulting in sludging in the microcirculation. In turn, this causes tissue hypoxia, ischemia, acidosis, and more sickling.

The gene for HbS is autosomal recessive. Patients who are **heterozygous** (sickle cell trait) are generally asymptomatic except under extreme stress (severe dehydration, temperature or pressure change), but do tend to be **susceptible to urinary tract infections**. On the other hand, those who have sickle cell disease (homozygous) are highly susceptible to vaso-occlusion and pain crises. Because these patients are functionally asplenic after early childhood, they are also at risk for many infections, especially by encapsulated organisms. In fact, **the highest rate of mortality occurs in children between the ages of 1 and 3 years as a consequence of sepsis**. Sickle crises may be hematological, septic, and vasoocclusive (Table 38-1).

During the assessment of patients with sickle cell disease, the history should focus on **identifying any precipitating causes and any complications**. Pain that is different from previous pain crises may be an indicator of a serious or life-threatening condition. A rapid assessment of the vital signs and a careful physical examination are important, because serious complications may have nonspecific manifestations. The clinician should be concerned if the patient has a fever, severe abdominal pain, respiratory or neurological symptoms, joint swelling, pain that is not relieved by usual measures, or priapism.

Vasoocclusive crises are the most common complications and may be precipitated by infection, stress, cold, dehydration, or high altitude, although the majority have no reported etiology. The **mechanism** is **sludging of red blood cells in the microcirculation leading to ischemia and infarction**. Musculoskeletal or abdominal pain are common. Intravenous hydration, oxygen, and pain control constitute the primary management. **Infants may present with sickle dactylitis (hand-and-foot syndrome) as a consequence of ischemia and infarction of the bone marrow of extremities**. A high index of suspicion must be maintained for sepsis, intraabdominal processes that can mimic vasoocclusive crisis (appendicitis, cholecystitis, mesenteric ischemia, pancreatitis), or osteomyelitis. **Fever or bandemia should raise the suspicion of infection.**

Acute chest syndrome usually presents with **chest pain, fever, hypoxia, and a new pulmonary infiltrate on x-ray**. The workup of ACS should include a complete blood count, reticulocyte count, urinalysis, blood and sputum cultures, arterial blood gas, and chest x-ray. Although finding an infiltrate on chest x-ray is important in diagnosing ACS, it is not uncommon for the initial x-ray to be normal. If pulmonary thromboembolism is suspected, a V/Q scan, conventional angiography, or CT angiography can be performed. However, each modality has its drawbacks. V/Q scan may be nondiagnostic because of baseline lung abnormalities, whereas the contrast load involved in angiography can induce sickling. Treatment of ACS involves supplemental oxygen, IV hydration, and analgesia with nonsteroidal antiinflammatory drugs or narcotics. Because it is often difficult to determine whether ACS has

Table 38-1

SICKLE CELL CRISES

TYPE OF CRISIS	COMMENTS	DIAGNOSIS	TREATMENT
Vasoocclusive crises	Precipitants: infection, dehydration, stress, fatigue, cold, high altitude		
Musculoskeletal pain	Commonly in low back, femur, tibia, humerus	Exam: normal or may have local tenderness	Hydration, analgesia
Abdominal pain	Pain usually acute onset, poorly localized, and recurrent; broad differential includes hepatobiliary, splenic, or renal disease	Exam: no peritoneal signs; complete blood count, liver function tests	Treat underlying etiology, supportive care*
Acute chest syndrome	Pleuritic chest pain, cough, dyspnea	Exam: fever, tachypnea, rales; pulse oximetry, chest x-ray, arterial blood gas, ventilation-perfusion (V/Q) scan, angiography	Treat underlying etiology, supportive care, supplemental oxygen, antibiotics, anticoagulation
Central nervous system crisis	Headache, neurological deficit, seizure, mental status changes; usually infarct in children and hemorrhage in adults	CT scan, lumbar puncture, MRI	Exchange transfusion

Priapism	Painful erection without sexual stimulation caused by sickling in corpus cavernosum	Exam: engorged, painful penis	Supportive care, exchange transfusion, aspiration of corpus cavernosum, intrapenile injection of vasodilator, urologic consultation
Dactylitis	Swelling of hands and/or feet; usually occurs before 2 years of age	Painful edema of hands and/or feet	Supportive care, warm compresses
Renal crisis	Usually asymptomatic; may have flank pain	Urinalysis shows hematuria or tissue	Supportive care
Hematological crises			
Splenic sequestration	Rapid onset of fatigue, listlessness, pallor, abdominal pain; most common in children <6 years of age	Exam: hypovolemia, splenomegaly; severe anemia or significant drop in hemoglobin	Correction of hypovolemia, packed red blood cell (PRBC) transfusion, exchange transfusion, splenectomy
Aplastic crisis	Precipitants: Parvovirus B19 infection, folic acid deficiency, phenylbutazone	Significant drop in hemoglobin with low reticulocyte count	IV fluids, PRBC transfusion; usually self-limited
Infectious crises	Common organisms: encapsulated (*Haemophilus influenzae*, *Streptococcus pneumoniae*), *Salmonella typhi*, *Mycoplasma pneumoniae*, *Escherichia coli*, *Staphylococcus aureus*	Exam: fever; complete blood count, urinalysis, blood and sputum and urine cultures (as indicated), chest x-ray	Broad-spectrum antibiotics

* Supportive care includes hydration and analgesia.

an infectious or noninfectious cause, **empiric antibiotics are recommended**. When thromboembolism is strongly suspected, the patient should receive anticoagulation. In severe cases, exchange transfusion may be indicated.

Stroke or central nervous system (CNS) crises can occur in all age groups, typically presenting as acute onset of hemiparesis, seizures, transient ischemic attacks, vertigo, cranial nerve palsies, or even unexplained coma. Cerebral infarction or subarachnoid hemorrhage may be present. These are usually painless events, abrupt in onset, and diagnosed by CT imaging or magnetic resonance imaging (MRI).

Hematological crises, characterized by abrupt drop in hemoglobin levels and generalized weakness and fatigue, are comprised of **two mechanisms: splenic sequestration and aplastic crisis.** Acute splenic sequestration usually presents in young children with splenomegaly and hypovolemia, sometimes preceded by a viral infection. The treatment is supportive, but occasionally necessitates splenectomy. **Aplastic crisis** confers a **high mortality rate**, associated with **erythropoietic failure in the bone marrow**. Often parvovirus B19 is implicated, and extremely low hemoglobin levels (with normal platelet and leukocyte counts) may be encountered. The treatment is supportive and sometimes necessitates blood transfusion.

Infectious crises can present as overwhelming sepsis, particularly with **encapsulated organisms.** *Streptococcus pneumoniae* sepsis is the most **common cause of death in children** with sickle cell disease. Thus, the **pneumococcal vaccine is administered to all children with sickle cell disease (SCD) at 24 months of age.** *Haemophilus influenzae* and *Salmonella* species are also common culprits. Unexplained fever in any patient with SCD, particularly children, should prompt immediate attention, and assessment for serious bacterial infection: complete blood count (CBC), chest radiograph, urinalysis, pulse oximetry, and cultures of the blood and urine. Broad-spectrum antibiotic therapy, such as intravenous ceftriaxone, is often used as the workup is in progress.

Comprehension Questions

[38.1]   A 3-year-old black female is brought into the ED by her mother for being pale and irritable. The girl is known to have sickle cell disease. Which of the following tests would help to differentiate an aplastic crisis from a vasoocclusive crisis?

    A. Reticulocyte count
    B. Platelet count
    C. Peripheral smear
    D. Hemoglobin level
    E. Lack of menses

[38.2] A 2-year-old male with sickle cell disease is being seen by his primary care doctor. Which of the following would make the most impact on mortality risk?

A. Screening urine culture
B. Bone radiograph to assess for osteomyelitis
C. Pneumococcal vaccination
D. Chest radiograph to assess for acute chest syndrome
E.   Usually diagnosed by elevated cardiac enzymes

[38.3] A 12-year-old black female is brought into the ED at the direction of her primary care physician. The patient's mother informs you that the patient has sickle cell disease. Which one of the following findings would be most concerning to you?

A. Fever
B. Pain that is typical of past crises
C. Mild abdominal pain
D. Hematuria

[38.4] Which of the following is most accurate concerning acute chest syndrome?

A. V/Q scans are always helpful in distinguishing between an infectious and noninfectious cause
B. It can be caused by pulmonary infection or infarction
C. It can be ruled out with a normal chest x-ray
D. Antibiotics should not be given until the patient is proven to have an infection

Answers

[38.1]   **A.** The reticulocyte count is low in aplastic crisis, but elevated or normal with a vasoocclusive crisis.

[38.2]   **C.** Pneumococcal sepsis is the leading cause of death in children ages 1 to 3 years. Thus, pneumococcal vaccine would be critical in its prevention.

[38.3]   **A.** The clinician should be worried if the patient has a fever, severe abdominal pain, respiratory or neurological symptoms, joint swelling, pain that is not relieved by usual measures, or priapism.

[38.4]   **B.** ACS can be caused by pulmonary infection or infarction.

CLINICAL PEARLS

❖ Sickle cell disease can manifest in any organ system and has a wide variety of clinical presentations ranging from mild to life-threatening.

❖ Because patients with sickle cell disease are functionally asplenic after early childhood, they are at risk for infection by encapsulated organisms (e.g., *Haemophilus influenzae, Streptococcus pneumoniae*).

❖ ACS is the leading cause of death in patients with sickle cell disease. Having a low threshold of suspicion in patients presenting with respiratory complaints is vitally important.

❖ Treatment of ACS involves supplemental oxygen, IV hydration, analgesia, empiric antibiotics, and possibly anticoagulation.

❖ Aplastic crisis has a very high mortality, associated with an abrupt fall in hemoglobin, relatively normal leukocyte and platelet count.

REFERENCES

Fixler J, Styles L. Sickle cell disease. Pediatr Clin North Am 2002;49(6):1193–210.

Freeman L. Sickle cell disease and other hemoglobinopathies: approaches to emergency diagnosis and treatment. Emerg Med Pract 2001;3(12):1–24.

Lee P. Sickle cell disease. In: Stobo JD, Hellmann DB, Ladenson PW, Petty BG, Thomas TA, eds. The principles and practice of medicine. New York: McGraw-Hill, 1996:327–47.

Paganussi PJ, Mayer T, Kou M. Sickle cell disease. In: Tintinalli JE, Kelen GD, Stapczynski JS, eds. Emergency medicine, 6th ed. New York: McGraw-Hill, 2004:1382–6.

Stobo JD, Hellmann DB, Ladenson PW, Petty BG, Thomas TA, eds. The principles and practice of medicine. New York: McGraw-Hill, 1996:718–22.

A 38-year-old homeless man is found sleeping under a bridge the night after a severe snow storm. He is easily aroused and complains of numbness in both hands and feet. He reports that the numbness was proceeded by a "pins and needles" sensation. He admits to being a smoker (20 pack-years), heavy drinker and a type II diabetic for at least 10 years. On examination, he is thin, malnourished with poor dentition. His blood pressure is 110/70 mmHg, heart rate is 70 beats per minute, and his temperature is 35°C (95°F). His hands and feet are hard, pale, and cold and have decreased sensation to light touch.

◆ **What is your next step?**

◆ **Most likely diagnosis?**

◆ **What is your next step in treatment?**

ANSWERS TO CASE 39: Frostbite and Hypothermia

Summary: A 38-year-old homeless man who has been exposed to freezing temperatures and has hard, cold, and pale hands and feet. Although his complaint of numbness could be related to many things, he has been exposed to freezing temperatures for an extended period of time.

 Next step: Transfer to emergency department and prevent further systemic heat loss. Remove any wet or constrictive clothing. Wrap patient in warm, dry blankets. The affected areas should be immobilized and insulated and kept away from dry heat sources.

Most likely diagnosis: Frostbite and hypothermia.

Next step in treatment: Rapid rewarming, by immersing the affected extremities in gently circulating water that is carefully maintained at a temperature of 40 to 42°C (104 to 108°F).

Analysis

Objectives

1. Be able to recognize frostbite and initiate prehospital treatment.
2. Discern between frostnip and superficial and deep frostbite.
3. Know the treatment for frostbite.

Considerations

This patient has numerous risk factors for peripheral neuropathy, including diabetes and alcoholism. Frostbite occurs when the skin and body tissues are exposed to cold temperature for a prolonged period of time. He does give this history. While in the ED he would also be evaluated for other causes for his numbness; however, in light of his situation, the rewarming process would not be delayed to minimize soft tissue injury. Anyone who is exposed to freezing temperatures for a prolonged period of time can develop frostbite. People who are at increased risk include diabetics, smokers, those exposed to windy weather, which increases the rate of heat loss from skin, people with peripheral vascular disease and peripheral neuropathy or Raynaud disease.

APPROACH TO FROSTBITE

Definitions

Deep frostbite: involves death of skin, subcutaneous tissue, and muscle or deep tendons and bones.

Frostnip: the mildest form of frostbite and is marked by tissue blanching and decreased sensitivity.

Hypothermia: core body temperature less than 35°C (95°F).

Superficial frostbite: involves the skin and subcutaneous tissues, which are white, waxy, and anesthetic, have poor capillary refill, and are painful on thawing.

Clinical Approach

Normal Physiology   The human cold response is aimed at maintaining the core body temperature and the viability of the extremities. The central thermostat, which orchestrates temperature regulation in the body resides in the preoptic region of the anterior hypothalamus. Peripheral cooling of the blood activates the preoptic anterior hypothalamus, which leads to a cascade of events including catecholamine release, thyroid stimulation, shivering thermogenesis and peripheral vasoconstriction. Heat loss is reduced by peripheral vasoconstriction mediated by sympathetic stimulation and catecholamine release. In addition, shivering maintains or augments body heat, but only for a few hours, because of the depletion of glycogen, which is the source of heat during shivering. The extremities are protected by the "hunting reaction," which consists of irregular, 5- to 10-minute cycles of alternating periods of vasodilation and vasoconstriction that protect the extremities against sustained periods of vasoconstriction. If the body is exposed to cold of prolonged duration or magnitude and the core body temperature is threatened, then this mechanism is abandoned, the so called life-versus-limb mechanism.

Pathophysiology   **Maintenance of core temperature takes precedence over rewarming of the extremities**. So when the body is exposed to cold of a magnitude or duration significant enough to disrupt the core body temperature, continuous and intense vasoconstriction occurs promoting frostbite to the exposed tissue. **Frostbite occurs when tissue temperatures are less than 0°C (32°F).** There are two mechanisms for tissue damage: architectural cellular damage from ice-crystal formation and microvascular thrombosis and stasis. The initial phase of frostbite, the "prefreeze phase," is characterized by tissue temperatures dropping below 10°C (50°F), and cutaneous sensation being lost. There is microvascular vasoconstriction and endothelial leakage of plasma into the interstitium. Crystal formation does not occur until tissue temperatures drop below 0°C (32°F). During the "freeze–thaw" phase, extracellular ice-crystals form. In an attempt to maintain osmotic equilibrium, water leaves the cells causing cellular dehydration and intracellular hyperosmolality. This leads to cellular collapse and demise. The third phase is the "progressive microvascular collapse" phase. Red cells sludge and form microthrombi during the first few hours after the tissues are thawed. The exact mechanism is unclear. Hypoxic vasospasm, hyperviscosity, and direct endothelial damage all adversely affect flow. Ultimately there is plasma leakage and arteriovenous shunting resulting in thrombosis, increased tissue pressure, ischemia and necrosis. Table 39-1 lists the classifications of frostbite.

Table 39-1

CLASSIFICATION OF FROSTBITE

	DIAGNOSIS	TREATMENT	SEQUELAE
Frostnip	Tissue blanching and decreased sensation	Rapid rewarming in a water bath at 40–42°C (102–104°F)	None
Superficial Frostbite	Skin and subcutaneous tissue are white, waxy, anesthetic, have poor capillary refill, and are painful on thawing; may also have erythema, edema, and superficial vesicles	Rapid rewarming in a water bath at 40–42°C (102–104°F)	No deep injury ensues; healing occurs in 3–4 weeks
Deep Frostbite	Death of skin, subcutaneous tissue, muscles, tendons, or bones; tissue appears frozen and hard; on rewarming there is no capillary filling	Rapid rewarming as above; IV analgesics; admit to surgical service; updated tetanus; elevate affected extremity, prevent weight bearing, sterile dressing, separate digits with cotton wool, and protect extremities from maceration; occasionally amputation	Pain; paresthesia; anesthesia; thermal sensitivity; hyperhidrosis; Raynaud syndrome; atrophy; edema/lymphedema; compartment syndrome; rhabdomyolysis; tenosynovitis; stricture; osteoarthritis; necrosis; amputation

Source: Tintinalli JE, Kelen GD, Stapczynski JS, eds. Emergency medicine, 6th ed. New York:1175–79.

Therapy The ultimate goal of prehospital treatment is preservation of life. Often the **frostbite and hypothermia coexist so prevention of further systemic heat loss is the priority**. Field rewarming of frozen tissue is rarely done unless the possibility of evacuation does not exist. There is a direct relationship between the length of time the tissue is frozen and the extent of cellular damage. Field rewarming should not be performed if there is any potential for interrupted or incomplete thawing. **Tissue refreezing is disastrous**.

In the ED, a thorough history should be obtained including ambient temperature, wind velocity, duration of exposure, type of clothing worn, medication history, and preexisting medical problems that could affect tissue loss. **After stabilizing the core temperature** and addressing associated conditions, **rapid thawing** should be initiated. Most patients will be **dehydrated** and so intravenous fluids (crystalloid) are administered. **Rapid rewarming of frozen or partially thawed tissue is accomplished by immersion in gently circulating water that is carefully maintained at a temperature of 40 to 42°C (102 to 104°F).** Rewarming is continued until the tissue is pliable and distal erythema is noted, usually about 10 to 30 minutes. Active, gentle motion is encouraged but direct tissue massage should be avoided. Because tissue rewarming is very painful, producing throbbing, burning pain, and tenderness, **parenteral analgesics** should be administered. Sensation is often diminished after thawing and then disappears with bleb formation. Sensation does not renormalize until after healing is complete.

After thawing, the injured extremities should be elevated to minimize swelling. Sterile dressings should be applied and involved areas handled gently. Digital exercises are encouraged to help avoid venous stasis. Treatment also includes NSAIDs, topical aloe vera, possible debridement of clear blisters while leaving the hemorrhagic ones alone, and tetanus vaccine if indicated. Antibiotics are also often given. Amputation is often delayed for up to 3 weeks, because the extent of tissue injury is difficult to initially assess.

Comprehension Questions

[39.1] A 22 year-old male was on a snow ski trip and was reported missing by his friends. He was found buried in snow after being missing for 8 hours. What should be your initial step?

A. Rapid rewarming until he can be life flighted to nearest hospital

B. Check for airway, breathing, circulation, and then maintain core body temperature by removing wet clothes and wrapping in warm, dry blankets

C. Immediately place on rescue bed and pull down mountain to first aid station

D. Leave him in the snow for insulation and call for immediate transport

[39.2] A 16-year-old backpacker was lost in the woods for 12 hours in the snow. He appears to have suffered frostbite to the cheeks, hands, and feet. What should your next step be?

A. Rapid thawing in room temperature water at the first aid station on the ski resort
B. Begin rapid rewarming with water 40 to 42°C (103 to 104°F), while waiting for EMS
C. Place patient next to radiant warmer and give warm fluids
D. Transport to nearest emergency department and begin rapid rewarming there

[39.3] A 14-year-old boy wandered into the woods chasing after his dog, and lost his bearings. When he was finally found, he was brought into the ED with severe frostbite of the fingers of both hands. Originally, they appeared very blue, and now, they are beginning to become black, and have still not regained sensation 24 hours later. Which of the following describes the most appropriate time to wait before deciding on amputation of the affected fingers?

A. 24 hours after the episode
B. 48 to 72 hours after the episode
C. 3 to 7 days after the episode
D. 10 to 14 days after the episode
E. 2 to 3 weeks after the episode

Answers

[39.1] **B.** Initial step in any emergency should be the ABCs—airway, breathing, and circulation. In this case, you also want to prevent any further systemic heat loss.

[39.2] **D.** Rapid rewarming in the field is rarely practical; instead, you should transport to the nearest ED where complete rapid rewarming can be performed.

[39.3] **E.** Generally, 3 weeks is required to assess viability of tissue after frostbite to see whether amputation is required. Tissue thought to be necrotic sometimes can become viable.

CLINICAL PEARLS

❖ Because hypothermia and frostbite often occur simultaneously, prevention of further systemic heat loss is the highest priority.

❖ Field rewarming is rarely warranted because of the potential for incomplete or interrupted rewarming. Injured parts should be protected, core temperature stabilized, and patient transferred to ED for rapid rewarming in gently circulating water of 40 to 42°C (102 to 104°F).

REFERENCES

Ahya SN, Flood K, Subramania P. The Washington manual of medical therapeutics, 30th ed. Philadelphia: Lippincott Williams & Wilkins 2001:541.

Danzl DF. Frostbite. In: Rosen P, Barkin R, eds. Emergency medicine, concepts and clinical practice, 4th ed. St. Louis: Mosby-Year Book, 1998:953–62.

Olin JW. Other peripheral arterial diseases. In: Goldman L, Bennett JC, eds. Cecil textbook of Medicine. 21st ed. Philadelphia: WB Saunders 2000.

A group of teenagers was swimming at the lake, when one of the boys failed to surface after diving off a platform. He was quickly found and rescued by another swimmer from the lake bottom. The patient was noted to be apneic, and cardiopulmonary resuscitation (CPR) was initiated by one of the bystanders. After the paramedics arrived, the patient was noted to have spontaneous shallow respirations, weak palpable pulse, and Glasgow Coma Scale (GCS) score of 7 (eyes 1, verbal 2, motor 4). The paramedics intubated the patient and transported him to your facility. In the emergency department, the patient has an initial pulse rate of 70 beats per minute, blood pressure of 110/70 mmHg, spontaneous respiratory rate of 12 breaths per minute, temperature of 35.6°C (96.1°F), GCS score of 6 (eyes 1, verbal 1, motor 4), and oxygen saturation of 92 percent on 100 percent FiO_2.

◆ **What are the complications associated with this condition?**

◆ **What are the best treatments for this patient?**

ANSWERS TO CASE 40: Drowning and Near-Drowning

Summary: A teenage boy presents with near-drowning following a diving accident at a lake.

◆ **Complications**: Submersion results in a global hypoxic-ischemic event primarily affecting the brain, lungs, and heart. This can result in noncardiogenic pulmonary edema, hypoxic encephalopathy, respiratory and metabolic acidosis, dysrhythmias, acute tubular necrosis (rare) and hemodilution or hemoconcentration (rare). Late potential complications include pneumonia, acute lung injury (ALI), acute respiratory distress syndrome (ARDS), and empyema.

◆ **Best treatments**: Most important treatment is delivered in the prehospital setting. The ABCs of emergency management must be followed. Rapid correction of hypoxia, acidosis, and hypotension are critical following the initial ABCs. The goal of resuscitation should be aimed at preventing further anoxic brain injury. Aggressive respiratory support, including **intubation**, and **ventilatory assistance** should be applied early on. IV access is mandatory, and fluids should not be withheld. Cardiac arrhythmias should respond to correction of hypoxemia. If not, then they should be treated using standard measures. Maintain cervical spine stabilization until spinal trauma is ruled out. Bronchoscopy may be necessary to remove large particulate matter or secretions in selective patients.

Analysis

Objectives

1. Learn the pathophysiology of freshwater and saltwater drowning.
2. Become familiar with the epidemiology and prevention of drowning.
3. Learn the special problems associated with cold water submersion injury and submersion complications in contaminated water.

Considerations

By report this teenage boy had been diving and swimming with his friends prior to being found unresponsive underwater. Precipitating causes of the submersion event, such as **drugs, alcohol, head injury, cardiac arrest, seizures, and attempted suicide or homicide, must be considered in any patient who is found unresponsive in water**. Given that the patient had been **diving**, it is conceivable that **cervical spine injury or head injury** could have preceded the submersion process; therefore cervical spine stability should be maintained until injuries can be ruled out radiographically. Similarly, any external signs of head trauma should prompt early computed tomography (CT) evaluation following cardiopulmonary stabilization.

The initial management is correction of the hypoxemia. However, after initial resuscitation, careful physical examination should be performed to identify other possible injuries. His initial radiographic evaluations should include, chest radiography, and cervical spine x-rays, followed by head CT after initial stabilization. Once the cardiopulmonary condition has been stabilized and radiographic survey completed, this patient should be admitted to the ICU where continued cardiopulmonary monitoring and mechanical ventilation support can be provided. In addition, bowel rest, nasogastric decompression, and gastric pH control should be provided. **One-third to one-half of near-drowning victims will develop a fever during the first 48 hours following submersion, and in approximately 80 percent of patients the fever resolves spontaneously without antibiotics.**

APPROACH TO DROWNING

Definitions

Drowning: death secondary to asphyxia by submersion in a liquid, usually water, or death within 24 hours of a submersion incident.

Immersion syndrome: a traditional term that refers to the sudden death that occurs after submersion in very cold water, probably resulting from dysrhythmias induced by vagal stimulation.

Near-drowning: a submersion incident that results in survival of the victim, or results in death greater than 24 hours after a submersion incident.

Submersion incident: a simple descriptive term that does not imply a prognosis.

Clinical Approach

Epidemiology and Prevention   Even though the number of drownings has decreased over the past 20 years, it continues to be a leading cause of injury deaths among children and adolescents. It is second only to motor vehicle accidents in causing accidental deaths in persons between the ages of 5 and 44 years. More than 4500 persons die from drowning in the United States each year. Although there is no agency that actively collects data on submersion incidents, it is estimated that its incidence is 2 to 20 times the reported number of drownings.

Risk factors for drowning include age, gender, and race. The incidence of drowning is bimodal in distribution, with toddlers and teenagers being the most vulnerable. Males are more likely to die of drowning than females in all age groups. **Teenage boys (15 to 19 years old) are likely to be victims because of an association with risk-taking behavior, alcohol intoxication, and drug use.** Common sites of drowning for teens and adults are in lakes, rivers, and saltwater bodies. The other group at high risk for drowning is the **toddler** (0 to 2 years old). These deaths predominantly occur in bathtubs and water-containing structures around the home, with the majority occurring in children ages 7 to 15 months. These deaths are often the result of the toddler having inadequate or brief lapses of supervision. The residential swimming pool is a common submersion site for toddlers, where it is the most common site of drowning for victims who are younger than 5 years of age. **Most pool submersions occur at the child's home**, often **within the first 6 months of pool exposure**. Other submersions occur in sinks, buckets, tubs, toilets, and washers. Children can fall headfirst into a bucket and cannot right themselves owing to their relatively cephalic center of gravity and their insufficient body mass to tip it over. **Hot tubs and spas also pose special hazards**, as many have **suction devices** that can entrap the child.

The drowning rate for black children who are older than the age of 4 years is lower than that of white children, whereas the rate for black and white children 0 to 4 years of age is nearly identical. This is possibly a result of the lack of recreational water exposure to inner-city and lower socioeconomic children.

Although certain medical illnesses can predispose individuals to submersion injury, the precise frequency is difficult to determine. Epilepsy has been well documented to increase the risk of drowning and near-drowning with up to a tenfold increased risk of submersion injury. Epileptic children with other associated handicaps are at even greater risk. Epilepsy-associated drowning occurs predominately in bathtubs and swimming pools. Patients with undiagnosed long QT syndrome have an increased risk of immersion injury, and it has been suggested that sudden exposure to cold water may trigger syncopal episodes in these individuals.

Child abuse and homicide by submersion do occur. In situations suspected of abuse, a judicious history and physical exam along with an understanding of normal childhood developmental capabilities is of the utmost importance. Approximately 1 in 30 child homicides is caused by intentional drowning. Up to 8 percent of drowning and near-drowning episodes in children younger than 5 years old are inflicted. Eighty-five percent of intentional bathtub drownings involve children 15 to 30 months of age.

With the rapidly increasing number of swimming pools, freshwater recreation vehicles, the potential for increasing numbers of drownings and near-drownings is growing. An increased awareness and the institution of preventative measures can help to decrease the incidence. These efforts must focus on education of parents, children, and physicians. Preventive measures include legislation requiring adequate fencing, decreasing the use of alcohol when boating and swimming, and increasing the number of citizens trained in CPR. It is well documented that alcohol plays a significant role in drowning accidents. In a recent United States survey, 70 percent of males and 66 percent of females reported the use of alcohol while participating in aquatic activities during the previous year. Water safety education for children, teenagers, and parents that encourages wearing flotation devices and never swimming alone should be reinforced in the school, community, and physician's office.

Teenagers should be encouraged to learn CPR and receive counseling regarding alcohol and drug use.

Pathophysiology of Freshwater and Saltwater Drowning   While there are some physiological differences in the effects of fresh- and saltwater immersion, the usual sequence of events in all instances begins with voluntary apnea, and with the rise in PaO_2 and $PaCO_2$; involuntary breathing occurs leading to water entry into the lungs and worsening hypoxemia.

"Dry drowning" is a phenomenon seen in approximately 15 percent of submersion victims, and is a consequence of **persistent laryngospasm** causing obstructive asphyxia. Injuries in these individuals are initially related to decreased oxygen tension resulting in global hypoxemia; however, with the persistence of laryngospasm, negative pressure pulmonary edema (forced inspiration against a closed glottis) develops where increased capillary endothelium permeability occurs with surfactant disruption, leading to ALI or ARDS. The initial treatment for near-drowning victims remains the same regardless of whether the submersion injury occurred in fresh- or saltwater. However, it is worthwhile to note the pathophysiological differences and their effects on subsequent hospital management.

Management   One of the most critical elements in the successful management of submersion victims is prompt and effective basic life support delivery in the prehospital setting. **The Heimlich maneuver**, which was once applied to facilitate the removal of water from the lungs and airway is **no longer recommended because of unproven effectiveness in water removal and the high rate of associated aspiration induced by this maneuver.**

Early intubation is recommended for all apneic patients. Intravenous fluids consisting of lactated Ringer solution or normal saline should be initiated in most victims. Except in the hypoglycemic patients, **glucose-containing solution administration is contraindicated**, because its administration in animals with incomplete cerebral ischemia produces worse neurological outcome.

It has been reported that approximately 93 percent of near-drowning victims arriving at the hospital with a spontaneous pulse survive without serious sequelae, therefore suggesting that some submersion victims may be discharged without hospitalization. "Secondary drowning" refers to infrequent occurrence of respiratory deterioration that has been reported in pediatric patients more than 12 hours after the submersion event, and the possible evolution of this process has traditionally prevented the discharge of near-drowning victims from the ED. Recent retrospective data have suggested that children who presented to the ED with a GCS score =13, normal physical examination, normal respiratory effort, and room air O_2 saturation >95 percent at 4 to 6 hours after ED presentation, may be safely discharged from the ED.

Cold Water Submersion Injury   Sustained immersion in cold water is thought to be advantageous by inducing the *diving reflex* and producing *hypothermia.* In the diving reflex, blood is shunted away from the victim's peripheral tissues to the heart and brain, leading to a decrease in metabolism and thus reducing possible anoxic injury. The protective effects of this reflex may partially account for reports of complete neurological recovery in children after prolonged submersion. Hypothermia has been theorized to be protective because of the induction of global hypometabolic state, along with the generalized vasoconstriction leading to the conservation of oxygen and glucose from peripheral tissues for brain metabolism.

There should be clear distinction between "cold" and "ice" water. The rare survivor of prolonged submersion has usually been in freezing temperature water (<5°C [41°F]), and has typically sustained core body temperatures that have fallen extremely rapidly to <28 to 30°C (82.4 to 86°F). However, in most drownings, surface cooling alone occurs and is unlikely to decrease body temperature fast enough to give neuroprotection. Another theory regarding the cerebral protection of ice-water drownings is that victims of ice-water submersions are more likely to have involuntary respiration and a greater likelihood of aspiration or fluid rebreathing. In such a case, it may be possible for the brain to cool to a protective level (<30°C [86°F]) provided that the water aspirated is icy and cardiac output lasts long enough for sufficient heat exchange to occur. However, once cell death has occurred (at 5 to 6 minutes), hypothermia gives no further benefit and is considered a poor prognostic sign.

Cold water also has potentially harmful effects, most significantly **cardiac irritability** leading to **ventricular fibrillation and death, sinus bradycardia, atrial fibrillation, exhaustion, and altered mental status.** There are also complications that occur with rewarming efforts. During initial rewarming, the core body temperature may actually drop before increasing. This afterdrop may occur because of the venous return of colder blood from the extremities, or by the conduction of heat from the warmer core to cooler surface layers. In patients who have severe hypothermia, afterdrop may further worsen respiratory, cardiac or neurologic function or induce arrhythmias. One way to avoid this complication is to focus on core rewarming. Active core rewarming measures include administration of warmed intravenous fluids (36 to 40°C [96.8 to 104°F]), heated humidified inspired oxygen (40 to 44°C [104 to 111.2°F]), and warmed gastric, bladder, or peritoneal lavage. More aggressive methods include hemodialysis, extracorporeal rewarming (venovenous or arteriovenous), and cardiopulmonary bypass. Another complication is rewarming shock, associated with vasodilation and increased metabolic needs and victims with borderline cardiovascular function are unable to respond adequately. Hypotension, metabolic acidosis, tissue ischemia, and other consequences of shock may therefore be exacerbated during rewarming.

Submersion in Contaminated Water　　Contaminated bodies of water such as lakes, streams, ponds, and rivers, and the presence of particulate contaminants such as mud, sand, sewage, and bacteria, may pose special problems. These particles can obstruct the smaller bronchi and bronchioles and greatly increase the risk of aspiration and infection. There are also unusual microorganisms to be considered, such as *Naegleria fowleri*, specific to the drowning medium and geographic region. *Aeromonas* pneumonia has also been identified as a common pathogen in near-drowning victims. If fever, leukocytosis, and radiographic evidence of pneumonia persist, *Aeromonas* should be considered as a possible source. Antibiotics are generally reserved for obvious sewage contamination or unusual bacteria. One-third to one-half of near-drowning victims will have a fever during the first 48 hours after their submersion, and it resolves spontaneously (without antibiotics). Pulmonary infections, either bacterial or fungal, may be related to aspiration during resuscitation, as this has been reported to occur in approximately 25 percent of the patients. Broad-spectrum antimicrobial therapy should be considered in victims with persistent fever, worsening pulmonary or general clinical status, or proven evidence of pulmonary infection.

Comprehension Questions

[40.1] Which of the following patients may be appropriately discharged from the ED after several hours of observation?

A. A 3-year-old boy found face-down in the swimming pool, requiring 4 minutes of CPR, has a return of normal vital signs, with GCS score of 15, and mild respiratory distress.

B. A 12-year-old boy found unconscious and submerged in a swimming pool after striking his head on the bottom. His chest x-ray (CXR) and head CT are normal. His GCS score is 14. He is complaining of headache and no respiratory symptoms.

C. A 6-year-old boy who was washed into the ocean by a large wave and was rescued by a bystander. No CPR was required, and the boy had an initial GCS score of 14 and normal vital signs. CXR and physical examination are normal. Room air O_2 saturation is 95 percent.

D. A 3-month-old boy who was brought to the ED after accidental submersion in the bathtub. The physical examination is unremarkable except for bruising over both arms and ankles. His CXR is normal and his room air O_2 saturation is 98 percent.

[40.2] Which of the following is *least likely* to be a factor contributing to submersion-induced pulmonary injury?

A. Surfactant washout leading to alveolar collapse
B. Laryngospasm leading to negative pressure pulmonary edema
C. Aspiration of gastric contents during resuscitation
D. Hypoventilation secondary to hypercapnia

[40.3] A 24-year-old surfer is found submerged in the water for 5 minutes, and after CPR is alert, oriented, and has normal vital signs. He is brought into the ED with normal vital signs. His lungs are clear on auscultation and the oxygen saturation is 97 percent on room air. The chest radiograph appears normal. What is the most likely explanation for the lack of pulmonary findings?

A. Saltwater will not exhibit the same water-immersion findings as freshwater
B. The clinical and radiographic findings usually lag behind by 12 to 24 hours
C. The patient likely experienced "dry drowning"
D. The patient likely was face-up for the majority of time unaccounted for

Answers

[40.1] **C.** Although the boy described in choice A is stable, his initial requirement for 4 minutes of CPR places him at a great risk for pulmonary and neurological sequelae. The patient described in B has minimal respiratory symptoms, but his injury mechanism and current findings are concerning for issues related to closed head injury that may require further observation and interventions. The patient described in D is stable from the submersion standpoint, but the physical findings described suggest possible intentional injury that may need further elucidation.

[40.2] **D.** Each of the other answers (A, B, and C) are all potential mechanisms contributing to submersion-related pulmonary injury.

[40.3] **C.** Dry-drowning caused by laryngospasm, which leads to hypoxemia and unconsciousness, occurs in approximately 10 percent of immersion victims. The laryngospasm is not associated with large amounts of water aspirated into the lungs.

CLINICAL PEARLS

❖ Drugs, alcohol, head and cervical spine injury, cardiac arrest, seizures, and attempted suicide or homicide must be considered in any patient who is found unresponsive in water.

❖ One-third to one-half of near-drowning victims will develop a fever during the first 48 hours following submersion; in approximately 80 percent of patients the fever resolves spontaneously without antibiotics.

❖ Except in the hypoglycemic patients, glucose-containing solution administration is contraindicated, because its administration in incomplete cerebral ischemia may worsen neurological outcome.

❖ Active core rewarming is probably the best technique to resuscitate the hypothermic drowning victim.

❖ *Aeromonas* pneumonia is a common pathogen in near-drowning victims.

❖ If fever, leukocytosis, and radiographic evidence of pneumonia persist, *Aeromonas* should be considered as a possible source. Antibiotics are generally reserved for obvious sewage contamination or unusual bacteria.

REFERENCES

Causey AL, Tilelli JA, Swanson ME. Predicting discharge in uncomplicated near-drowning. Am J Emerg Med 2000;18:9–11.

Kuo DC, Jerrard DA. Environmental insults: smoke inhalation, submersion, diving, and high altitude. Emerg Med Clin N Am 2003;21:475–97.

Weinstein MD, Kriegr BP. Near-drowning: epidemiology, pathophysiology, and initial treatment. J Emerg Med 1996;14:461–7.

A 47-year-old woman complains of a severe headache of abrupt onset of 8 hours duration. The pain is diffuse, throbbing and worsened when she went outside into the sunlight to drive to the hospital. She denies any recent fever, neck pain, numbness, weakness, vomiting, and any change in vision. She was concerned because she has never had a headache as strong as this before. Her past medical and family histories are unremarkable. She does not take any medications, does not smoke, and only drinks alcohol socially.

On examination, her temperature is 36.9°C (98.4°F), blood pressure 136/72 mmHg, heart rate 88 beats per minute, and respiratory rate of 16 breaths per minute. She is not in any acute distress but appears to be mildly uncomfortable, and does not want to move her head. Her pupils are equal and reactive bilaterally. There is no evidence of papilledema on fundoscopic examination. Movement of her neck causes her some increased discomfort. Her neurological exam is normal, including cranial nerves, strength, light touch sensation, deep-tendon reflexes, and finger-to-nose. The computed tomography (CT) scan of her head is normal.

◆ **What is the most likely diagnosis?**

◆ **What is the next diagnostic step?**

ANSWERS TO CASE 41: Headache

Summary: This is a 47-year-old woman with acute onset of "the worst headache of her life."

◆ **Most likely diagnosis:** subarachnoid hemorrhage.

◆ **Next diagnostic step:** CT scan of the head.

Analysis

Objectives

1. Learn to differentiate emergent, urgent, and less urgent causes of headache.
2. Understand the treatment of various types of headache.

Considerations

This 47-year-old woman has an acute onset of severe headache, described **as the "worse headache of her life."** The acute onset as well as severity are very suspicious for subarachnoid hemorrhage. Location of the headache is not very specific, and this patient has diffuse pain. Headache is a very common chief complaint in the emergency department (ED), accounting for 1 to 6 percent of visits. When evaluating patients with headaches, the clinician's goals are to identify those with serious or life-threatening conditions and to alleviate pain. This particular patient has a severe headache and some nuchal rigidity. She is not febrile, which makes meningitis less likely. Subarachnoid hemorrhage is likely given the sudden onset, and severity of the headache. The physical examination should be focused for nonneurological causes of headache including sinuses palpated for tenderness, temporal arteries palpated for tenderness or reduced pulsations (temporal arteritis), and a thorough eye examination assessing pupils, visual acuity, and fundoscopic examination, followed by a detailed neurological examination. This patient's CT scan of the head is unremarkable, which does not rule out subarachnoid hemorrhage. CT scan is often performed to rule out a cerebral mass lesion before performing lumbar puncture (LP). **Erythrocytes in the cerebral spinal fluid (CSF), or a xanthochromic CSF is diagnostic, but may take up to 12 hours to appear. In other words, a negative LP in the face of clinical suspicion may necessitate repeat LP.**

APPROACH TO HEADACHE

Up to 6 percent of ED visits are by patients with headache. Headaches can be caused by many intracranial and extracranial processes. One of the easiest ways to classify them is to separate them into primary and secondary causes. Primary headaches account for most cases and include migraine, tension-type, and cluster headaches. Secondary headaches are the result of some other disease process (e.g., infection, tumor). Headaches can also be subdivided into emergent, urgent, and nonurgent categories. Emergent headaches have a critical etiology that mandates immediate identification and treatment (e.g., meningitis, subarachnoid or other intracranial bleed, hypertensive encephalopathy). While urgent headaches can still be serious and require timely diagnosis and therapy, they are not immediately life-threatening. Examples are stroke, temporal arteritis, brain tumor, pseudotumor cerebri, migraine, and cluster headaches. In general, nonurgent causes are benign and easily reversible. This category includes tension-type and postlumbar puncture headaches.

As in most cases, the history is vitally important. The history should focus on the nature of the pain (location, severity, character, timing), any associated symptoms or precipitants, past medical history (including medications), and family history. **Ominous** historical findings include a sudden onset, the **"worst headache of life,"** headaches dramatically **different from past episodes**, **immunocompromise**, **new onset after age 50 years**, and **onset with exertion**.

A complete physical examination with a detailed neurological evaluation can also help to separate the emergent from other causes. Abnormal vital signs can be a harbinger of life-threatening conditions. Other warning signs include altered mental status, meningeal signs, focal neurological deficits, and a rash suspicious for meningococcemia. Some types of headache have classic historical or exam findings that will aid in narrowing the differential (Table 41-1).

Because there is no routine workup of headaches, testing must be based on clinical suspicion (Table 41-2). In general, CT imaging of the head is warranted for new-onset or worst headaches (especially if the patient is older than age 50 years, immunocompromised, or has a history of cancer). Other indications include headache with altered mental status, fever or meningeal signs, focal neurological deficits, evidence of increased intracranial pressure, history of trauma, and anticoagulant use. In general, management includes stabilizing any life-threatening conditions, controlling pain, and addressing any underlying disease or specific etiologies.

Subarachnoid Hemorrhage

Subarachnoid hemorrhage **(SAH)** has an annual incidence of 1 in 10,000 Americans, **usually affecting younger patients**. The median age is 50 years. The presentation can be very subtle, often with a normal neurological examination, with little or no nuchal rigidity, normal level of consciousness, and normal vital signs. Nevertheless, **the mortality associated with SAH approaches 50 percent.** Thus, it is vital for the ED physician to maintain a high index of suspicion in a patient with acute onset of severe headache. CT scan is usually the initial imaging test, and although the newer high-resolution CT imaging modalities have higher sensitivity, **no imaging procedure can definitively rule out SAH.** The **lumbar puncture revealing xanthochromic CSF is considered the gold standard of diagnosis.** Thus, many

Table 41-1
CLASSIC HISTORICAL AND EXAM FINDINGS

ETIOLOGY	HISTORY	EXAM
Subarachnoid hemorrhage (SAH)	"Thunderclap" onset, "worst headache of life"	Retinal hemorrhages; meningismus
Meningitis		Fever, meningismus, altered mental status.
Hypertensive encephalopathy	Diffuse, throbbing headache; worse in morning	Diastolic blood pressure >120–130 mmHg, altered mental status, papilledema
Migraine	Unilateral, throbbing headache with nausea, photophobia, or phonophobia; may be accompanied by visual, motor, or sensory disturbances; more common in women	
Cluster	Severe, unilateral periorbital pain with lacrimation, rhinorrhea; worse at night; attacks "clustered" in short time period; more common in men	Ipsilateral conjunctival injection, ptosis, miosis
Temporal arteritis	Pain over temporal artery; visual problems, jaw claudication; fever malaise, weight loss; worse at night; more common in women >50 years old	Tenderness or induration of temporal artery; optic nerve edema
Brain tumor	Headache with nausea and vomiting; worse in morning	Papilledema
Pseudotumor cerebri	Headache with diplopia; classically young obese female with irregular menses	Papilledema
Tension-type	"Band-like" headache	Pericranial muscle tenderness
Postlumbar puncture	Worse upon standing, better when lying down	

Table 41-2
DIAGNOSTIC TESTS AND TREATMENT

ETIOLOGY	DIAGNOSTIC TESTS	TREATMENT
Subarachnoid hemorrhage	CT scan, lumbar puncture (LP) if CT negative (look for xanthochromia)	Neurosurgical consult, control hypertension, analgesia, nimodipine
Meningitis	LP	IV antibiotics
Hypertensive encephalopathy	CT scan, rule out other end-organ damage	Control hypertension (nitroprusside, labetalol)
Migraine		Nonsteroidal antiinflammatory drugs (NSAIDs), antiemetics (metoclopramide, prochlorperazine), serotonin agonists (sumatriptan), ergot alkaloids (DHE); narcotics if refractory.
Cluster		Oxygen (nonrebreather), 4% intranasal lidocaine, oral triptans, DHE
Temporal arteritis	Erythrocyte sedimentation rate; consider temporal artery biopsy	Steroids to prevent blindness; NSAIDs
Brain tumor	CT scan; consider CT with contrast or MRI	If elevated intracranial pressure, neurosurgical consultation, hyperventilation, osmotic agents, steroids
Pseudotumor cerebri	LP with opening pressure	Repeated LPs, steroids, acetazolamide
Tension-type		Stress reduction, NSAIDs, muscle relaxants; narcotics if refractory
Postlumbar puncture		Hydration, lying flat, NSAIDs, narcotics, caffeine, epidural blood patch

authorities advocate performing a lumbar puncture on all patients suspected of having SAH, even in the face of a normal CT scan. Neurosurgical evaluation is important once the diagnosis of SAH is established. Treatment usually involves an antiseizure medication, and a calcium channel blocker such as nimodipine (Nimotop) 60 mg every 6 hours which may decrease the cerebral arterial spasm. Angiographic evaluation is usually undertaken to assess for possible surgical intervention of lesions such as berry aneurysms. Prognosis generally correlates with neurological status and intracranial pressure.

Cerebral Causes

Viral or bacterial meningitis can cause severe headache. Again lumbar puncture is the best method of assessing for these infections. Immunocompromised states such as human immunodeficiency virus (HIV) may cause the symptoms to be subtle. Pre-LP CT imaging does not necessarily need to be performed in the face of a normal neurological examination, normal level of consciousness, and absence of papilledema. Stroke or transient ischemic attack (TIA) may present as headache, but usually there is a history of or continued neurological deficit. The headache that accompanies brain tumors is classically described as being worse in the morning, associated with nausea or vomiting, but is only seen in a very small fraction of the time. Persistent atypical headache (such as new onset after age 50 years), severe, or associated with even subtle cognitive or neurological function should be investigated, usually with CT imaging.

Temporal Arteritis

Temporal arteritis **(TA)** almost always occurs in patients **older than age 50 years**, and **more commonly in women**. It is systemic arteritis, which presents as severe and throbbing, located over the frontotemporal region. Often, the temporal artery has a diminished pulse, or is tender, or is throbbing. **The diagnosis is established by fulfilling three of the following: age older than 50 years, new-onset localized headache, decreased pulse or tenderness over the temporal artery, an erythrocyte sedimentation rate (ESR) exceeding 50 mm/h, and abnormal artery biopsy. Vision loss is at stake** and immediate treatment should include **prednisone 40 to 60 mg/d** and urgent referral.

Primary Headache Syndromes

Migraine headaches are common, usually with onset in the teenage years or twenties, with women being more often affected than men. The mechanism is likely a primary response of the brain tissue to a trigger leading to brainstem pathway dysfunction (rather than the previous theory of vasospasm). Often auras can precede the headache, which are thought to be primary neuronal dysfunction. Migraine without aura is the most common variety, usually slow in onset, unilateral, and throbbing. Family history is often positive. Migraine with aura is similar, but with an aura usually within 60 minutes of the headache; the aura usually consists of visual symptoms (lights flashing or scotomata), hemiparesthesias, or aphasia that are completely reversible. Treatment principles include placing the patient in a dark, quiet room, and intravenous hydration if the patient is dehydrated. Pharmacological treatment includes dihydroergotamine (DHE), a serotonin (5-HT) nonspecific agonist, sumatriptan, a selective 5-HT agonist; or dopamine antagonists such as metoclopramide chlorpromazine, or prochlorperazine. Intravenous dexamethasone 20 mg after standard migraine therapy may reduce recurrences. In general, opiates are used less often.

Tension headaches are extremely common, usually bilateral, nonpulsating, "band-like" around the forehead to the occiput, usually not associated with nausea or vomiting. Treatment include nonsteroidal antiinflammatory drugs (NSAIDs) or, if severe, similar therapy as with migraine headaches. **Cluster headaches** are rare, more common in **men, and usually have their onset after 20 years of age.** They typically present as **unilateral, severe, orbital or temporal pain, often associated with ipsilateral lacrimation, nasal congestion, rhinorrhea, miosis, or ptosis.** They tend to occur in clusters, on the same side for several weeks and then remit for months or years. High-flow oxygen is usually effective, and DHE and sumatriptan have some efficacy.

Comprehension Questions

[41.1] Several patients have been brought into the ED with a chief complaint of headache. The triage nurse asks you which you think should be seen first. Which of the following patients is likely to be the most urgent situation?

    A. A 52-year-old man with headache of 8 hours duration, and blood pressure of 210/120 mmHg

    B. A 32-year-old woman with severe throbbing headache involving the right side of her head

    C. A 32-year-old woman who underwent an outpatient bilateral tubal ligation under spinal anesthesia and now complains of severe bilateral headache, especially with sitting up

    D. A 35-year-old woman with severe headache and a diagnosis given to her of pseudotumor cerebri

[41.2] A 22-year-old woman complains of headache of 2 hours duration that is described as unilateral and throbbing with nausea, photophobia, and phonophobia. Which of the following is the most likely diagnosis?

    A. Cluster headache

    B. Brain tumor

    C. Migraine headache

    D. Tension-type headache

[41.3] A 34-year-old woman is brought into the ED for "the worst headache of her life." She has some lethargy, photophobia, and nuchal rigidity. A lumbar puncture is performed after examining her eye grounds. What finding in cerebrospinal fluid is most concerning for subarachnoid hemorrhage?

A. Red blood cells
B. White blood cells
C. Elevated opening pressure
D. Xanthochromia

Answers

[41.1] **A.** Hypertensive encephalopathy is a type of emergent headache, and likely to be the most urgent of the cases presented.

[41.2] **C.** Migraine headaches are described as unilateral and throbbing with nausea, photophobia, or phonophobia.

[41.3] **D.** Xanthochromia in cerebrospinal fluid is most concerning for subarachnoid hemorrhage.

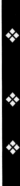

CLINICAL PEARLS

❖ Ominous historical findings include a sudden onset, the "worst headache of life," headaches dramatically different from past episodes, immunocompromise, new onset after age 50 years, and onset with exertion.

❖ Diagnostic testing must be based on clinical suspicion. For example, if there is a concern for a subarachnoid hemorrhage, a CT scan of the head and lumbar puncture are warranted.

❖ In general, management includes stabilizing any life-threatening conditions, controlling pain, and addressing any underlying disease or specific etiologies.

REFERENCES

Davis V. Headache. In: Hamilton GC, Sanders AB, Strange GR, Trott AT, eds. Emergency medicine: an approach to clinical problem-solving. Philadelphia: WB Saunders, 2003:535–51.

Godwin SA, Villa J. Acute headache in the ED: evidence-based evaluation and treatment options. Emerg Med Pract 2001;3(6):1–32.

Mick NW, Peters JR, Silvers SM. Blueprints in emergency medicine. Malden, MA: Blackwell Publishing, 2002:139–142.

Schull M. Headache and facial pain. In: Tintinalli JE, Kelen GD, Stapczynski JS, eds. Emergency medicine, 5th ed. New York: McGraw-Hill, 2000:1422–9.

A 16-year-old boy is found having a seizure on a hot summer day. The paramedics state they found him in an apartment without any air-conditioning. They established an IV of normal saline prior to arrival and obtained a fingerstick glucose of 146 mg/dL. Because he was postictal during transport, they were unable to obtain any other history about past medical problems, medications, or allergies.

On arrival in the emergency department (ED), his temperature is 41.1°C (106°F), blood pressure is 157/92 mmHg, heart rate is 156 beats per minute, and respiratory rate is 28 breaths per minute. He is extremely warm to touch. He is combative, moaning and flailing his arms and legs at staff. His pupils are mid-range and reactive to light. His mucous membranes are dry. His neck is supple. The rest of his exam is unremarkable except for his tachycardia.

◆ **What is the most likely diagnosis?**

◆ **What is the best initial treatment?**

ANSWERS TO CASE 42: Heat Stroke

Summary: This is a 16-year-old boy with a seizure who is hyperthermic, tachycardic, tachypneic, and has altered mental status.

◆ **Most likely diagnosis:** seizure secondary to heat stroke.

◆ **Best initial treatment:** management of the ABCs and rapid cooling.

Analysis

Objectives

1. Recognize the clinical signs and symptoms associated with heat-related illness.
2. Understand the management and treatment of heat-related illness.

Considerations

When evaluating hyperthermic patients, the clinician must first determine whether the patient suffers from a primary heat illness. The next step is to decide whether the patient has a mild, self-limiting form of heat-related illness or life-threatening heat stroke. Because **heat stroke has a mortality of 10 to 20 percent even with treatment,** it is essential to diagnose and begin therapy immediately. This patient has severe heatstroke, as evidenced by his altered mental status and seizure.

APPROACH TO HEAT-RELATED ILLNESSES

The body's ability to maintain thermal homeostasis depends on a variety of internal (physiological) and external (behavioral and environmental) factors. As a general rule, when the body gains heat faster than it can be eliminated, heat-related illness follows. Risk factors for developing heat illness include ambient heat and humidity, extremes of age, strenuous exercise, cardiovascular disease, dehydration, obesity, impaired mentation, and various drugs (e.g., diuretics, anticholinergics, antihistamines, phenothiazines, cyclic antidepressants, sympathomimetics, alcohol).

The spectrum of heat-related illness varies in severity from benign to severe. Table 42-1 describes the minor syndromes. In contrast to these benign entities, **heat stroke is characterized by a loss of thermoregulation, tissue damage, and multiorgan failure.** Classically, patients present with **hyperpyrexia (temperature >41°C [106°F]),** central nervous system (CNS) dysfunction (e.g., altered mental status, seizure, focal neurological deficits), and anhidrosis.

Diagnosis

Diagnosing heat stroke is largely a matter of ruling out other causes of hyperthermia with concomitant CNS dysfunction. The differential includes alcohol

Table 42-1
MINOR HEAT ILLNESSES

DIAGNOSIS	CAUSE	SYMPTOMS	TREATMENT
Heat edema	Vasodilation and pooling of fluids in dependent areas	Mild swelling of hands and feet	Self-limited; elevate legs, use of support hose; no diuretics
Heat rash	Blockage of sweat gland pores, may have secondary staphylococcal infection	Pruritic, erythematous, maculopapular rash on clothed areas	Antihistamines for itching, loose-fitting clothing; chlorhexidine cream, dicloxacillin, or erythromycin if infected
Heat cramps	Salt depletion (often from drinking only water)	Severe muscle cramps in fatigued skeletal muscles (usually calves, thighs, shoulders) during or after strenuous exercise	Fluid and salt replacement, rest
Heat syncope	Vasodilation, decreased vasomotor tone, volume depletion	Postural hypotension and syncope	Removal from heat source, rehydration, rest
Heat exhaustion	Water and salt depletion	Sweating, weakness, fatigue, headache, nausea, dizziness, malaise, lightheadedness, temperature usually <40°C (104°F)	Rest, volume, and salt replacement

withdrawal; salicylate toxicity; phencyclidine, cocaine, and amphetamine toxicity; tetanus; sepsis; neuroleptic malignant syndrome; encephalitis, meningitis, and brain abscess; malaria; typhoid fever; malignant hyperthermia; anticholinergic toxicity; status epilepticus; cerebral hemorrhage; diabetic ketoacidosis; and thyroid storm.

Laboratory studies should include complete blood count, electrolytes, blood urea nitrogen (BUN)/creatinine, glucose, liver enzymes, coagulation studies, urinalysis, urine myoglobin, and arterial blood gas. An electrocardiogram (EKG) should be considered if the patient has syncope or a history of cardiovascular disease. Chest radiographs are useful to rule out aspiration or any pulmonary infection. CT scan of the head and/or lumbar puncture may also be needed.

Treatment

In treating heat stroke, the clinician should strive to stabilize the **ABCs, commence rapid cooling, replace fluid and electrolyte losses, and treat any complications.** The goal is to cool the patient to 40°C (104°F) to avoid overshoot hypothermia. Initial measures consist of moving the patient from the hot environment and removing clothing. The most effective means of cooling is **evaporative, using cool mist and fans. Alternatives are ice packs to the groin and axillae, cooling blankets, ice water immersion, peritoneal lavage, and cardiopulmonary bypass.** Antipyretics are not effective in this scenario.

In addition, **shivering can be controlled with benzodiazepines or phenothiazines.** Benzodiazepines can also be used to treat any seizures. If the laboratory studies reveal evidence of rhabdomyolysis, mannitol and alkalinization of the urine are other considerations. The most common complications of heat stroke are rhabdomyolysis, renal failure, liver failure, disseminated intravascular coagulation, heart failure, pulmonary edema, and cardiovascular collapse.

Comprehension Questions

[42.1] Which of the following is *not* a symptom or sign of heat exhaustion?

    A. Nausea

    B. Headache

    C. Sweating

    D. Altered mental status

[42.2] A 33-year-old man is found comatose in the noon-hour on a hot summer day. His core temperature is 41.7°C (107°F). The ED physician orders evaporative cooling measures and ice packs. The patient begins to shiver intensely. Which of the following is the best next step?

A. Continued observation
B. Short-acting benzodiazepine
C. Begin intravenous cooling solution
D. Increase the number of ice bags

[42.3] A 70-year-old man is brought into the ED complaining of headache and fatigue. His blood pressure is 100/70 mmHg, heart rate is 100 beats per minute, and core temperature is 40.3°C (104.5°F). After applying ice bags, his core temperature is down to 38°C (100.4°F). Which of the following is the best next step?

A. Observation for 4 to 6 hours and then, if stable, discharge home
B. Continue ice bags until the core temperature is 36.7°C (98°F).
C. Admission to the hospital to observe for complications
D. Administer cold gastric lavage

Answers

[42.1]   **D.** Altered mental status is not a symptom or sign of heat exhaustion. Heat exhaustion can present with sweating, weakness, fatigue, headache, nausea, dizziness, malaise, or lightheadedness.

[42.2]   **B.** Benzodiazepines are first-line therapy for shivering or seizures in heat stroke.

[42.3]   **C.** All patients with severe heat exhaustion or heat stroke, particularly those who are older, should be admitted.

CLINICAL PEARLS

❖ Heat stroke is distinguished from other heat illnesses by a loss of thermoregulation, tissue damage, and multi-organ failure. Classically, these patients present with hyperpyrexia and CNS dysfunction.

❖ Because heat stroke has a mortality of 10 to 20 percent even with treatment, it is essential to diagnose and begin therapy immediately.

❖ The treatment of heat stroke consists of stabilizing the ABCs, rapid cooling, replacing fluid and electrolyte losses, and treating any complications (e.g., shivering, seizures, rhabdomyolysis).

REFERENCES

Guisto JA. Heat illness. In: Hamilton GC, Sanders AB, Strange GR, Trott AT, eds. Emergency medicine: an approach to clinical problem-solving. Philadelphia: WB Saunders, 2003:301–12.

Mick NW, Peters JR, Silvers SM. Blueprints in emergency medicine. Malden, MA: Blackwell Publishing, 2002:299–300.

Stobo JD, Hellmann DB, Ladenson PW, Petty BG, Thomas TA. The principles and practice of medicine. New York: McGraw-Hill, 1996:965–6.

Walker JS, Hogan JE. Heat Emergencies. In: Tintinalli JE, Kelen GD, Stapczynski JS, eds. Emergency medicine, 5th ed. New York: McGraw-Hill, 2000:1235–42.

Wexler RK. Evaluation and treatment of heat-related illness. Am Fam Phys 2002;65:2307–14.

You are in the emergency department when two patients arrive by paramedics. By report, the two men in their twenties were victims of lightning injury while playing golf. Eyewitnesses at the scene report that the victims were standing several feet apart, when one of the men was struck directly by lightning that resulted in both men immediately falling to the ground and becoming unconscious. One of the victims was found pulseless at the scene and cardiopulmonary resuscitation (CPR) was initiated by a bystander. The second man was noted to be unconscious for several minutes after the incident and has remained confused. On examination, one victim has extensive soft-tissue burns over his back, and he is intubated and ventilated without spontaneous respirations. No palpable pulse is identified and fine ventricular fibrillation appears on the electrocardiogram (EKG) monitor. The second victim is awake with a pulse rate of 80 beats per minute, blood pressure of 130/80 mmHg, respirations of 18 breaths per minute, Glasgow Coma Scale (GCS) score of 13, with no identifiable external sign of injury.

◆ **What are the complications of lightning injury?**

◆ **How are the complications identified?**

ANSWERS TO CASE 43: Lightning and Electrical Injury

Summary: Two victims present to the emergency department following lightning injuries. One patient with cardiac arrest appears to have been a victim of a direct lightning strike, while the second victim appears to have minimal external signs of injury.

 Lightning-related complications: cardiac injury, usually in the form of arrhythmia, neurological damage, burns, spinal cord injury, and respiratory arrest.

 Identification of complications: thorough and careful physical examination and electrocardiography will identify arrhythmia and cutaneous burns. Computed tomography (CT) scan of the head is indicated in all patients with severe lighting injury and those with abnormal neurological examination. Spinal protection and immobilization are necessary until injury is ruled out, and aggressive, persistent resuscitation according to advanced life support protocol is indicated, including airway control and ventilation support until spontaneous respiration is restored.

Analysis

Objectives

1. Learn to recognize and treat the immediate and late complications associated with electrical injury and lightning injury.
2. Learn to recognize the spectrum of injury associated with lightning and electrocution.
3. Understand the relationship between Ohm's law and injuries produced by electric current.

Considerations

One patient suffered a direct lightning strike and is in cardiac arrest. Because of its massive direct current countershock, lightning is capable of inducing depolarization of the entire myocardium leading to cardiac standstill. **Immediate cardiac arrest is the most common cause of death after a lightning strike.** However, respiratory arrest may also occur, either as a consequence of paralysis of the respiratory center in the medulla, or as a consequence of tetany of the respiratory muscles from electric current passing through the thorax. Many patients will regain cardiopulmonary function if timely, aggressive, resuscitation efforts are able to sustain circulation while organ systems recover.

Given the first patient's young age and lack of comorbidities, there is a greater likelihood for response to resuscitation efforts than in victims with cardiac arrest from other traumatic causes. The heart's inherent automaticity renders it possible for spontaneous recovery if immediate defibrillation and tissue oxygenation is maintained. The second patient, although hemodynamically stable, has suffered a high-risk electrical injury with loss of consciousness. Head and/or spinal injury could be present as a consequence of being "thrown" by the lightning strike. He requires evaluation with CT scan of the head, EKG, spinal immobilization and evaluation, and initial observation in the ICU for close monitoring of the cardiopulmonary status.

APPROACH TO LIGHTNING AND ELECTRICAL INJURY

Although lightning strike is a rare phenomenon, **this injury is associated with a 25 percent fatality rate, and more than 70 percent of those who survive have permanent injuries**. Lightning strike is responsible for approximately 100 deaths annually in the United States. Electrical injury, excluding lightning, is responsible for more than 500 deaths annually, with approximately 20 percent of its victims being younger than age 18 years. The effects of electrical injury are related to the intensity and magnitude of the electric current. According to **Ohm's Law**, the current flow (amperage) is directly related to the voltage and inversely related to the resistance in the current's pathway, represented by the following formula: **current (amperage) = voltage/resistance.** Because of their low resistance, **nerves, blood vessels, mucous membranes and muscle are the preferred pathways for electric current passage and are most susceptible to electrical and lightning injury.** Bones, fat, tendon, and skin have relatively high resistance, and therefore sustain less damage during electric and lightning injuries. The probable path of the electrical current should be assessed; for example, **burns on both hands indicates a path likely through the heart, which has a poor prognosis.**

Electrical current exists in two forms: **alternating current (AC)** and **direct current (DC).** AC involves electrons flowing back and forth in cycles, whereas in DC, the electron flow occurs in only one direction. Alternating current (AC) is more dangerous because it may cause tetanic muscle contractions and the "locking on" phenomenon, preventing the victim from releasing the electrical source and prolonging the exposure to the current. Lightning strike is a form of DC electrical injury with extremely high voltage and amperage, but short duration of exposure. During lightning injury, the electrons flow in only one direction, thereby typically inducing a single intense muscle contraction that "throws" its victim and causes simultaneous fractures and spinal injury. There are four types of lightning injury (Table 43-1).

Pathophysiology

Electrical injury can cause direct necrosis of the myocardium, ischemic injury as a result of vasoconstriction caused by excess catecholamine release, or disturbances in the cardiac rhythm. Even low currents can produce arrhythmias, including asystole and ventricular tachycardia. Late dysrhythmias are uncommon in previously healthy patients, but can be produced by patchy myocardial necrosis and injury to the sinoatrial (SA) node. Lightning is able to induce cardiac standstill by depolarizing the entire myocardium. Because of the inherent automaticity of the heart, normal sinus rhythm often spontaneously returns.

Table 43-1
TYPES OF LIGHTNING INJURY

Direct strike: the most serious type; when the major path of lightning current travels through the victim

Side flash: when the current is discharged from a victim or object of direct strike onto a nearby person

Ground current or stride potential: when the lightning strikes the ground and then enters the victim's body from one foot and exits via the opposite foot

Flashover phenomenon: when the force of nearby lightning causes expansion and implosion of surrounding air, causing a blast effect

Clinical Considerations

Cardiac Effects   All victims of lightning strike and high-voltage electric injury should have immediate **EKG** monitoring and cardiopulmonary support to maintain tissue perfusion as needed. A cool, extremity with diminished sensation and pulse is usually caused by vasoconstriction and nerve ischemia, which may or may not resolve spontaneously. Because extremity compartment syndrome may develop, reexamination with **compartment pressure** measurements are indicated in selective patients. Aggressive treatment by **fasciotomy** is indicated when elevated compartment pressures are identified. Victims of electrical injury with no loss of consciousness or physical findings who are asymptomatic and have normal EKGs can be safely discharged home.

Neurological Effects: Pathophysiology   Nerve damage is common after electrical injury, but no one condition is pathognomonic. Approximately 75 percent of patients struck by lightning will have transient loss of consciousness and brief extremity weakness or paresthesia. Lightning victims often have **keraunoparalysis**, a temporary paralysis with loss of sensation that typically involves lower limbs. Strength and sensation return to normal within a few hours. Other physical findings common in electrical injury are confusion, amnesia, headache, visual disturbance, and seizure. Direct spinal cord injury has been reported after hand-to-hand flow with damage to C_4-C_8.

The most serious effect, especially common after lightning strike, is injury to the respiratory control center in the medulla, resulting in respiratory arrest. In addition, lightning and electrical injury victims often have fixed and dilated pupils as a result of autonomic responses, and this should not interpreted as a sign of nonsurvivability until cerebral function is fully assessed.

Neurological Effects: Clinical Considerations   As in any apneic trauma victim, the **airway, oxygenation, and ventilation** should be restored immediately. **CT scan of the head** is indicated in patients with neurological findings or loss of consciousness to evaluate for possible intracranial pathology. **Spinal immobilization** should be continued until neurological exam is normal or injury is ruled out radiographically. Most victims of electrical and lightning injury without cardiac arrest will survive, but should be counseled that persistent sequelae, including memory deficits, sleep disturbances, dizziness, fatigue, headaches, and attention deficits may occur.

Skin: Pathophysiology   Burns are common after high-voltage electrical injury, but are less often seen after lightning strike because of instantaneous exposure time. Victims of electrical injury have "flash burns" caused by heat generated by the electrical current, or "flame burns," usually as a consequence of ignition of clothing. Because of its instantaneous exposure time, burns are less common after lightning injury. Lightning strike can cause partial-thickness linear burns in areas of high sweat concentration and low resistance, which result in a transient fern-like skin pattern called the **Lichtenberg Figure** that is pathognomonic of lightning. In children, the most common mode of electrical injury is from chewing or biting electrical cords, which manifests as perioral edema and eschar formation.

Skin: Clinical Considerations   Thorough **physical exam** will reveal any cutaneous manifestations of electrical injury. Early **intravenous access** should be established for fluid management as soon as possible in any burned patient. Fluids should be titrated to adequate urine output. Severe injuries will require admission to a specialized burn unit. Children may have excessive bleeding from the labial artery as a consequence of **perioral** burn.

Special Considerations   Other injuries associated with electrical and lightning injuries include **fractures** from severe muscle contraction or blunt trauma after exposure. Upper limb and spinal fractures are common. The kidneys are particularly vulnerable to anoxic damage that accompanies electrical injury, where **rhabdomyolysis** is common. However, rhabdomyolysis is rare after lightning injury. **Rupture of the tympanic membrane** occurs in up to 50 percent of lightning victims. **Cataracts** often present as a late sequelae of lightning strike. **Curling ulcers** are common in burn victims, and preventative treatment for these stress ulcers should be initiated at admission.

Comprehension Questions

[43.1] A 12-year-old boy sustained an electrical injury to the left arm. There is an obvious entry point in the left index finger, and circumferential second- and third-degree burns to the forearm. An escharotomy has been performed, but the hand remains cool with decreased sensation and no Doppler signal in the palmar arch. Which of the following is the most appropriate next step in management?

    A. Arteriogram of the left brachial artery
    B. Fasciotomy of the left forearm
    C. Left brachial artery exploration
    D. Splint, elevate, and observe

[43.2] A 49-year-old man was fixing the electrical wiring in his house as a remodeling project and neglected to shut off the electricity at the electrical box. He suffered a substantial electrical injury primarily on the right hand, and was taken by paramedics to the ED. Which of the following is most likely to be true regarding electrical injury?

A. Cataract formation usually only occurs when there is a contact point on the head
B. Renal failure is usually a result of direct electrical injury to the kidney
C. With high-voltage injuries, dysrhythmia usually develops 24 to 48 hours after injury
D. Even with minor cutaneous involvement, major internal injury can occur

[43.3] A 13-year-old male and his friend were curious about the inner workings of high-voltage transformers. After scaling the fence around one such complex near their school, one of the boys touched the transformer, believing that because he was wearing rubber-soled tennis shoes, he would be immune to electrical shock. He suffered a significant jolt of electricity at 10,000 V. Which of the following organ systems is most susceptible to high-voltage injuries?

A. Bones, tendons, and muscles
B. Skin, brain, and fat
C. Fat, heart, and skeletal muscle
D. Blood, nerves, and mucous membranes

[43.4] A 45-year-old accountant was getting into his car on the top of his high-rise office building during a thunderstorm. Suddenly, a lightning strike occurred, throwing him to the ground. Which of the following is most accurate regarding complications of his injuries?

A. Tetanic contractions are commonly caused by its AC current
B. The instantaneous duration of exposure lessens cutaneous burn risk compared to other high-voltage electrical injuries
C. Rhabdomyolysis is a common delayed sequelae
D. Respiratory arrest is caused by paralysis of thoracic muscles

Answers

[43.1] **B.** This patient with circumferential forearm burn has evidence of an ischemic hand despite incising the burn eschar. Fasciotomy is indicated to relieve compartment pressure, which is compressing the arterial supply.

[43.2]   **D.** Even with minor cutaneous involvement, major internal injury can occur. The renal failure following electrical shocks generally occurs as a result of myoglobinuria. Although dysrhythmia is common after electrical injury, it almost always develops *immediately* after exposure. Cataract formation may occur even when there is no contact point on the head.

[43.3]   **D.** In high-voltage injuries, the electricity tends to follow the path of least resistance. Blood, nerves, and mucous membranes are frequently injured after electrical exposure because of their low resistance. Fat, bones, and tendon have high resistance.

[43.4]   **B.** Because of instantaneous exposure, burns are relatively rare in lightning injury. Lightning is DC current, and respiratory arrest is usually a result of injury to the respiratory control center in the medulla. Rhabdomyolysis is common after high-voltage electrical injury, but rare after lightning strike.

CLINICAL PEARLS

❖   Victims of lightning strike should be treated with aggressive ventilatory and circulatory support until cerebral function can be assessed, because many patients will recover function with time.

❖   Typical signs of brain death, fixed/dilated pupils and apnea, do not necessarily indicate brain death in electrical victims. Moreover, typical triage criteria for mass casualty situations do not apply to electrical injury.

❖   Even with small outward sign of injury, major internal damage is common.

❖   Children may have excessive bleeding from chewing on electrical cords.

REFERENCES

Cherington M. Neurologic manifestations of lightning strikes. Neurology 2003;2:182–5.

Fish RM. Electric injury part III: cardiac monitoring indications, the pregnant patient, and lightning. J Emerg Med 2000;18:181–7.

Fontanarosa PB. Electrical shock and lightning strike. Ann Emerg Med 1993;22:112–21.

Koumbourlis AC. Electrical injuries. Crit Care Med 2002;30:S424–30.

A 10-year-old boy with sickle cell disease presents to the emergency department (ED) in the midst of presumed sickle cell crisis manifested as severe abdominal pain, pleuritic chest pain, dyspnea, and fever. His initial hemoglobin is 9 g/dL, white blood cell count (WBC) is 15,500 cells/mm³, and chest x-ray reveals a nonspecific infiltrate in the left lung field with a small left pleural effusion. The electrocardiogram reveals sinus tachycardia. Following treatment with intravenous fluid, supplemental oxygen by nasal canula, parenteral analgesics, and empiric broad-spectrum antibiotic therapy, the patient complains of worsening dyspnea and chest pain, requiring increasing oxygen supplementation by facemask and eventual endotracheal intubation. At this juncture, exchange transfusion therapy is contemplated.

 What are the complications associated with blood transfusions in this setting?

◆ **What are ways to reduce the incidence of transfusion-related complications?**

ANSWERS TO CASE 44: Transfusion Reaction

Summary: A 10-year-old boy with sickle cell crisis associated with severe respiratory symptoms (acute chest syndrome). The patient continues to have significant respiratory symptoms despite supportive care, and therefore exchange transfusion therapy is considered.

 Transfusion complications: transfusion reactions and transfusion-related infections

 Ways to reduce transfusion-related complications: strict adherence to patient identification, specimen handling, and blood product storage protocols, and thorough review of transfusion history

Analysis

Objectives

1. Develop an understanding of the epidemiology and basic pathophysiology of transfusion reactions.
2. Become familiar with the evaluation and treatment of acute, life-threatening transfusion complications.
3. Learn several indications for blood product pretreatment (leukoreduction, washing, irradiation).
4. Gain an appreciation for the full range of possible complications of transfusion therapy.

Considerations

Because sickle cell disease predisposes the patient to chronic anemia, it is more than likely that this particular patient has had an extensive history of transfusions; therefore, a thorough review of the transfusion history is vital. If the patient or the medical records indicates prior occurrence of minor transfusion reactions, then premedication with antihistamines and/or antipyretics may be useful. As a group, patients who are homozygous for sickle hemoglobin are at markedly increased risk of suffering complications from transfusion therapy, including transfusion-related infections (approximately 10 percent are infected with hepatitis C virus), and noninfectious etiologies related to alloimmunization (affecting up to 50 percent of sickle cell patients). The increased risks of alloimmunization are primarily related to recurrent antigen exposure and phenotypic dissimilarities between blood cells in the predominately white-donated blood supply and African American sickle cell patients.

To reduce the risk of transfusion-related complications, blood banks have intensified the cross-matching process for transfusions in sickle cell patients, with a demonstrable decrease in rates of alloimmunization. **Leukocyte-reduced packed red blood cells (PRBC) are recommended for patients**

with sickle cell disease and other patients requiring recurrent transfusions. Additional benefits include a reduced rate of human leukocyte antigen
(HLA) alloimmunization and possible decreased rates of febrile nonhemolytic transfusion reactions (FNHTRs).

APPROACH TO TRANSFUSION COMPLICATIONS

Conceptually, transfusion complications are best categorized into (a) acute
immune-mediated reactions, (b) delayed immune-mediated reactions, (c) non-
immunologic complications, and (d) infectious complications.

Acute Immune-Mediated Reactions

Acute Hemolytic Transfusion Reactions   Acute hemolytic transfusion
reactions occur in 1:25,000 transfusions and cause death in 1:470,000 transfusions. The **majority of acute hemolytic transfusion reactions** is due to
errors made during the processing of the blood, either at the patient bedside
or in the blood bank. The majority of these reactions may be avoided with
meticulous specimen processing, patient identification, and transfusion guidelines. Onset of reaction is **immediate, presenting with a combination of
hypotension, tachypnea (often with the sensation of chest constriction),
tachycardia, fever, chills, nausea, hemoglobinuria, and body pain (joints,
lower back, legs).** Hemolysis can be either intravascular (more severe) or
extravascular and is directed towards donor red blood cells (RBCs), usually
mediated by preformed antibodies (anti-A, anti-B) within the recipient's
serum. Because the causative antibodies to ABO group antigens are preexisting in susceptible individuals, no prior alloantigen exposure is necessary for
acute hemolysis to occur. However, recent sensitization to other alloantigens
(such as an Rh-negative patient being exposed to Rh-positive blood) can result
in similar pathology if a subsequent blood transfusion contains the same
alloantigen(s). Given the potential for new alloantibody formation, a blood
sample from the recipient should only be used for cross-matching assays within 48 hours from the time of collection.

Immediate management of suspected cases includes stopping the transfusion
and changing the IV tubing or using alternative access sites to initiate aggressive
crystalloid infusions, aiming to **maintain urine output above 1 to 1.5 mL/kg/h
for 24 hours.** The remainder of the transfusion and a sample of the patient's
blood should be sent to the blood bank for testing. The sequelae of acute hemolysis include **acute tubular necrosis (ATN), disseminated intravascular coagulation (DIC), and myocardial ischemia** (as a consequence of hemodynamic
instability). DIC may be confirmed by the presence of **hemoglobinuria and
plasma-free hemoglobin.** The definitive diagnosis of acute hemolytic transfusion reactions is made with **direct antiglobulin test** (DAT, also known as the
direct Coombs assay), which detects antibody or complement bound to the surface of donor RBCs in a sample of the recipient's blood (see Table 44-1).

Table 44-1

MANAGEMENT STEPS FOR TRANSFUSION REACTION

TRANSFUSION REACTION SUSPECTED	TRANSFUSION REACTION CONFIRMED	BACTERIAL CONTAMINATION SUSPECTED/ CONFIRMED	SUSPECTED/ CONFIRMED ANAPHYLAXIS	HEMODYNAMICALLY STABLE WITH MINOR TRANSFUSION REACTION
1. Stop transfusion 2. ABC 3. New IV tubing and crystalloid infusion 4. Inotrope/pressor as needed 5. Antihistamine and/or antipyretics as needed 6. Workup (plasma hemoglobin, urine myoglobin, DAT, repeat cross-match, Gram stain and culture, confirmation of paperwork)	In addition to column 1 1. Initiate brisk diuresis (fluid and/or diuretics) 2. Monitor coagulation status (CBC, PT/PTT, fibrinogen, FDP) 3. Monitor renal functions (BUN, Cr) 4. Monitor for hemolysis (bilirubin, LDH, haptoglobin)	1. Consider or initiate early, empiric IV antibiotics 2. Send appropriate cultures 3. Monitor coagulation, hepatic, and renal status	1. Administer epinephrine* and corticosteroids, with or without antihistamines 2. Test for anti-IgA antibody in recipient	1. Stop transfusion 2. Transfusion reaction workup, especially in first-time recipient 3. Administer antihistamine and/or antipyretics as indicated 4. Institute moderate fluid diuresis as tolerated

*Epinephrine dose is 10 mL of 1:100,000 solution or 1 mL of 1:10,000 solution.

Abbreviations: ABC, airway, breathing, and circulation; BUN, blood urea nitrogen; CBC, complete blood count; Cr, creatinine; DAT, direct antiglobulin test; FDP, fibrogen degradation products; LDH, lactate dehydrogenase; PT/PTT, prothrombin time/partial thromboplastin time.

Source: Santen S. Transfusion therapy. In: Tintinalli JE, Kelen GD, Stapczynski JS, eds. Emergency Medicine, 6th ed., New York:McGraw-Hill, 2004; pp 1348–54.

Febrile Nonhemolytic Transfusion Reactions These reactions occur with approximately 0.5 to 1 percent RBC units, 2 percent apheresis platelet unit, and 5 to 30 percent donor-pooled platelets. **FNHTRs constitute the most common and least-worrisome complications of blood product transfusion.** Patients may present with fever, chills, rigors, headache, malaise, and tachycardia, but **without hemodynamic instability and respiratory compromise.** Fever production is believed to occur as the result of cytokines present in transfused blood products or by antibodies against leukocytes (leukoagglutinins) present in recipient or donor blood. Because prior foreign leukocyte exposure is required for leukoagglutinin formation in the recipient, **fever in a first-time transfusion recipient should be treated as an acute hemolytic reaction until proven otherwise.** Conversely, prior episodes of FNHTR indicate an increased risk of recurrence.

Depending on the severity, management may include stopping the transfusion, administration of an antipyretic, and patient reassurance. Patients with a history of febrile reactions can be premedicated with antipyretics. **Antipyretic premedication** is a matter of preference, but **should be generally avoided in first-time transfusion recipients, because fever is more likely to represent serious sequelae in these patients.** Severe rigors associated with FNHTR can be treated with meperidine. Because FNHTR is a diagnosis of exclusion, samples of patient's blood and the transfusate should be sent to rule out a hemolytic reaction or bacterial contamination. Prestorage leukoreduction has not been proven to reduce the incidence of FNHTR; however, the use of leukoreduced blood in patients with a history of FNHTR is still widely practiced.

Allergic Transfusion Reactions The incidence of these allergic reactions is approximately 1 to 3 percent of transfusions. These reactions are caused by recipient antibodies (immunoglobulin [Ig] E) against donor serum proteins, and may range from urticaria to frank anaphylaxis. Urticaria can be managed symptomatically with antihistamines and by briefly stopping the transfusion until symptoms resolve. Mild allergic reactions do not necessitate discontinuing the transfusion, as symptoms are not strictly dose related. Patients prone to develop these reactions can be premedicated with antihistamines to prevent the development of mild allergic reactions.

Frankly anaphylactic reactions to blood products are rare (1:20,000 to 1:170,000) and can occur within seconds of transfusion initiation. Anaphylactic reactions are IgE-mediated and occur, in most cases, as the result of **genetic deficiency of IgA in the recipient,** resulting in the production of anti-IgA IgE. Other less-common causes of anaphylaxis include reactions caused by IgE against allergens in the transfused blood, and the passive transfer of reactive IgE from donor to the recipient. **Patients with known IgA deficiency should be given RBCs and platelets that have been thoroughly washed free of plasma proteins. Plasma component transfusions in IgA-deficient patients should be obtained from IgA-deficient donors.**

Anaphylaxis should be managed by urgent attention to ABCs (airway, breathing, circulation), accompanied by the administration of **epinephrine, antihistamines, and corticosteroids**, along with the immediate discontinuation of the transfusion. **Patients taking angiotensin-converting enzyme (ACE) inhibitors** will have more severe anaphylactic reactions (i.e., severe angioedema) because of their **inability to degrade bradykinin**, a normal substrate of ACE and a key player in the anaphylactic cascade.

Transfusion-Related Acute Lung Injury Transfusion-related acute lung injury (TRALI), with an estimated incidence of 1:4500 transfusions, is an underrecognized **life-threatening complication of transfusion**. TRALI is thought to be **mediated by antileukocyte antibodies**, resulting in systemic inflammation and neutrophil-mediated lung injury. The onset is generally within 6 hours of exposure to plasma-containing transfusion products, with most cases occurring within 1 to 2 hours. Random donor platelet transfusions (pooled platelets) are responsible for the majority of cases. Patients with hematological malignancies and cardiac disease appear to be at increased risk of developing TRALI for unclear reasons. Fever, tachycardia, and dyspnea are the most common presenting symptoms. **The hallmark of this complication is respiratory distress with the presence of diffuse, bilateral alveolar and interstitial infiltrates on radiographic imaging.** TRALI may be easily confused with acute pulmonary edema secondary to volume overload. Because **TRALI patients have normal to low left-heart pressures, pulmonary artery catheters may be useful for differentiating between TRALI and pulmonary edema**. The management of this condition consists of stopping the transfusion and immediate attention to the ABCs, which may include intubation and mechanical ventilation. Respiratory impairment usually resolves within 48 to 72 hours in survivors (roughly 10 percent mortality rate). Radiographic abnormalities may persist for up to 7 days. Leukoreduction is not an effective preventative strategy. The exact pathogenesis of TRALI remains undetermined.

Delayed Immune-Mediated Reactions

Delayed Hemolytic Transfusion Reaction Delayed hemolytic transfusion reactions (DHTRs) can occur in either the intravascular or extravascular spaces, but are notably less severe than their acute hemolytic counterparts. The incidence is about 1:1,000 transfusions. The mechanisms of DHTR are related to recipients having developed antibodies against RBC alloantigens from prior foreign RBC exposures, most often through transfusions or pregnancies.

Unlike acute hemolytic reactions, however, which require high circulating levels of reactive antibodies, these **alloantibodies are present only at low levels prior to transfusion**. Following exposure to these alloantigens, antibody generation is slowly increased over the following days, gradually resulting in hemolysis of the donor RBCs. **Symptoms associated with DHTR are mild to nonexistent**. Patients typically present with a mild fever, recurrent anemia, and a positive DAT up to 2 weeks following transfusion. No specific therapy is warranted aside from repeat transfusion. Because alloantibodies responsible for DHTR are present at such low levels prior to transfusion, these generally escape detection by standard cross-matching methods. As such, these reactions are largely unpreventable.

Graft-Versus-Host Disease   Transfusion-related graft-versus-host disease (GVHD) is a rare disorder where donor leukocytes engraft successfully in the recipient's bone marrow, which over time may lead to a severe graft-mediated reaction against the recipient's tissues, including the bone marrow. It is **fatal in >90 percent of cases.** Symptoms of GVHD develop on average 1 to 2 weeks following transfusion and include fevers, maculopapular rashes, hepatitis, diarrhea, nausea, vomiting, weight loss, and pancytopenia leading to sepsis and death. **Immunocompromised recipients are especially at risk for GVHD, therefore blood products administered to these patients should be subjected to gamma irradiation** to render remaining leukocytes incapable of proliferation. Furthermore, blood products donated by first-degree relatives or between patients with matched HLA haplotypes have an increased risk of donor leukocyte engraftment because of homology between donor and recipient HLA genes; therefore, **blood product donations by first-degree relatives should be irradiated prior to transfusions.**

Posttransfusion Purpura   Posttransfusion purpura is rare a complication, characterized by sudden thrombocytopenia occurring 5 to 10 days following transfusion of any blood product. The pathophysiology involves native platelet destruction, mediated by antibodies to the platelet antigen (PLA) 1. Anti-PLA1 antibodies develop in patients previously exposed to foreign platelets through transfusion or pregnancy. Patients usually present with spontaneous bleeding (mucous membranes, epistaxis, hematochezia, hematuria). **Nine percent of patients may develop intracranial hemorrhage**. Treatment involves administration of intravenous immunoglobulin, corticosteroids, plasma exchange therapy, and transfusion with **PLA1-negative platelets**. If left untreated, the thrombocytopenia usually resolves spontaneously within 2 weeks of onset.

Alloimmunization   Alloimmunization refers to the formation of new antibodies against antigens on donated cells. **The formation of alloantibodies against HLA surface molecules may render patients refractory to platelet transfusions**, thus supporting the administration of leukoreduced blood for patients who will likely need exogenous platelets in the future. The presence

Table 44-2
TRANSFUSION-RELATED INFECTIOUS RISKS

INFECTIOUS AGENT	ESTIMATED UNITS AT RISK	TRANSMISSION RATE	OTHER
Viruses			
Human immunodeficiency virus (HIV) 1 and 2	1:1,900,000	90%	Substantial risk reduction because of nucleic acid testing
Human T-cell leukemia virus (HTLV) 1 and 2	1:641,000	30%	Causes adult T-cell leukemia and transverse myelopathy
Hepatitis A virus (HAV)	1:1,000,000	90%	
Hepatitis B virus (HBV)	1:137,000	70%	Chronic disease develops in <10%
Hepatitis C virus (HCV)	<1:1,000,000	90%	Substantial risk reduction because of nucleic acid testing; chronic disease develops in >50%
Parvovirus B19	1:3,300–1:40,000	Unknown	Severe reactions in sickle cell patients
Cytomegalovirus (CMV)	6-12%	Unknown	Main risk is to immunocompromised and low-birth-weight infants; risk reduced substantially with leukoreduction
Epstein-Barr Virus (EBV)	Unknown	Unknown	Same as for CMV

Bacteria			
Red blood cells	1:30,000	6% (sepsis)	Rare
Random donor platelets	1:500 (per 5 units)	20% (sepsis)	Transmission rates are proportional to platelet storage time (maximum shelf life is 120 hours)
Apheresis platelets	1:2,400	20% (sepsis)	
Parasites			
Trypanosoma cruzii	1:42,000 to 1:1,000,000	<10%	Regional variation
Malaria, babesiosis	Less than 1:1,000,000	<10%	Currently rare in the United States

of alloantibodies is primarily responsible for the increased rates of transfusion complications seen in repeat transfusion recipients.

Infectious Complications

The most frequent and concerning infectious complication of transfusion therapy is bacterial contamination, which can be detected in up to 2 percent of blood products. The most commonly isolated organism in refrigerated products (i.e., RBCs) is *Yersinia enterocolitica*, which can grow at temperatures as low as 1°C (33.8°F). Other cryophilic organisms include *Pseudomonas, Enterobacter,* and *Flavobacterium*. Platelets, which are stored at room temperature (22 to 24°C [71.6 to 75.2°F]), are more likely to develop gross contamination than are refrigerated products. *Staphylococcus* and *Salmonella* are often reported in fatal cases of platelet transfusion-mediated sepsis. Signs and symptoms may include fevers, rigors, chills, rash, hypotension, and even shock accompanied by sepsis. Symptoms may develop immediately or over several hours. Suspected cases of contamination should be managed with respiratory and circulatory support, immediate discontinuation of the transfusion, and broad-spectrum antibiotic therapy. Because it is difficult to distinguish some of the immune-mediated transfusion reactions from bacterial transmission, **any transfusion that causes hypotension in the setting of fever warrants immediate testing of the donor blood with Gram stain and culture, in addition to standard workup for hemolytic reactions**.

Comprehension Questions

[44.1] A hemodynamically stable 40-year-old man with gastrointestinal (GI) bleeding and hemoglobin of 6 g/dL is receiving packed RBC transfusion. Soon after the initiation of blood transfusion, the patient becomes confused, develops urticaria, and is subsequently unresponsive with a systolic blood pressure of 60 mmHg. Which of the following agents may have worsened this patient's condition?

A. The use of lisinopril (an ACE inhibitor)
B. Atenolol
C. Lactated Ringer solution
D. Morphine sulfate

[44.2] A 60-year-old woman with chronic anemia caused by a myelophthisic process presents to the emergency room from her oncologist's office with a hemoglobin of 6 g/dL. She notes feeling very lethargic over the past week, and had some mild chest discomfort while climbing stairs in her house last night. A type- and cross-match is performed for 2 units of packed erythrocytes, which are given without incident and marked improvement in her symptoms is seen. While going over discharge instructions with the emergency physician, the patient notes that she feels feverish and slightly short of breath. Over the next several minutes her dyspnea worsens markedly. Vital sign measurement reveals an oxygen saturation of 93 percent, a heart rate of 120 beats per minute, and a blood pressure of 95/55 mmHg. The patient continues to deteriorate from a respiratory standpoint despite supplemental oxygen, requiring endotracheal intubation. A portable chest radiograph shows evidence of diffuse bilateral infiltrates. Which of the following statements is most accurate regarding this patient's condition?

A. This patient's left ventricular end-diastolic pressure is likely to be elevated.
B. This condition has a mortality rate of up to 90 percent.
C. Diuretic therapy is unlikely to be effective.
D. Radiographic abnormalities develop several days after the onset of clinical manifestations.

Answers

[44.1] **A.** Patients taking ACE inhibitors may experience a more severe anaphylactic reaction than other patients because of their inability to degrade bradykinin; however, these agents do not confer an increased risk of anaphylaxis. Patient misidentification is the leading preventable cause of transfusion reactions.

[44.2] **C.** Patients with TRALI are not volume overloaded, but rather suffer from increased capillary permeability at the level of the pulmonary vasculature. As such, they have normal to low left-side heart pressures, and will only be harmed by diuretic therapy because of the potential to cause organ hypoperfusion. Mortality rates are around 10 percent. Radiographic abnormalities are present almost immediately, and persist for several days after the resolution of clinical manifestations.

REFERENCES

Goodnough et al. Transfusion medicine (parts 1 and 2). *N Engl J Med* 1999;340:438–47, 525–33.

Snyder EL. Transfusion reactions. In: Hematology: basic principles and practice, 3rd ed. Churchill-Livingstone, 2000.

A 17-year-old boy is brought to the emergency department (ED) by his soccer coach after he developed the acute onset of right testicular pain while at practice. The patient doesn't remember getting kicked or hit during practice and denies any fever, dysuria, and penile discharge. He does not have any abdominal pain or vomiting.

On exam, he is afebrile with normal vital signs. He is in mild distress because of the pain. His abdomen is benign. On visual inspection, he has right scrotal erythema and swelling, although no penile lesions or discharge. Because his scrotum is so diffusely tender, it is difficult to examine it more closely, although there is no testicular rise when his inner thigh is stroked. His urinalysis shows 3 to 5 white blood cells (WBC)/high-power field (hpf).

◆ **What is the most likely diagnosis?**

◆ **What is the most appropriate next step?**

ANSWERS TO CASE 45: Scrotal Pain

Summary: This is a 17-year-old boy who presents with acute onset of right testicular pain without trauma.

 Most likely diagnosis: testicular torsion.

 Most appropriate next step: urological consultation. Manual detorsion can be attempted while awaiting the consultant.

Analysis

Objectives

1. Learn the differential diagnoses for acute scrotal pain.
2. Recognize the clinical signs and symptoms of testicular torsion.
3. Understand the diagnostic and therapeutic approach to suspected testicular torsion.

Considerations

The differential diagnosis of acute testicular pain includes testicular torsion, epididymitis, and torsion of the testicular appendages. Because of the risk of ischemia and infarction of the testes, testicular torsion is the priority condition that must be promptly recognized and treated. This patient is 17 years old without a history of trauma. Teens during puberty are especially at risk of testicular torsion because of high hormonal stimulation. This patient's history of acute onset, especially associated with vigorous physical activity, is classic. The involved testis is firm, tender, and located higher in the scrotum on examination, and the cremasteric reflex is absent, again consistent with testicular torsion. When the clinical presentation is unclear, Doppler flow studies of the intratesticular blood flow may be helpful. This patient, however, has a clear-cut diagnosis, and time is of the essence.

APPROACH TO SCROTAL PAIN

Definitions

Epididymitis: infection of the epididymis, which is a fine tubular structure about 5 m long compressed into an area of 5 cm. Chlamydia or gonorrhea are often causative in men younger than age 35 years, whereas coliforms are the etiology in older men.

Fournier gangrene: polymicrobial necrotizing infection of the perineal subcutaneous fascia particularly seen in diabetic males (Fig. 45-1). Aggressive emergent surgical debridement is necessary as a life-saving measure.

Testicular torsion: twisting of the testicular and spermatic cord leading to ischemia and infarction of the affected testes if untreated.

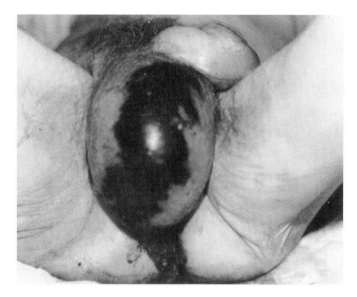

Figure 45-1. Fournier gangrene of the scrotum. (Reproduced with permission from Scheider RE. Male gential problems. In: Tintinalli JE, Kelen GD, Stapczynski JS, eds. Emergency medicine, 6th ed. New York: McGraw-Hill, 2004: 615.

> **Torsion of the appendages:** twisting of one of four pedunculated structures of the testes: appendix testes (most commonly affected), appendix epididymis, paradidymis, and vas aberrans. These structures have no physiological purpose and classic finding is "blue dot sign."

Clinical Approach

When any male presents with scrotal pain, testicular torsion must be considered. Prompt diagnosis and therapy are vital because delays can lead to ischemia, loss of the testicle, and impaired fertility. In general, the maximum survival time of the testis is 4 hours after the onset of ischemia, but clinical parameters are often unreliable. Patients with testicular torsion often have a congenital "bell clapper" deformity, which allows the epididymis and testicle to hang freely and rotate in the scrotum. When torsion occurs, the spermatic cord becomes twisted, cutting off the blood supply to the testicle. Although torsion can occur at any age, it is most common in the neonatal period and around puberty.

When obtaining the history, the clinician should focus on the onset and duration of pain and any associated symptoms, such as nausea and vomiting, fever, urethral discharge, and dysuria. It is also important to inquire about any previous episodes and any recent trauma. A typical patient with testicular torsion presents with the sudden onset of severe pain in the lower abdomen, inguinal area, or testicle. It is often preceded by strenuous physical activity or trauma. Past episodes that resolved spontaneously are not uncommon.

Table 45-1

DIFFERENTIAL DIAGNOSES FOR ACUTE SCROTAL PAIN

DIAGNOSIS	COMMENTS	CLINICAL FINDINGS	TREATMENT
Epididymitis	Gradual onset; may have fever, irritative voiding symptoms; <35 years old, usually sexually transmitted disease-related; >35 to 40-years-old, caused by coliform bacteria	Localized tenderness over epididymis, urethral discharge; pain better with scrotal elevation; Doppler US: increased blood flow	Antibiotics, analgesia, bed rest with scrotal elevation and scrotal support
Torsion of the appendix testis	Testicular appendage has no physiological purpose	"Blue dot" sign; Doppler US: normal or increased blood flow	Analgesia, scrotal support; usually resolves in 10–14 days
Strangulated inguinal hernia		Inguinal and scrotal swelling, signs of intestinal obstruction	Surgery
Idiopathic scrotal edema	Prepubertal males; sudden onset; little or no pain	Erythema, scrotal edema, nontender testis and epididymis	Resolves spontaneously in 2–5 days
Testicular tumor	Usually asymptomatic, but acute pain may be caused by hemorrhage into tumor	Enlarged, irregular, tender testis; Doppler US needed	
Fournier gangrene	Polymicrobial infection causing necrotizing fasciitis of perineal, genital, or perianal regions; risk factors: diabetes, immunocompromise	Scrotal pain, perineal erythema and swelling → induration, local cyanosis, and blistering; signs of sepsis; US: diffuse swelling and thickening of scrotum	Surgical debridement, antibiotics
Orchitis	Usually seen as an extension of epididymitis or with mumps, viral illnesses, or syphilis	Bilateral testicular swelling and tenderness	Symptomatic and disease-specific therapy

On exam, the clinician should pay close attention to any abdominal findings, scrotal swelling or edema, penile discharge or rash, inguinal lymphadenopathy, and testicular tenderness or masses. Classically, a torsed testicle is diffusely tender and swollen with an abnormal (horizontal) lie. There is usually a loss of the cremasteric reflex on the affected side. **However, no historical or exam findings can definitively distinguish testicular torsion from other disease processes.**

Testicular torsion is largely a clinical diagnosis, and no diagnostic tests should delay urological evaluation and surgical exploration. Often, the testis is swollen and the physical findings are obscured. If the diagnosis is uncertain, color-flow Doppler ultrasound (US) or radionuclide scintigraphy may be helpful. The utility of these studies is limited by their availability and timeliness. In addition, scintigraphy does not provide any anatomical information and, therefore, cannot differentiate epididymitis from torsion of the appendix testis. Many times, leukocytes are found in the urine of men with testicular torsion. This finding should not distract the clinician from the diagnosis.

Treatment

When the diagnosis of testicular torsion is considered, prompt urological consultation is mandatory. **Definitive treatment involves emergent surgical exploration, detorsion, and orchiopexy.** While awaiting urological consultation, the clinician may attempt manual detorsion. Because most torsions occur in a lateral to medial manner, the testis should initially be turned in a medial to lateral direction like **"opening a book."** Successful detorsion results in significant pain relief. If the pain worsens, however, the maneuver should be tried in the opposite direction. The differential diagnosis for acute scrotal pain includes several benign and emergent conditions (Table 45-1).

Comprehension Questions

[45.1] A 22-year-old baseball player comes into the ED complaining of 12 hours of severe right testicular pain. He denies a history of trauma. On examination, his right testis is diffusely tender and indurated, and does not change with patient position. He has a cremasteric reflex on the right side. Which of the following is the best next step?

A. Continued observation
B. Oral antibiotics
C. Bed rest, ice to scrotum, and elevation of the scrotum
D. Surgical exploration of the scrotum

[45.2] A 32-year-old jogger is brought into the emergency department with the acute onset of severe left testicular pain. A diagnosis of testicular torsion is made, and manual detorsion is successfully accomplished. Which of the following is the most appropriate advice to this patient?

A. Likely no further therapy is needed
B. Surgical exploration may be needed if another episode of torsion occurs
C. Surgical correction will be needed but does not necessarily need to be done urgently
D. Surgical exploration still needed to be performed and should occur within 24 hours

Match the probable diagnoses (A to F) to the clinical scenario in questions [45.2] to [45.6]:

A. Torsion of the appendix testes
B. Testicular torsion
C. Epididymitis
D. Orchitis
E. Testicular malignancy
F. Acute prostatitis

[45.3] A 24-year-old male complains of severe left scrotal pain increasing over 24 hours. Urinalysis shows 25 WBC/hpf, and Doppler flow shows increased intratesticular flow.

[45.4] A 58-year-old man complains of urgency, dysuria, lower back pain, and pain with ejaculation.

[45.5] A 14-year-old boy complains of 2 days of testicular pain. On examination, there appears to be tender nodule of the testes. Transillumination reveals a small blue spot of the affected area.

[45.6] A 28-year-old man complains of heaviness in his scrotum. On examination, there is a firm, nontender mass involving his right testis.

Answers

[45.1] **D.** The clinical history is consistent with testicular torsion. The presence of a cremasteric reflex does not rule out the disease. Emergency scrotal exploration is the procedure of choice when the history, physical, and imaging tests do not rule out testicular torsion.

[45.2] **C.** Derotation of the torsed testis converts an emergent surgical correction procedure into an elective one. Manual derotation is not definitive therapy.

[45.3] **C.** The Doppler ultrasound finding consistent with epididymitis is increased or preserved blood flow. Also epididymitis usually has a slower onset of pain.

[45.4]   **F.** Acute prostatitis usually occurs in older patients. Urinary urgency, hesitancy, frequency, perineal pain with ejaculation are common symptoms. The causative organism is *Escherichia coli* in the majority of cases, and treatment of choice is ciprofloxacin 500 mg twice daily for 30 days.

[45.5]   **A.** Torsion of the testicular appendages classically presents as a tender testicular nodule, and upon transillumination, a "blue dot" may be seen. Color Doppler flow is increased or normal. Management is observation, because the process will resolve in time.

[45.6]   **E.** Testicular carcinoma classically presents as an asymptomatic scrotal mass.

CLINICAL PEARLS

❖ Testicular torsion should always be considered in the differential diagnoses of acute scrotal or abdominal pain.

❖ No single historical or exam findings can definitively distinguish testicular torsion from other processes.

❖ Time is testicle. If testicular torsion is suspected, prompt urological consultation is mandatory.

❖ Definitive treatment of testicular torsion is surgery. Manual detorsion may be attempted as a temporizing measure.

REFERENCES

Freeman L. Male genitourinary emergencies: preserving fertility and providing relief. Emerg Med Pract 2000;2(11):4–14.

Haynes BE, Bessen HA, Haynes VE. The diagnosis of testicular torsion. JAMA 1983;249:2522.

Mick NW, Peters JR, Silvers SM. Blueprints in emergency medicine. Malden, MA: Blackwell Publishing, 2002:119–20.

Schneider RE. Male genitourinary problems. In: Tintinalli JE, Kelen GD, Stapczynski JS, eds. Emergency medicine, 5th ed. New York: McGraw-Hill, 2000:633–6.

It is approximately 2 AM, when a woman presents to the emergency department (ED) with her 3-year-old son. According to the mother, the patient had been playing and fell off the upper level of his bunkbed earlier in the evening. On examination, the child is somnolent. His pulse rate is 110 beats per minute, blood pressure is 100/85 mmHg, respiratory rate is 28 breaths per minute, and Glasgow Coma Scale (GCS) score is 11 (eye opening 2,verbal 5, motor 4). There is presence of soft-tissue contusion over the left frontal scalp and ecchymosis over the left periorbital region. The chest is clear with bilateral breath sounds. The abdomen is mildly distended and tender throughout. The patient's left thigh is markedly swollen and tender, and all his extremities are mottled and cool.

 What is the most likely mechanism responsible for this patient's clinical picture?

 What are the next steps in the management of this patient?

ANSWERS TO CASE 46: Pediatric Trauma

Summary: A 3-year-old boy presents several hours after an unwitnessed fall, with somnolence and external signs of head injury. In addition to the contusions on the scalp, his abdomen is distended and tender, left thigh is swollen and tender, and his skin is mottled and cool.

 Most likely responsible mechanism: this child has multiple injuries, possibly secondary to intentional trauma.

 Next steps in management: pediatric trauma resuscitation and evaluation to include administration of intravenous fluids, a thorough examination, and a computed tomography (CT) scan of the head and abdomen. **Protection of the child by reporting potential child abuse, and admission to the hospital.**

Analysis

Objectives

1. Become familiar with the evaluation and management of a pediatric patient with multiple severe injuries presenting in shock.
2. Recognize the signs in the presentation of a child that are consistent with a battered child and become familiar with the appropriate response.

Considerations

The presentation of this child should raise concerns for multiple reasons, and it is vitally important to appropriately prioritize your attention to these concerns. The first priority should be concern over his medical condition, not the mechanism of the injury. This patient's vital signs presented in the case scenario are not out of the range of normal for his age (Table 46-1). Despite the normal vital signs, his general presentation indicates the potential for multisystem injuries, and putting that together with the findings of mottled and cool skin indicate that this child is in **hemorrhagic shock until proven otherwise**. The vital signs of an injured child can be within normal ranges for an extended period of time secondary to an excellent ability to compensate physiologically for hypovolemia. However, when the limits of that compensatory reserve are reached, the ability of a child to tolerate shock is poor and his condition will likely decline very rapidly.

The secondary concern regarding this child is the manner in which he presented suggesting potential abuse. Factors that raise these concerns include the **delay in presentation**, the extent of **the injuries that appear much more severe than can be accounted for by the history**, the **age** of the child, and the **unwitnessed report** of the injury. All 50 states have mandatory child abuse reporting laws for the treating physician. Regardless of the management plan, this child should be placed in a protected environment (admitted), and a report

Table 46-1

NORMAL VITAL SIGNS BY AGE GROUP

AGE GROUP (YEARS)	HEART RATE (BEATS/MIN)	BLOOD PRESSURE (mmHG)	RESPIRATORY RATE (BREATHS/MIN)
0–1	120	80/40	40
1–5	100	100/60	30
5–10	80	120/80	20

of suspected abuse should be submitted. However the treating physician's suspicions or emotions should not delay the child's medical care (which is the first responsibility). Accurate and complete evaluations and documentation of your findings in an unbiased manner is the first important step. Confrontations with family members in the midst of a trauma room evaluation are rarely fruitful, and can hamper your efforts to care for the child.

APPROACH TO THE PEDIATRIC TRAUMA PATIENT

A **systematic and expeditious approach** to any children with unknown injury mechanisms or mechanisms capable of producing multisystem injury should include a rapid survey for all potential injuries, **consideration of the need for intubation, administration of intravenous fluids, and the prevention of heat loss. CT scan of the head and abdomen** may be obtained for further evaluation as needed, and the patient should be prepared for operative care as indicated. In those patients with multiple injuries identified, prioritizing the most life-threatening problem is of paramount importance. Even when intracranial hemorrhage may be suspected on the basis of physical presentation, the immediate threat to most children with multisystem injury is hypovolemic shock from abdominal injury and other hemorrhagic sources. Addressing blood loss source is critical not only for the correction of hemorrhagic shock but for the prevention of secondary brain injury in these patients.

The guidelines found in the advanced trauma life support (ATLS) and advanced pediatric life support (APLS) manuals should be followed in the initial management of injured children. **The initial priorities** are the assessment and maintenance of **airway, oxygenation, and ventilation.** Determination for immediate intubation is dependent on the initial evaluation of the child and the resources available. Certainly, if there is any **airway compromise**, or if the **neurological status** raises concern of airway protection (a **GCS score <9**; Table 46-2), then **intubation is mandatory**. If the airway is not compromised and the GCS score is adequate, then the decision for elective intubation may be determined by the level of patient cooperation and the timely completion of potentially lifesaving diagnostic studies such as CT imaging.

Table 46-2
PEDIATRIC GCS VERBAL SCORES

5	Appropriate words or social smile; fixes and follows
4	Cries, but consolable
3	Persistently irritable
2	Restless, agitated
1	None

The circulation and the neurological status should be the next priorities. Approximately 90 percent of pediatric patients presenting with blunt trauma are successfully managed without operative intervention. However, the **initial signs of shock, including tachycardia, skin changes, and lethargy, represent a loss of approximately 25 percent of the child's blood volume** (Table 46-3). The likelihood of injury requiring operative control of hemorrhage is much greater in these children, and careful attention should be paid to the amount of fluid or blood that is required to maintain stable vital signs. A large-bore IV should be started, and two sequential boluses of **20 mL/kg of warmed crystalloid solution** should be administered. If further fluids are required beyond this, then administration of packed red blood cells (10 mL/kg) should be considered. Evaluation of the **abdomen by ultrasound (if unstable) or CT scan** should be performed to determine the extent of injuries. **If the vital signs worsen** during the attempt to obtain a head and abdominal CT scan, this should be abandoned and a **laparotomy performed** to control any hemorrhage.

There is no doubt that the child in this case presents a considerable challenge. Not only does the possibility of abuse evoke strong emotions that are difficult to ignore during the evaluation, there is potential of multiple life threatening injuries that must be prioritized. A systematic and efficient approach, with focus on the most immediate of concerns cannot be emphasized enough (Table 46-4).

Approach to the Battered Child

In 1962, Kempe described a syndrome of repeated child abuse. In many hospitals, his name is now used as a code to describe the pediatric inpatient that requires high visibility protection and psychological support because of suspected child abuse. Since the publication of Kempe's article, it has become increasingly more apparent that child abuse is a substantial problem in our society. According to the national clearinghouse for child abuse and neglect, there were an estimated 1300 fatalities in 2001 secondary to child abuse. Mandatory reporting laws now exist in all states.

Table 46-3

SYSTEMIC RESPONSES TO BLOOD LOSS IN THE
PEDIATRIC PATIENT

<25% BLOOD VOLUME LOSS	25–45% BLOOD VOLUME LOSS	>45% BLOOD VOLUME LOSS
Weak, thready pulse; increased heart rate	Increased heart rate	Hypotension, tachycardia to bradycardia
Lethargic, irritable, confused	Change in the level of consciousness, dulled response to pain	Comatose
Cool, clammy	Cyanotic, decreased capillary refill, cold extremities	Pale, cold
Minimal decrease in urinary output; increased specific gravity	Minimal urine output	No urine output

Source: ATLS Manual, American College of Surgeons, 1997:297.

Table 46-4

INITIAL MANAGEMENT OF THE INJURED CHILD

Primary survey	Establishment of a reliable airway
	Ventilation
	Establishment of large-bore IV lines
	Support of circulation
	Rapid assessment of neurological status
Secondary survey	Diagnostic studies

	Establishment of surgical priorities
	    Mass lesion in the brain
	    Chest and abdominal injuries
	    Peripheral vascular injuries
	    Fractures

Source: Oneill JA, Principles of Pediatric Surgery, St. Louis: Mosby, 2003:783.

There are very few other things encountered by physicians that will evoke such strong distasteful emotions, making one think that reporting of these cases would not be a significant problem. However, to report a case of child abuse, the physician must first recognize it as such. The subtleties of recognizing child abuse, and the fear of making incorrect accusations of caregivers that appear well-meaning can make this a difficult issue. The reporting and protection of the battered child is further confounded by the legal requirements for appropriate and complete documentation by the physician, which often is lacking if suspicions of abuse were not entertained upon initial presentation.

Intentional injury accounts for approximately 10 percent of all trauma cases in children younger than 5 years old. While this figure may be alarming, it also suggests that the vast majority of trauma in children is actually accidental. There are several key aspects of the history, physical exam, and presentation of the child that should alert the practitioner to the possibility that the trauma was not accidental. Table 46-5 lists suggestive characteristics that should alert the practitioner to abuse. Skin and soft-tissue injuries are the most common injury encountered in child abuse cases. This is followed by fractures, which often are multiple or repetitive. The third most common problem with child abuse is head injury. Unfortunately, this is also the injury with the highest mortality. Finally, visceral injuries account for 10 to 15 percent of abuse cases. These include hollow visceral perforations, and duodenal or mesenteric hematomas, as well as liver, spleen, and kidney fractures.

Currently, there is no federal standard regarding the legal requirements for reporting of child abuse. However, all states have mandatory reporting legislation for suspected child abuse that includes health care workers, school personnel, social workers, and law enforcement officers. Very few states recognize the physician patient communication privilege as exempt from these reporting requirements. Most states impose either a fine or imprisonment penalty on individuals that knowingly or willfully fail to report abuse. However, several states also impose penalties for false reports of child abuse.

When intentional injury is suspected in a pediatric trauma case, the appropriate child protective agency should be notified after the child's medical condition is addressed. During the investigational process, it is often incumbent on the medical personnel to provide a high-visibility protected environment for the child. Although it is often emotionally tempting for the physician to become involved in the investigational process, it is important at this stage to **maintain focus on the medical condition**. This becomes particularly important in terms of adequate documentation. A **complete, unbiased, and well-recorded history and physical** examination can be vital in the protection of the child at a later date.

Particularly important information includes detailed descriptions of the reported mechanism of the injury, the time of the injury and any delay in presentation, the presence of witnesses, conflicts and inconsistencies. A complete physical exam should be documented and should include pictures or diagrams of all bruises, documentation of the color of each bruise, a

Table 46-5
PATTERNS SUGGESTING PHYSICAL ABUSE

Presentation	Age younger than 3 years (limited ability to communicate)
	Significant delay between injury and presentation

	Presence of risk factors
	  Chronic illness
	  Premature birth
	  Congenital deficiencies
	  Mental delay

History	Unwitnessed injury
	Injuries not consistent or more significant than suggested by the history
	Evasive responses
	Reported self-injury not consistent with the child's stage of development
Physical	Multiple injuries
	Signs of prior injuries and fractures
	Injuries and different stages of healing

	Pattern of injuries
	  Demarcated buttock scalding injuries
	  Retinal hemorrhage
	  Multiple bruises
	  Hand or whip marks
	  Cigarette burns

Table 46-6
MUSCULOSKELETAL MANIFESTATIONS OF ABUSE

Spiral fractures attributed to falls

Subperiosteal calcification with no history of injury

Multiple fractures in various stages of healing

Bucket-handle fractures or epiphyseal–metaphyseal separation and fragmentation from pulling or shaking forces

Unexplained fractures associated with chronic subdural hematomas

Source: Oneill JA, Principles of Pediatric Surgery, St. Louis: Mosby, 2003.

complete neurological exam, and a genital exam. An eye exam for retinal hemorrhages should be performed because this is often encountered with cerebral trauma and the "shaken baby syndrome." Radiographic evaluations should be performed on all extremities to search for patterns of previous injury (Table 46-6). Any reports from previous admissions (including from other hospitals) should be referenced.

Comprehension Questions

[46.1] A 3-year-old boy is brought into the ED with multiple bruises, abrasions, and several deep lacerations over the flank region. The parents state that he fell out of his bed. Which of the following is the most important next step in this patient?

    A. Reporting these injuries to Child Protective Services
    B. Firmly, but without judgment, confront the parents with the discrepancy of the story and the injuries
    C. Take accurate pictures of the injuries and seal them in an evidence envelope
    D. Evaluate the ABCs and any urgent injuries
    E. Station guards in front of the exits of the building to prevent the parents from leaving

[46.2] An 11-month old baby is brought into the ED after rolling down a staircase while still buckled into the infant car seat. The baby is crying, but is consolable by his mother. His heart rate is 116 beats per minute and blood pressure 80/40 mmHg at rest. The physical examination reveals only slight bruising over the knees. The abdomen is nontender. Which of the following is the best next step?

    A. CT scan of the abdomen to assess for intraperitoneal hemorrhage
    B. Chest radiograph to assess for pleural hemorrhage
    C. Continued observation and reassurance
    D. IV access and infuse normal saline 10 mL/kg

[46.3] A 4-year-old girl is brought into the emergency room for multiple blunt trauma that was reportedly inflicted by stepparents. Which of the following injuries is most likely to cause mortality?

    A. Ruptured spleen
    B. Head injury
    C. Punctured lung
    D. Ruptured intestines with sepsis

Answers

[46.1]   **D.** The first and foremost priority is on the patient's medical condition, and as normal, initially addressing the ABCs. Child protective services probably do need to be notified, and the injuries do need to be documented. In general, the parents should not be confronted, but rather asked about their story.

[46.2]   **C.** The normal heart rate and blood pressure levels of a child are substantially different from that of any adult. These values are normal for an infant.

[46.3]   **B.** Head injury is the most common cause of death due to blunt trauma to a child.

CLINICAL PEARLS

❖ The first priority in evaluating a child with suspected abuse is the ABCs.

❖ The most life-threatening injury in intentional child injury is head injury.

❖ Soft-tissue and skin injuries are the most common child injury.

REFERENCES

American College of Surgeons. Advanced trauma life support. Chicago: Author, 1997.

Boyce MC, Melhorn KJ, Vargo G. Pediatric trauma documentation: adequacy for assessment of child abuse. Arch Pediatr Adolesc Med 1996;150(7):730–2.

DiScala C, Sege R, Li G, Reece R. Child abuse and unintentional injuries: a 10-year retrospective. Arch Pediatr Adolesc Med 2000;154(1):16–22.

Kempe CH, Silverman FN, Steele BF, et al. The battered child syndrome. JAMA 1962;181:17–24.

O'Neill JA. Child abuse. In: O'Neill JA, ed. Principles of pediatric surgery. Saint Louis: Mosby, 2003.

A 72-year-old woman is transported by paramedics from the scene of a motor vehicle crash (MVC) to your emergency department. By the paramedics' account, the patient was the restrained driver of a vehicle that pulled out into traffic from the curbside, resulting in side-impact collision to the driver-side door. The patient was initially unconscious but regained consciousness prior to paramedics' arrival. In the field, her pulse rate was 90 beats per minute, blood pressure 120/70 mmHg, respiratory rate 28 breaths per minute, and Glasgow Coma Scale (GCS) score of 13. She is noted to have ecchymoses and swelling of the left forearm and left leg. In the emergency center, her temperature is 35.8°C (96.4°F), blood pressure 110/70 mmHg, pulse rate 90 beats per minute, respiratory rate 24 breaths per minute, and GCS score 12. A 10-cm scalp laceration of the left frontal-parietal region was noted. The patient's cervical spine is immobilized, and tenderness is present along the entire neck. Her left lateral chest wall is tender with soft tissue ecchymosis and diminished breath sounds. Her abdomen is nontender and her pelvis appears stable. The examination of her extremities reveals soft tissue ecchymosis and swelling on the left forearm and hand along with abrasions, ecchymoses, tenderness, and diminished movements in both legs.

◆ **What indicators suggest a poor outcome in this patient?**

◆ **What is your therapeutic approach?**

ANSWERS TO CASE 50: Geriatric Trauma

Summary: A 72-year-old woman is brought to the hospital following a motor vehicle collision with lateral impact. She has a scalp laceration and evidence suggestive of left chest injury.

 Indicators of poor outcome: the patient's age, chest injury, and hypothermia.

 Therapeutic approach: early recognition of injuries, aggressive monitoring, supportive care, and pain reduction are important in improving outcome in high-risk, geriatric trauma patients.

Analysis

Objectives

1. Know the differences in the prognosis and clinical presentation of trauma in geriatric patients.
2. Become familiar with approaches that may help improve outcome in geriatric trauma patients.

Considerations

Aside from the patient's age, the initial presentation of this patient revealed a hemodynamically stable patient with perhaps minor soft tissue injuries and possible rib fractures from a low-speed MVC. However, given this patient's age and the mechanisms of injury, her expected outcome may be poor. Several problems should raise strong concerns during the primary survey. The blood pressure level of 110/70 mmHg and pulse rate of 90 beats per minute appear normal at first glance, but may actually represent shock. Older patients often have baseline blood pressure readings that are considerably higher (a general **rule of thumb is systolic pressure of 100 + age during normal stressed conditions**). **The left chest wall soft-tissue injury and diminished breath sound are highly suggestive of rib fractures and pneumothorax, and should be assessed rapidly with chest radiograph.** Her initial GCS score of 13 is extremely concerning, and may indicate closed head injury, hypoxia, or inadequate cerebral perfusion; the initial treatment should include supplemental oxygen by 100 percent nonrebreather mask. Once the primary and secondary survey have been completed, parenteral analgesics for pain control and measures to maintain body heat should be the next priorities, because pain, vasoconstriction, and shivering contribute to increase afterload and increase oxygen consumption demand and potential cardiac morbidity. The most difficult problem in the early management of this patient is completion of the necessary diagnostic studies, while maintaining adequate monitoring, pain control, and minimizing heat dissipation.

The initial evaluation should include assessment of tissue perfusion, such as measuring urine output, serum lactate, and/or base deficits. Given the initial findings and the mechanism of injury, this patient is a candidate for admission to an intensive care unit, where cardiopulmonary monitoring, chest physiotherapy, and pain control can be provided. Rib fractures in individuals older than age 65 years carry a twofold increased mortality rate and several-fold increased pulmonary infection rate, partially because of atelectasis; thus, epidural analgesia for pain control should be considered.

Older patients often have coexisting medical problems that may impact the response to the acute injuries. Details surrounding the initial injuring events are frequently relevant (e.g., medication reactions, chest pains, strokes). Nevertheless, the basic approach to trauma in the older patient is the same as the approach to the adult patient.

APPROACH TO GERIATRIC TRAUMA

Physiological Changes

The older age group is one of the fastest growing population sectors in the United States. Thus, the number of geriatric trauma incidents, arbitrarily defined as affecting those older than age 65 to 70 years, is expected to likewise increase. Injuries in these individuals are associated with higher mortality and longer hospital stay. Many physiological changes occur with aging (Table 47-1), including the progressive loss of myocyte number and increase in myocyte volume resulting in the ventricular stiffness and cardiac diastolic dysfunction. Furthermore, atherosclerotic changes cause large vessel stiffness and increased afterload. Additionally, aging contributes to diminution of cardiac beta-adrenergic response, leading to diminished heart rate response. Because of the age-related cardiovascular changes, **the elderly patient is much less capable of responding to increases in cardiac output** demands. **Myocardial infarction is the leading cause of death among 80-year-old patients in the postoperative and postinjury settings.** The elderly patient's limited ability to respond to stress and injuries has prompted some groups to apply age (>70 years) as the sole criteria for trauma team activation, and by adapting to this approach, these investigators have demonstrated significant reduction in geriatric trauma mortality.

Outcome Predictors in Geriatric Patients

Various groups have attempted to identify outcome predictors in geriatric trauma patients (Table 47-2). "High risk" patients can be identified based on mechanism, physiological parameters, and laboratory parameters. In the management of "high-risk" patients, early admission to the ICU, with earlier initiation of invasive hemodynamic monitoring, and aggressive resuscitation

TABLE 47-1
PHYSIOLOGICAL ALTERATIONS ASSOCIATED WITH AGING

Cardiovascular
  Loss of myocytes with reciprocal increase in myocyte volume and diminution in
  cardiac diastolic volume
  Large-vessel calcification with increase in afterload
  Diminished cardiac chronotropic response to beta-adrenergic stimulation
  Intimal hyperplasia and decreased vascular compliance result in decrease in arterial
  perfusion

Pulmonary
  Decrease in forced expiratory volume in 1 second (FEV_1) as a result of decrease in
  respiratory muscle strength and an increase in chest wall rigidity
  Decrease in functional respiratory alveolar surface area

Renal
  Diminution in renal size after age 50 years
  Glomerulosclerosis may occur as the result of degenerative processes such as
  hypertension and diabetes, leading to decrease in glomerular filtration rate

Hepatic
  Decrease in liver size after age 50 years
  Diminished and delayed regenerative capacity of the liver

Immunologic
  Impairment in T-lymphocyte–mediated immunity resulting in increased infection
  risks
  Inflammatory mediated responses are diminished (tumor necrosis factor-alpha,
  interleukin-1, interleukin-6, and leukocyte adhesion molecule expression) leading
  to diminished inflammatory responses

---

based on hemodynamic parameters are associated with a reduction in geriatric
trauma patient mortality. Thus, **expedited patient disposition to allow early
invasive monitoring** and **resuscitation** is helpful. Scalea and colleagues
showed that early resuscitation of the "high-risk" elderly trauma patients, with
goals directed at attaining **cardiac output of >3.5 L/min** and/or a **mixed
venous saturation of >50 percent,** led to an improvement in survival from 7
percent in historical control patients to 53 percent in the aggressively managed patients.

Given the overall poorer survival of geriatric trauma patients, some questions have been raised regarding the quality of life of the survivors. Long-term
studies of geriatric trauma patients indicate that majority of survivors return to
a level of previous independence. Factors associated with long-term **reduced
independence** include **hemodynamic shock upon admission, GCS score
≤7, age ≥75 years, head injury, and sepsis.**

TABLE 47-2
PREDICTORS OF MORBIDITY AND MORTALITY

Morbidity predictors
  Mechanisms
    Automobile–pedestrian collision
    Diffuse beating

  Physiological Parameters
    Systolic blood pressure <150

  Laboratory parameters
    Base deficit (< –6 mEq/L)
    Lactic acid (>2.4 mmol/L)

  Anatomic injuries
    Blunt chest trauma with rib fractures

Mortality Predictors
  Systolic blood pressure <90

  Hypoventilation (respiratory rate <10 breaths per minute)

  Glasgow Coma Scale-score = 3

Comprehension Questions

[47.1] A 70-year-old man is involved in a car accident and suffers some head and chest injury. Which of the following is the *least* reasonable endpoint in the resuscitation of this patient?

    A. Urine output >0.5 mL/kg/h
    B. Improvement in GCS score from 11 to 13
    C. Cardiac output of >6 L/min
    D. Decrease in capillary refill from 4 seconds to 2 seconds

[47.2] A 75-year-old man undergoes an exploratory laparotomy for significant blunt trauma of the abdomen after he was thrown from his truck in a motor vehicle accident. He seems to be hemodynamically stable following surgery. Which of the following is the most likely cause of death in the postoperative period?

    A. Sepsis
    B. Hemorrhage
    C. Acute respiratory distress syndrome (ARDS)
    D. Myocardial infarction
    E. Pulmonary embolism

[47.3] An evaluation of a 80-year-old woman who was a pedestrian struck by an automobile traveling at a speed of 20 miles per hour identified right tibia and fibula fracture, right pubic ramus fracture, and facial lacerations. Her vital signs are a pulse of 80 beats per minute, blood pressure of 120/70 mmHg, respiratory rate of 20 breaths per minute, and a GCS score of 15. Which of the following sequences of events is the most appropriate in management of this patient?

A. Computed tomography (CT) scan of the abdomen; plain x-rays of the pelvis, lower extremities, and spine; splinting of fractures; and invasive monitoring in the ICU

B. CT scan of the abdomen; splinting of fractures; invasive monitoring in ICU; and x-rays of the pelvis and lower extremities

C. Invasive monitoring in ICU; splinting of the fractures; and CT of abdomen.

D. Splinting of fractures; invasive monitoring in the ICU; and CT of abdomen; and x-rays of the extremities and pelvis

Answers

[47.1] **C.** Maintenance of urine output >0.5 mL/kg/h, improvement in mentation, and the improvement in peripheral perfusion as demonstrated by the capillary refill, are all reasonable indicators of clinical improvement. The monitoring of cardiac output is useful as an assessment of patient response, but 6 L/min cardiac output is greater than the expected response in most injured patients (3.5 L/min).

[47.2] **D.** Myocardial infarction is the most common cause of death in the perioperative or postinjury period in the geriatric patient.

[47.3] **B.** The sequence of events outlined is most appropriate for immediate identification of possible intraabdominal hemorrhagic source in a patient with injury mechanism capable of producing multiple injuries. When this life-threatening problem is ruled out, the next step is early invasive monitoring in the ICU, while simultaneous efforts are made to identify other non–life-threatening injuries.

CLINICAL PEARLS

❖ A general rule of thumb for the expected systolic pressure is 100 + age during normal stressed conditions

❖ Myocardial infarction is the leading cause of death among 80-year-old patients in the postoperative and postinjury settings.

❖ Goal-directed therapy in geriatric trauma tends to improve outcomes.

REFERENCES

Aalami OO, Fang TD, Song HM, et al. Physiologic features of aging persons. Arch Surg 2003;138:1068–76.

Scalea TM, Simon HM, Duncan AO, et al. Geriatric blunt multiple trauma: improved survival with early invasive monitoring. J Trauma 1990;30:129–36.

Victorino GP, Chong TJ, Pal JD. Trauma in the elderly patient. Arch Surg 2003;138:1093–98.

Listing of Cases

Listing by Case Number

Listing by Disorder (Alphabetical)

LISTING BY CASE NUMBER

LISTING OF CASES (BY ALPHABETICAL ORDER)

❖ INDEX

Note: Page numbers followed by f indicate figures; those followed by t indicate tables.